1000 SBAs and EMQs for Medical Finals

First edition authors
Neel Sharma

2nd Edition
CRASH COURSE

SERIES EDITORS

Philip Xiu
BA, MA, MB BChir, MRCP
GP Registrar, Yorkshire Deanery

Shreelata Datta
MD, MRCOG, LLM, BSc (Hons), MBBS
Honorary Senior Lecturer
Imperial College, London,
Consultant Obstetrician and Gynaecologist
King's College Hospital
London, UK

FACULTY ADVISORS

Juhu Joseph
FRCS (Tr & Orth)
Consultant Orthopaedic & Trauma Surgeon, Northumbria Healthcare NHS
Foundation Trust

Vidhya Nair
MBBS, FRCP
Consultant in Elderly Medicine
Leeds Teaching Hospitals NHS Trust

1000 SBAs and EMQs for Medical Finals

Philip Xiu
BA, MA, MB BChir, MRCP
GP Registrar, Yorkshire Deanery

ELSEVIER

ELSEVIER

Senior Content Strategist: Jeremy Bowes
Senior Content Development Specialist: Alex Mortimer
Project Manager: Andrew Riley
Design: Christian Bilbow

First edition 1998
Second edition 2019

ISBN: 978-0-7020-7384-7
eISBN: 978-0-7020-7352-6

Notices

Practitioners and researchers must always rely on their own experience and knowledge in evaluating and using any information, methods, compounds or experiments described herein. Because of rapid advances in the medical sciences, in particular, independent verification of diagnoses and drug dosages should be made. To the fullest extent of the law, no responsibility is assumed by Elsevier, authors, editors or contributors for any injury and/or damage to persons or property as a matter of products liability, negligence or otherwise, or from any use or operation of any methods, products, instructions, or ideas contained in the material herein.

your source for books,
journals and multimedia
in the health sciences
www.elsevierhealth.com

Working together
to grow libraries in
developing countries

www.elsevier.com • www.bookaid.org

The
publisher's
policy is to use
**paper manufactured
from sustainable forests**

Printed in Great Britain
Last digit is the print number: 10 9 8 7 6 5 4 3 2

Series Editors' foreword

The *Crash Course* series was conceived by Dr Dan Horton-Szar who as series editor presided over it for more than 15 years – from publication of the first edition in 1997, until publication of the fourth edition in 2011. His inspiration, knowledge and wisdom lives on in the pages of this book. As the new series editors, we are delighted to be able to continue developing each book for the twenty-first century undergraduate curriculum.

The flame of medicine never stands still, and keeping this all-new fifth series relevant for today's students is an ongoing process. Each title within this new fifth edition has been re-written to integrate basic medical science and clinical practice, after extensive deliberation and debate. We aim to build on the success of the previous titles by keeping the series up-to-date with current guidelines for best practice, and recent developments in medical research and pharmacology.

We always listen to feedback from our readers, through focus groups and student reviews of the Crash Course titles. For the fifth editions we have reviewed and re-written our self-assessment material to reflect today's 'single-best answer' and 'extended matching question' formats. The artwork and layout of the titles has also been largely re-worked and are now in colour, to make it easier on the eye during long sessions of revision. The new on-line materials supplement the learning process.

Despite fully revising the books with each edition, we hold fast to the principles on which we first developed the series. Crash Course will always bring you all the information you need to revise in compact, manageable volumes that still maintain the balance between clarity and conciseness, and provide sufficient depth for those aiming at distinction. The authors are junior doctors who have recent experience of the exams you are now facing, and the accuracy of the material is checked by a team of faculty editors from across the UK.

We wish you all the best for your future careers!

Shreelata Datta and Philip Xiu

Prefaces

Author

This book provides a practical, no-nonsense approach to tackling the medical finals exam, in a format that is written specifically for the exam. Each chapter address one speciality in medicine or surgery and begins with easier questions before moving onto harder Ebel classified questions. The detailed answer explanations provides you with a good grounding of the most common topics covered, as well as harder topics to distinguish the distinction level canditates.

I have been at the coalface of exams and teaching and as such have recent knowledge of the stresses that exams can cause. The solution is to cover as much of the most common areas that are tested by the examiners, and to see as many possible permutations of common exam clinical scenarios as possible, which this book covers with its 1000 questions in both SBAs and EMQs. As in clinical practice, I have toiled over this book and gained great satisfaction from producing it, and then gratefully and humbly watch it be markedly improved and corrected by the Faculty Editors Dr Nair and Mr Joseph. Both of which have carefully screened over each word, and without whom the book would not have been possible.

I am indebted to those who have taught me, those who have worked with me and most importantly, those I have been priviliged enough to care for.

All that remains is to wish you the very best of luck.

Philip Xiu

Faculty Advisors

The purpose of this book is to cover medical and surgical cases which may feature in final exams.

We hope you find it a useful revision aid which will stimulate your thirst for learning and help you get through finals!

We wish you the best of luck!

Juhu Joseph and Vidhya Nair

Series Editors' acknowledgements

We would like to thank the support of our colleagues who have helped in the preparation of this edition, namely the junior doctor contributors who helped write the manuscript as well as the faculty editors who check the veracity of the information.

We are extremely grateful for the support of our publisher, Elsevier, whose staffs' insight and persistence has maintained the quality that Dr Horton-Szar has set-out since the first edition. Jeremy Bowes, our commissioning editor, has been a constant support. Alex Mortimer and Barbara Simmons our development editors have managed the day-to-day work on this edition with extreme patience and unflaggable determination to meet the ever looming deadlines, and we are ever grateful for Kim Benson's contribution to the online editions and additional online supplementary materials.

Contents

HAEMATOLOGY

Haemoglobin	
Male	135–177 g/L
Female	115–165 g/L
Mean corpuscular haemoglobin (MCH)	27–32 pg
Mean corpuscular haemoglobin concentration (MCHC)	32–36 g/dL
Mean corpuscular volume (MCV)	80–96 fL
Packed cell volume (PCV)	
Male	0.40–0.54 L/L
Female	0.37–0.47 L/L
White blood count (WBC)	$4–11 \times 10^9$/L
Basophil granulocytes	$<0.01–0.1 \times 10^9$/L
Eosinophil granulocytes	$0.04–0.4 \times 10^9$/L
Lymphocytes	$1.5–4.0 \times 10^9$/L
Monocytes	$0.2–0.8 \times 10^9$/L
Neutrophil granulocytes	$2.0–7.5 \times 10^9$/L
Platelet count	$150–400 \times 10^9$/L
Serum B_{12}	160–925 ng/L (150–675 pmol/L)
Serum folate	2.9–18 µg/L (3.6–63 nmol/L)
Red cell folate	149–640 µg/L
Red cell mass	
Male	25–35 mL/kg
Female	20–30 mL/kg
Reticulocyte count	0.5–2.5% of red cells ($50–100 \times 10^9$/L)
Erythrocyte sedimentation rate (ESR)	<20 mm in 1 hour

COAGULATION

Bleeding time (Ivy method)	3–9 min
Activated partial thromboplastin time (APTT)	23–31 s
Prothrombin time	12–16 s
International Normalized Ratio (INR)	1.0–1.3
D-dimer	<500 ng/mL

LIPIDS AND LIPOPROTEINS

Cholesterol	3.5–6.5 mmol/L (ideal <5.2 mmol/L)
HDL cholesterol	
Male	0.8–1.8 mmol/L
Female	1.0–2.3 mmol/L
LDL cholesterol	<4.0 mmol/L
Triglycerides	
[H^+]	35–45 nmol/L
pH	7.35–7.45

BIOCHEMISTRY (SERUM/PLASMA)

Alanine aminotransferase (ALT)	5–40 U/L
Albumin	35–50 g/L
Alkaline phosphatase	39–117 U/L
Amylase	25–125 U/L
Aspartate aminotransferase (AST)	12–40 U/L
Bicarbonate	22–30 mmol/L
Bilirubin	<17 µmol/L (0.3–1.5 mg/dL)
Calcium	2.20–2.67 mmol/L (8.5–10.5 mg/dL)
Chloride	98–106 mmol/L
C-reactive protein	<10 mg/L
Creatinine	79–118 µmol /L (0.6–1.5 mg/dL)
Creatine kinase (CPK)	
Female	24–170 U/L
Male	24–195 U/L
CK–MB fraction	<25 U/L (<60% of total activity)
Ferritin	
Female	6–100 µg/L
Male	20–260 µg/L
Postmenopausal	12–230 µg/L
α-Fetoprotein	<10 kU/L
Glucose (fasting)	4.5–5.6 mmol/L (70–110 mg/dL)
γ–Glutamyl transpeptidase (γ–GT)	
Male	11–58 U/L
Female	7–32 U/L
Glycosylated (glycated) haemoglobin (HbA_{1c})	3.7–5.1%
Iron	13–32 µmol /L (50–150 µg/dL)
Iron–binding capacity (total) (TIBC)	42–80 µmol /L (250–410 µg/dL)
Magnesium	0.7–1.1 mmol/L
Osmolality	275–295 mOsm/kg

Phosphate	0.8–1.5 mmol/L
Potassium	3.5–5.0 mmol/L
Prostate–specific antigen (PSA)	≤4.0 µg/L
Protein (total)	62–77 g/L
Sodium	135–146 mmol/L
Urate	0.18–0.42 mmol/L (3.0–7.0 mg/dL)
Urea	2.5–6.7 mmol/L (8–25 mg/dL)

BLOOD GASES (ARTERIAL)

P_aCO_2	4.8–6.1 kPa (36–46 mmHg)
P_aO_2	10–13.3 kPa (75–100mmHg)
Male	0.70–2.1 mmol/L
Female	0.50–1.70 mmol/L
Bicarbonate	22–26 mmol/L

Introduction

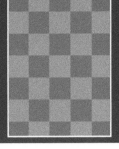

Crash Course: 1000 SBAs and EMQs for Medical Finals, is intended to provide medical students, with a convenient tool for assessing and improving their knowledge of medicine.

There are actually more than 1000 questions in the book; which are similar in both complexity and format to the medical finals level questions you might expect (i.e., suitable for use in a Final MB qualifying examination).

We have graded the questions in the rough ratio of difficulties that a student might face in finals; this allows the student to choose which ones to tackle.

The explanations for each of the questions not only goes into detail as to why the answer option is correct, but also expands the subject matter to suggest why other answers are wrong.

PURPOSE OF MEDICAL FINALS EXAMINATIONS

The aim of medical finals is to measure the clinical competence (i.e., professional knowledge, skills and attitudes) against a defined criteria and standards. To pass finals, students should demonstrate safety and competence at the level of a day 1 Foundation Programme Year 1 (FY1) doctor.

Contrary to many student's fears, ranking of candidates is only a secondary objective.

Elements of competence

Competence can be divided up into three distinct categories:
Knowledge – demonstrating factual regurgitation and applied clinical reasoning
Skills – clinical skills and communication skills
Attitudes – and professional behaviour
This can be summarized in Miller's triangle:

Cognition is tested at the base of the triangle: 'Knows' and 'Knows how' and this is tested primarily by written/computer-based assessments, whereas Behaviour is tested under the apex of the triangle 'Shows how' and 'Does' and these are tested under performance or hands on assessment.

This book will address the extended matching questions (EMQs) and single best answer (SBA) component.

How do medical schools compare?

Currently, medical finals for each medical school are different. Each school has their own curriculum syllabus and uses different methods of examination, which means that students at different universities may not be directly comparable. The questions can be drawn from a local bank of questions and a percentage from the Medical Schools Council Assessment Alliance (MSCAA) question bank (questions contributed by all UK Medical Schools and used across the UK).

Reliability and validity of finals

Assessment of competence and knowledge should thus be based across all of Miller's triangle, to get an accurate assessment of a student's performance. This sampling method crosses methodologies (in content, in time, across examiners and patient feedback), which leads to higher validity and reliability of a student's performance.

This book will focus on the written part of medical finals, namely that of SBA and EMQs.

SINGLE BEST ANSWER (SBA)

SBA style questions are the most popular means of written assessment in both undergraduate and postgraduate medical examinations.

Anatomy of an SBA

They have a stem or vignette, describing the problem. They present five options all of which are plausible, but one of which is clearly correct. The options should be homogeneous (i.e., all the options should be diagnoses, investigations or mechanisms) and not a mix.
Stem: They have a stem or vignette, describing the problem.
Lead-in: The lead-in asks the question.
Answer options: There are 5 answer options for each question item.
Example:
Stem: A term baby is born with a vitelline duct still present. Her baby check was normal and she was discharged 2 days after birth. She remains well until she attends university at 19 years of age, when she develops colicky abdominal pain.
Lead-in: What is the likely cause?
Answer options:
    a. Appendicitis
    b. Meckel Diverticulum
    c. Exomphalos
    d. Gastroschisis
    e. Atresia
Answer: B

EXTENDED-MATCHING QUESTIONS (EMQs)

EMQs are a popular method of assessment in undergraduate and postgraduate medical examinations. This self-assessment book will provide you with a mixed set of EMQs divided by themes that most commonly appear in your exams.

The most important skill in answering EMQs successfully is in choosing the correct option out of a list of very similar symptoms or signs.

Anatomy of an EMQ

Themes: EMQs are divided into themes, which defines the subject of the question.
Answer options: There can be between 8 to 15 answer options for each question item, and some answers can be used more than once.
Lead-in: The lead-in defines the task.
Stems: They have a stem or vignette describing the problem. For each item question, select one lettered option that is most closely associated with the question. Example:
Theme:
   Fatigue
Options:
   A. Acute leukaemia
   B. Anaemia of chronic disease
   C. Congestive heart failure
   D. Depression
   E. Epstein–Barr virus infection
   F. Folate deficiency
   G. Glucose 6-phosphate dehydrogenase deficiency
   H. Hereditary spherocytosis
   I. Hypothyroidism
   J. Iron deficiency
   K. Lyme disease
   L. Microangiopathic haemolytic anaemia
   M. Miliary tuberculosis
   N. Vitamin B12 (cyanocobalamin) deficiency
Lead-in:
   For each patient with fatigue, select the most likely diagnosis.
Stems:
   1. A 19-year-old woman has had fatigue, fever, and sore throat for the past week. She has a temperature of 38.3°C, cervical lymphadenopathy and splenomegaly. Initial laboratory results show a white blood cell count of 18×10^9/L (80% lymphocytes, with many exhibiting atypical features). Serum aspartate aminotransferase (AST, GOT) activity is 200 U/L. Serum bilirubin concentration and serum alkaline phosphatase activity are within normal limits. **Answer: E**
   2. A 15-year-old girl has a two-week history of fatigue and back pain. She has widespread bruising, pallor, and tenderness over the vertebrae and both femurs. Full blood count shows haemoglobin concentration of 70 g/dL, leukocyte count of 2.0×10^9/L, and platelet count of 15×10^9/L. **Answer: A**

HINTS AND TIPS FOR THE TEST-SMART STUDENTS

Students who are knowledgeable about exam technique can pick up on cues in the question or options that lead them to the correct answer without having to use the full depth of their medical knowledge. The most important tricks that lead to this are listed below.

Grammatical cues

One or more options do not follow grammatically from the stem and lead-in. This occurs when question writers pay more attention to the correct answer than to the distractors. Usually, the correct answer makes grammatical sense but some or all of the distractors do not. This gives test-smart students clues on how to answer.

Logical cues

Occur when a subset of the options is collectively exhaustive. For example:
Crime is
   A   Spread evenly across all social classes
   B   Over-represented among the poor
   C   Over-represented among the middle-classes and rich
   D   An indication of psychosexual maladjustment
   E   Reaching a plateau of tolerability for the nation.

Options A, B and C include all possibilities, so the test-smart student could eliminate D and E.

Absolute terms

Sometimes there are absolute terms such as 'always' or 'never' in the options. These options are less likely to be true and can be eliminated by the test-smart student – in the real-world, things are rarely so cut and dried.

Long correct answers

The correct answer option is longer, more specific or more complete than the others.

Word repeats

The correct answer repeats a word or phrase used on the stem.

Convergence strategy

This one is tricky. Basically, this error occurs when the correct option is given the most elements in common with the other answers, i.e., it is not out at the extremes. A simple example of this occurs when the options are:

A Pencil and pen
B Pencil and highlighter
C Pencil and crayon
D Pen and marker

Then by simply counting, Pencil appears 3 times, Pen twice and the rest once each. So, the correct answer is more likely to be A as it contains the two most common words. Sounds ridiculous? Perhaps, but it does happen frequently so you have to take care to avoid it in your questions.

DIFFICULTY OF QUESTIONS

The questions are divided up into different levels of difficulties.

This book uses a modified Ebel method to divide the questions and rate them in difficulty. We used subject matter experts to rate questions according to their importance, categorising them as essential, important or acceptable.

Medical finals examiners will often have this sort of grid to define the percentage of questions that a borderline student should be able to answer correctly.

For example, we would expect that a borderline 'pass' student should answer 90% of all essential questions correctly, and 70% of all important questions, as opposed to 40%–50% of all acceptable questions which are there to stretch the most able of students.

Essential knowledge

Consists of essential knowledge, that all medical students must know before qualification. These consist of emergencies, and common management themes, to ensure that a student is safe to practice.

Important knowledge

Constitutes the bulk majority of questions, and these are important core topics which students should know in order to pass finals. Students should be getting the majority of these questions correct and these will form the bulk of any examination.

Acceptable knowledge

These are harder questions which stretch the most able of students. These comprise around 10%–20% of any chapter, and are designed to be able to distinguish the average student from the distinction level student. Some more esoteric diagnosis and management of rarer disease are covered here.

HOW DO SCHOOLS SET UP A HIGH QUALITY WRITTEN EXAM?

A team of experienced question writers generate a first draft of questions. These can be from consultants or registrars who are involved in teaching. The questions are then reviewed and refined at a meeting of the examiners.

More senior examiners conduct tertiary level review and select questions for inclusion in the test paper (using a blueprint syllabus) from the national MSCAA question bank.

The questions undergo refinement and review by speciality senior examiners who may request clarification or changes. This set of questions are then screened by a team of external examiners who are part of the quality assessment.

There may be final reviews before the questions are put into use for the exam.

HOW TO MAKE THE BEST USE OF THIS BOOK

Some students like to use the book to simulate the time restrictions imposed by medical finals; you should be aiming to allocate about one minute per question. You can attempt the questions in chunks of 10 or more. After answering chunks of questions, you should spend some time in reviewing the explanations at the end of the chapter.

Even if you got the question right, the explanations will help with surrounding topics and can help the student gain further marks in other questions.

Some students find it useful to check the explanations after doing each question, without time restrictions. This technique is good for the student that wants to use the book to 'learn' the most high-yield exam materials, in conjunction with their own notes.

ONLINE INTERACTIVE ASSESSMENT – EBOOK

Finally, do not forget to access/download your accompanying Student Consult eBook (which comes with the printed version of this book – instructions on the inside front cover). You can then access **all** the questions anywhere from your laptop or mobile device and choose either to read in the regular eBook format or to utilise the 'Interactive Assessment' tool, to help test yourself and monitor your progress.'

CONCLUSION

Whatever you choose to do, if you manage to finish the book it will put you in good stead for the real medical finals.

Good luck with your exams!

MEDICINE QUESTIONS

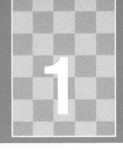

Cardiology 1

SINGLE BEST ANSWER (SBA) QUESTIONS

1. A 19-year-old university rower presents for the pre-Oxford–Cambridge boat race medical evaluation. He is healthy and has no significant medical history. However, his brother died suddenly during football practice at age 15. Which one of the following is the most likely cause of the brother's death?
   a. Aortic stenosis
   b. Congenital long QT syndrome
   c. Congenital short QT syndrome
   d. Hypertrophic cardiomyopathy (HCM)
   e. Wolff–Parkinson–White syndrome

2. A 65-year-old man presents to the heart failure outpatient clinic with increased shortness of breath and swollen ankles. On examination his pulse was 100 beats/min, blood pressure 100/60 mmHg and jugular venous pressure (JVP) +10 cm water. The patient currently takes furosemide 40 mg BD, spironolactone 12.5 mg, bisoprolol 2.5 mg OD and ramipril 2.5 mg BD. Which of the following is true?
   a. Diuretics reduce the degree of neurohormonal activation in heart failure
   b. Diuretics alone rarely provide rapid symptomatic relief
   c. Beta-blockers are contraindicated
   d. Treatment with spironolactone reduces mortality
   e. Angiotensin-converting enzyme (ACE) inhibitors are unlikely to induce hypotension if an adequate diuresis has been achieved with diuretics

3. A 73-year-old woman complains of sudden-onset chest pain. On examination you note her pulse is regular at 53 beats/min. You request an electrocardiogram (ECG) which demonstrates a time interval of 3 seconds between each consecutive P wave. What is the most likely diagnosis?
   a. Sick sinus syndrome
   b. First-degree atrioventricular (AV) block
   c. Mobitz type 1 block
   d. Mobitz type 2 block
   e. Complete heart block

4. A 63-year-old man complains of gradual-onset chest pain. On examination you note his pulse is regular at 60 beats/min. You request an ECG which demonstrates an increasing PR interval which eventually culminates in an absent QRS complex after the P wave. What is the most likely diagnosis?
   a. Sick sinus syndrome
   b. First-degree AV block
   c. Mobitz type 1 block
   d. Mobitz type 2 block
   e. Complete heart block

5. A 28-year-old man with no past medical history and not on medications presents to the emergency department with palpitations for several hours and was found to have supraventricular tachycardia. Carotid massage was attempted without success. What is the treatment of choice to stop the attack?
   a. Intravenous (IV) lignocaine
   b. IV digoxin
   c. IV amiodarone
   d. IV adenosine
   e. IV quinidine

6. A 75-year-old cigarette smoker with known ischaemic heart disease and a history of cardiac failure presents to the emergency department with a 6-hour history of increasing dyspnoea. His ECG shows a narrow complex regular tachycardia with a rate of 160 beats/min. What is the most appropriate initial step in patient care?
   a. His heart rate should be slowed using IV atenolol to aid in the diagnosis of the rhythm
   b. He should be given a single IV dose of lignocaine (50 mg) followed by an infusion at 4 mg/min
   c. He should be given IV adenosine to aid in the diagnosis of the rhythm
   d. His rhythm may represent a ventricular tachycardia and he should be immediately cardioverted
   e. He should not be given high flow oxygen

7. A 57-year-old man comes to his general practitioner (GP) concerned about his general health. He is particularly worried as there is a strong family history of heart disease. The GP performs an ECG which shows a prolonged PR interval of 0.3 seconds. What is the most likely diagnosis?
   a. Sick sinus syndrome
   b. First-degree AV block
   c. Mobitz type 1 block
   d. Mobitz type 2 block
   e. Complete heart block

8. A 75-year-old man is referred by the GP to the cardiology outpatient clinic. The patient has atrial fibrillation (AF) and hypertension. Examination reveals a blood pressure of 124/80 mmHg and his pulse

varies between 90 and 130 beats/min. His last echocardiogram (done 1 month ago) revealed left atrial chamber dimensions that are increased above normal. What is the most effective management?
a. Adenosine
b. No medication
c. Digoxin alone
d. Cardioversion
e. Digoxin, with warfarin

9. You are a house officer on call when a nurse bleeps you to review an ECG. The ECG demonstrates an intermittent absence of the QRS complex but no evidence of progressive PR interval increase. What is the most likely diagnosis?
a. Sick sinus syndrome
b. First-degree AV block
c. Mobitz type 1 block
d. Mobitz type 2 block
e. Complete heart block

10. A 48-year-old woman attends her GP for a routine health check. She was found to have high cholesterol (at 5.8 mmol/L) and high triglyceride level (at 2.7 mmol/L). She is a nonsmoker and consumes 10 units of alcohol per week. Her body mass index is 29 kg/m^2 and she is otherwise well with no personal or family history of illnesses. Clinical examination and vital signs were unremarkable. Her calculated QRISK is 12%. Which one of the following in her initial management is LEAST likely needed?
a. Low carbohydrate diet
b. High consumption of monounsaturated fats
c. Regular aerobic exercise
d. Start medical therapy with statins
e. Decrease body mass index to <25

11. You are a house officer on call when you are bleeped to see a patient complaining of dizziness. On further questioning the patient comments that he has blacked out on several occasions in the past. You perform an ECG which shows regular P and QRS complexes occurring independently of one another. What is the most likely diagnosis?
a. Sick sinus syndrome
b. First-degree AV block
c. Mobitz type 1 block
d. Mobitz type 2 block
e. Complete heart block

12. You are called to see a 48-year-old man who is found to be unresponsive by the nursing staff. You cannot obtain a palpable carotid pulse and the cardiac monitor shows ventricular fibrillation. What is the first appropriate measure?

a. Sodium bicarbonate 50-mg IV injection
b. Defibrillation with 200 J
c. One ampoule injection of IV calcium chloride
d. One ampoule injection of IV adrenaline
e. Carotid artery compression

13. You are a medical student attending a teaching session on ECG interpretation. The consultant tells you that a patient was admitted to the coronary care unit with an atrial rate of 300 beats/min and a ventricular rate of 150 beats/min. What is the most likely diagnosis?
a. Atrial flutter
b. First-degree AV block
c. Mobitz type 1 block
d. Mobitz type 2 block
e. Complete heart block

14. A 50-year-old lawyer presents to the cardiology outpatient clinic with recurrent episodes of dull central chest pain radiating up to her jaw and down her left shoulder, associated with sweating and nausea following exertion and alleviated by rest. She is a heavy smoker and her father died of a heart attack in his 40s. What is the most definitive diagnostic test in this case?
a. Echocardiography
b. Stress testing with echocardiography
c. Stress testing with myocardial perfusion scintigraphy
d. Coronary angiography
e. Electrocardiography during an attack

15. You are a house officer on call when you are asked to review a patient in the coronary care unit. You note that the patient has an atrial rate of 300 beats/min and a ventricular rate of 150 beats/min. The nurse says this is of new onset. Which management plan would you instigate first?
a. Sotalol
b. Radiofrequency catheter ablation
c. Procainamide
d. Lignocaine
e. Electrical cardioversion

16. A previously fit and well 36-year-old woman presents to her GP with a 2-month history of palpitations and sweats. These attacks come on suddenly and are unrelated to food intake, supine posture or exercise. She is a nonsmoker and does not drink alcohol. Which of the following investigations is the LEAST useful to evaluate this patient?
a. Thyroid function tests
b. Urinary collection for catecholamines
c. Holter monitor

d. Echocardiography
e. Upper gastrointestinal study

17. A 57-year-old Bangladeshi patient is admitted to accident and emergency (A&E) with palpitations. He speaks very little English but tells you he has a 'heart problem'. On examination you note his pulse is irregular at 145 beats/min. An ECG is performed which demonstrates no P waves. Which management plan would you instigate first?
a. Bisoprolol
b. Flecainide
c. Radiofrequency catheter ablation
d. Procainamide
e. Lignocaine

18. A 55-year-old man presents to a local district general hospital A&E with acute central chest pain, radiating to his neck and left shoulder, and associated with one episode of vomiting. His medical history includes hypertension and hyperlipidaemia. ECG and troponin show evidence of an acute myocardial infarction (MI). Primary percutaneous coronary intervention is unavailable within close distance; therefore a decision is made to perform thrombolytic therapy. This therapy is most beneficial when done within which of the following time limits from the onset of pain?
a. Within 2 days
b. Within 18 hours
c. Within 12 hours
d. Within 24 hours
e. Within 36 hours

19. A 37-year-old woman is complaining of palpitations following recent surgery. On examination her pulse rate is regular at 175 beats/min and blood pressure is stable at 125/70 mmHg. She tells you she was seen the night before by the on-call cardiologist for the same problem. Her past medical history includes asthma. You request an ECG which shows normal-shaped QRS complexes but no P waves. What is the next most appropriate step in management?
a. Adenosine
b. Verapamil
c. Carotid sinus massage
d. Direct current (DC) cardioversion
e. Flecainide

20. While on call you are bleeped to see a patient who has had a massive bleed PR. On examination you note he is drowsy with a blood pressure of 65/40 mmHg and pulse rate of 130 beats/min. While you obtain IV access, he arrests. The nurse calls the crash team and you commence cardiopulmonary resuscitation (CPR). After 2 minutes, you note QRS complexes on the cardiac monitor but no evidence of a pulse. What is the next most appropriate step in management?
a. Administration of colloid
b. DC shock 200 J
c. Amiodarone 300 mg IV
d. Adrenaline 1 mg IV
e. Atropine 1 mg IV

21. You are asked to review an 89-year-old arteriopath who complains of severe pain at rest in both feet, the toes of which are cold and purple. He has had a recent course of heparin and aspirin for suspected unstable angina. The major arterial pulses are present in the limbs, but there are areas of lace-like purplish discolouration on the skin over both knees. What is the most likely explanation for these findings?
a. Allergic reaction to the heparin
b. Cholesterol embolism
c. Haemorrhage from the anticoagulants
d. Heparin-induced thrombocytopaenia
e. Sepsis

22. A 65-year-old man has NYHA class III chronic heart failure. Despite conventional therapy with appropriate dosages of a diuretic, an ACE inhibitor and a beta-adrenergic blocker, his left ventricular ejection fraction hovers around 35%, and he continues to have shortness of breath on exertion. His latest urea and electrolytes test results were normal and you consider adding digoxin to his treatment regimen. Which one of the following is true regarding digoxin therapy in this situation?
a. A reasonable dosage is 0.50 mg/day orally
b. Serial drug levels are generally not necessary
c. A loading dose will be necessary
d. It is not likely to improve the ejection fractions
e. It is the treatment of choice if the patient's ECG shows AV block

23. A 42-year-old man presents with shortness of breath and haemoptysis. On examination you note a loud first heart sound (HS) and a rumbling mid-diastolic murmur at the apex. What is the most likely diagnosis?
a. Mitral stenosis
b. Mitral regurgitation
c. Aortic stenosis
d. Aortic regurgitation
e. Tricuspid stenosis

24. A 16-year-old boy athlete is brought to A&E after he collapsed during football training. On arrival, he appears alert and orientated. His vital signs and physical examination are normal. He remembers

feeling dizzy prior to collapsing but cannot recall much else. He is normally healthy and not on any regular medications. Blood tests have been sent. What is the most appropriate next step for this patient?
a. Admit him for cardiac monitoring
b. Request a neurology review
c. Order an ECG
d. Order electroencephalography (EEG)
e. Schedule a tilt-table test

25. A 55-year-old woman presents with shortness of breath on exertion and fatigue. On examination you note a soft first HS and a pansystolic murmur at the apex radiating to her axilla. What is the most likely diagnosis?
a. Mitral stenosis
b. Mitral regurgitation
c. Aortic stenosis
d. Aortic regurgitation
e. Tricuspid stenosis

26. A man has been diagnosed with essential hypertension by his GP and needs to commence on the appropriate treatment. In the treatment of essential hypertension, which of the following statements is true?
a. Alpha-blockers such as prazosin are unlikely to cause postural hypotension
b. Patients of Afro-Caribbean descent respond well to ACE inhibitors
c. ACE inhibitors are indicated if there is unilateral renal artery stenosis
d. Treatment with bendrofluazide may result in hypokalaemia
e. ACE inhibitors may cause ankle swelling as a side effect

27. An otherwise healthy 50-year-old male presents to the GP with palpitations and is noted to have an irregular heartbeat. He is otherwise fit and healthy. This resolves without treatment. Total duration was less than 2 hours. Full blood count, metabolic profile, thyroid studies, ECG and echocardiogram were all normal. Which one of the following would be the most appropriate treatment?
a. Aspirin
b. Clopidogrel
c. Do nothing
d. Dipyridamole
e. Warfarin

28. A 62-year-old man presents with angina and dyspnoea. On examination you note an ejection systolic murmur at the upper right sternal border radiating to his neck. What is the most likely diagnosis?
a. Mitral stenosis
b. Mitral regurgitation
c. Aortic stenosis
d. Aortic regurgitation
e. Tricuspid stenosis

29. A 50-year-old man has persistently elevated blood pressure of about 185/110 mmHg. He has been complaining of headaches for a few weeks but otherwise well. ECG reveals abnormal voltage changes and ST segment depression in the left ventricular leads. He was also found to have evidence of arteriovenous nipping on fundoscopy. What is the most appropriate management?
a. Advise weight loss and see again in 2 months
b. Arrange an exercise stress test
c. Hospitalize and give urgent IV antihypertensive medication
d. Begin oral antihypertensives and see in 2 months
e. Begin oral antihypertensives and see in 3 days

30. A 55-year-old woman presents with dyspnoea and orthopnoea. On examination you note a blowing early diastolic murmur at the left sternal edge. What is the most likely diagnosis?
a. Mitral stenosis
b. Mitral regurgitation
c. Aortic stenosis
d. Aortic regurgitation
e. Tricuspid stenosis

31. A 42-year-old man is reviewed in the outpatient cardiology department following a recent echocardiogram (echo). The echo demonstrates right ventricular dysfunction. On examination you note an elevated JVP in addition to a pansystolic murmur at the lower left sternal edge. What is the most likely diagnosis?
a. Mitral stenosis
b. Mitral regurgitation
c. Tricuspid regurgitation
d. Aortic stenosis
e. Aortic regurgitation

32. A 50-year-old Caucasian man sees his GP for a blood pressure check as he has recently been diagnosed with essential hypertension. His only other medical history is type II diabetes mellitus with no end-organ damage, which is well controlled on oral hypoglycaemic agents. His blood pressure has been 145/90 mmHg persistently despite diet and exercise for 3 months.

Which of the following is the first-line medication for blood pressure control in this patient?
a. Start on losartan
b. Start on bisoprolol
c. Start on thiazide diuretic
d. Start on nifedipine
e. Start on enalapril

33. A 62-year-old man presents with angina and dyspnoea. On examination you note a murmur at the right upper sternal border radiating to his neck. Which investigation is most likely to lead to a diagnosis?
a. Chest X-ray (CXR)
b. Echocardiogram
c. ECG
d. Coronary angiography
e. 24-hour ECG

34. A 42-year-old man presents with shortness of breath and haemoptysis. On examination you note a loud first HS and a rumbling mid-diastolic murmur at the apex. You request an echocardiogram and a CXR. The following are all features of the CXR in this condition EXCEPT?
a. Large right atrium
b. Large left atrium
c. Kerley B lines
d. Pulmonary venous hypertension
e. Narrowed carina

35. A 50-year-old man presents to the emergency department with a mild headache. He is known to have poorly controlled hypertension and is on multiple antihypertensive medications. On examination his blood pressure is 205/110 mmHg and there is no evidence of end-organ involvement. His headache is still present but there is no focal neurology identified. Which of the following is the least appropriate in the management of this patient's blood pressure?
a. Rapidly lowering blood pressure in the emergency department
b. Adjust treatment and follow-up within 24 to 48 hours of presentation in the community
c. Initiate a maintenance dose of an oral medication before discharge
d. Consider a short observation period before discharge
e. Discharge the patient, emphasizing the importance of close follow-up and compliance with medications

36. A 55-year-old man presents to A&E with shortness of breath and fatigue. On examination you note pitting oedema in both his lower limbs. You suspect

heart failure. Which investigation is most likely to demonstrate the aetiology?
a. CXR
b. Echocardiogram
c. ECG
d. Coronary angiography
e. 24-hour ECG

37. A 46-year-old woman presents with shortness of breath. She comments that she feels particularly breathless when lying down and uses five pillows to sleep at night. On examination her pulse rate is regular at 122 beats/min and her blood pressure is stable at 122/65 mmHg. You note bibasal crackles when listening to her chest. You suspect heart failure and order a CXR and echocardiogram. The following may all be features on her CXR EXCEPT?
a. Kerley B lines
b. Hilar haziness
c. Fluid in the left horizontal interlobar fissure
d. Upper lobe venous engorgement
e. Cardiomegaly

38. A 55-year-old banker is admitted to A&E complaining of sudden-onset shortness of breath. Following an echocardiogram, he is diagnosed with heart failure. What is the most likely aetiological cause for cardiac failure in the Western world?
a. Ischaemic heart disease
b. Hypertension
c. Valvular dysfunction
d. Cardiomyopathy
e. Arrhythmia

39. A 66-year-old man with heart failure secondary to previous MIs is on regular digoxin and furosemide without much effect. A recent echocardiogram shows global dysfunction. His renal function is normal. Which medication should be added to his management?
a. ACE inhibitors
b. Verapamil
c. Disopyramide
d. Phosphodiesterase inhibitors
e. Propranolol

40. A 65-year-old man presents with shortness of breath at rest. Physical examination reveals evidence of pitting oedema over the sacrum and leg oedema to the midthigh. An echocardiogram is requested which demonstrates an ejection fraction of 0.4. What is the next most appropriate step in management?
a. ACE inhibitor
b. Angiotensin II receptor antagonist
c. Beta-blocker

d. Calcium channel antagonist
e. Diuretic

41. A 72-year-old man with known cardiac failure comes to see his GP. He is currently on a diuretic. His GP decides to commence an ACE inhibitor. The following are all side effects of ACE inhibitors EXCEPT?
   a. Renal failure
   b. Hypokalaemia
   c. Rash
   d. Angioedema
   e. Cough

42. A 64-year-old man with known cardiac failure presents with acute shortness of breath and a cough productive of frothy pink sputum. He comments that he feels nauseous. On examination you note wheezes and crackles throughout his chest. What is the next most appropriate step in management?
   a. Glyceryl trinitrate (GTN) infusion
   b. Aminophylline
   c. Metoclopramide
   d. Furosemide
   e. Mechanical ventilation

43. A 44-year-old female comes to your office with chest pain of several days' duration. She describes the pain as sharp and stabbing, and indicates that it is located at the left sternal border; it is increased by coughing and palpation. There is no family history of heart disease, nor is there a personal history of diabetes, hypertension, smoking or hyperlipidaemia. A physical examination, an ECG and chest radiographs are all normal. Further diagnostic studies should include which of the following?
   a. A treadmill exercise test with ECG and blood pressure monitoring
   b. A stress echocardiogram
   c. Referral for cardiac catheterization
   d. Stress myocardial perfusion imaging
   e. No additional tests

44. A 53-year-old man comes to see his GP complaining of chest pain. The GP performs an ECG which demonstrates ischaemic changes. The following are all risk factors for ischaemic heart disease EXCEPT?
   a. Hyperlipidaemia
   b. Smoking
   c. Hypertension
   d. High homocysteine levels
   e. High dietary folic acid intake

45. A 23-year-old man who has recently recovered from an upper respiratory tract infection presents to the

A&E department with chest pain made worse on breathing. On examination he is febrile, and has a 'scratchy' sound heard on auscultation in systole and diastole. ECG reveals widespread saddle-shaped ST segment elevation. What is the most likely diagnosis?
   a. Unstable angina
   b. Hyperventilation syndrome
   c. Pulmonary emboli
   d. Evolving cardiac infarction
   e. Acute pericarditis

46. A 56-year-old woman presents to A&E complaining of sudden-onset central chest pain. She comments that it came on at rest. She is referred for an exercise test and coronary angiogram. The exercise test is stopped early due to chest pain and ST depression in the lateral leads. However, she has normal coronary arteries on the angiogram. What is the most likely diagnosis?
   a. Decubitus angina
   b. Prinzmetal angina
   c. Cardiac syndrome X
   d. Unstable angina
   e. Stable angina

47. A 55-year-old man has been recently diagnosed with hypertension and commenced on treatment. He attends his GP to find out more about the condition. Which of the following is the commonest cause of hypertension?
   a. Polycystic kidney disease
   b. Renin-producing tumour
   c. Undetermined cause
   d. Oral contraceptive pills
   e. Coarctation of aorta

48. You are on call in A&E when a patient with sudden-onset chest pain is admitted. You request an ECG which shows evidence of T-wave inversion in leads V2–V6 but no evidence of ST elevation. You prescribe aspirin, enoxaparin and clopidogrel. What is the most appropriate dose of enoxaparin?
   a. 40 mg once a day
   b. 20 mg once a day
   c. 1 mg/kg once a day
   d. 1.5 mg/kg twice a day
   e. 1 mg/kg twice a day

49. A previously fit and well 30-year-old gym instructor is admitted to hospital following a stab wound to the left side of his chest. He has a blood pressure of 80/45 mmHg and heart rate of 125 beats/min. Breath sounds are present throughout but his HSs are muffled. His JVP appears raised. What additional feature is most likely to be present in this patient?

a. Diastolic murmur over the praecordium radiating towards the left axilla
b. S3
c. Wide-split S2
d. An 18-mmHg blood pressure drop during inspiration
e. An 18-mmHg blood pressure drop during expiration

50. You are a house officer on call when you are asked to see a patient with chest pain. The patient tells you that he suffers from angina and this pain is similar to previous episodes of chest pain. An ECG is performed which rules out an MI. What is the next most appropriate step in management?
a. Atenolol
b. Glyceryl trinitrate (GTN)
c. Diltiazem
d. Nicorandil
e. Aspirin

51. An ECG is performed on a 45-year-old man as part of a routine medical check-up. His past medical history includes a previous MI some years ago. The ECG shows presence of Q waves. Q waves in inferior MI appear in which ECG leads?
a. I and II
b. II, III and aVF
c. V1, V2 and V3
d. I, aVF and V6
e. V4, V5 and V6

52. A 56-year-old man presents with central chest pain at rest. He comments that he feels short of breath and nauseous. An ECG demonstrates tall R waves, ST segment depression and tall T waves in leads V1 and V2. What is the most likely diagnosis?
a. Anterior myocardial infarct
b. Lateral myocardial infarct
c. Inferior myocardial infarct
d. Anterio-lateral myocardial infarct
e. Posterior myocardial infarct

53. A 21-year-old fit university student with no past medical history has sudden loss of consciousness 1 hour into a gym session. CPR is administered by bystanders. On arrival of the paramedics, he has regained consciousness. What is the most effective means of preventing sudden death in high-risk patients with asymptomatic HCM?
a. Amiodarone
b. An implantable cardioverter–defibrillator (ICD)
c. Chronic dual-chamber pacing
d. Metoprolol
e. Verapamil

54. A 42-year-old lawyer presents with sudden-onset chest pain. You suspect a myocardial infarct and explain to the patient that you need to measure a protein from his heart to confirm your suspicion. Which serum investigation is most likely to lead to a diagnosis?
a. Troponin
b. Creatine kinase
c. Myoglobin
d. Aspartate aminotransferase
e. Lactic dehydrogenase

55. Which ECG change would lead you to initiate thrombolytic therapy?
a. Right bundle-branch block
b. ST segment elevation in left ventricular leads
c. Widespread ST segment depression
d. Q waves in septal leads
e. Prolongation of the QT interval

56. A 32-year-old obese woman presents to the GP with sudden-onset crushing chest pain and nausea. The GP is concerned about a myocardial infarct and calls an ambulance. What is the next most appropriate step in management?
a. Metoprolol
b. Morphine
c. Metoclopramide
d. Aspirin
e. Streptokinase

57. A 45-year-old man attends the emergency department with worsening breathlessness and fevers. The medical team suspects a diagnosis of infective endocarditis. Which of the following is the most suggestive feature of infective endocarditis?
a. Appearing and changing murmurs
b. Erythema marginatum
c. Juxta-articular nodes
d. Atrial fibrillation
e. Lymphadenopathy

58. A 43-year-old man presents with central chest pain. He is diagnosed with an acute MI and referred for immediate angioplasty. The following are all late complications of a myocardial infarct EXCEPT?
a. Mitral valve regurgitation
b. Thromboembolism
c. Ventricular aneurysm
d. Pericarditis
e. Ventricular septal rupture

59. An elderly woman complains of abdominal distension, due to ascites, upper abdominal pain from an enlarged tender liver and flatulence. She is mildly jaundiced and has marked pitting of the legs.

Her arterial pulse is rapid and irregular, and she is sitting propped up in bed where it is evident that her face is cyanosed, and her jugular veins are engorged and pulsating in systole. She is passing little urine and the urine contains 2+ of protein. What is the most likely diagnosis?

a. Cirrhosis of the liver
b. Congestive heart failure
c. Malignant ascites
d. Nephrotic syndrome
e. Superior mediastinal obstruction

60. A 35-year-old IV drug abuser presents with night sweats and weight loss. On examination he is pyrexial with a temperature of 38.5°C. You suspect a diagnosis of infective endocarditis. Which of the following organisms is most likely to account for his condition?

a. *Streptococcus mutans*
b. *Streptococcus sanguis*
c. *Enterococcus faecalis*
d. *Staphylococcus aureus*
e. *Coxiella burnetii*

61. A 31-year-old woman presents with night sweats. On examination you detect a systolic murmur. She has severe gum and tooth decay and has recently had two teeth taken out. Which of the following organisms is most likely to account for her condition?

a. *Streptococcus mutans*
b. *Streptococcus sanguis*
c. *Enterococcus faecalis*
d. *Staphylococcus aureus*
e. *Coxiella burnetii*

62. A 40-year-old man with an underlying cardiac condition is about to undergo a root canal treatment with a new crown to be fitted in the dentist's office. Which one of the following conditions strongly warrants antibiotics prophylaxis?

a. Atrial septal defect
b. Ventricular septal defect
c. Previous coronary artery bypass grafting involving the use of the internal mammary arteries
d. Presence of a dual chamber pacemaker
e. None of the above

63. You are attending a seminar on infective endocarditis. The lecturer comments that some clinical features of the condition result from immune complex deposition. The following features are all the result of immune complex deposition EXCEPT?

a. Splenic abscess
b. Janeway lesions
c. Roth spots

d. Osler nodes
e. Splinter haemorrhages

64. A 35-year-old man complains of fatigue, night sweats and weight loss. On examination you note a systolic murmur and evidence of splenomegaly. Which investigation is most likely to lead to a diagnosis?

a. Serology testing
b. CXR
c. ECG
d. Full blood count
e. Blood cultures

65. A 31-year-old man presents with several months of shortness of breath and chest discomfort. An ECG shows evidence of T-wave flattening. You request an echocardiogram which demonstrates dilated ventricles with global hypokinesis. What is the most likely diagnosis?

a. Dilated cardiomyopathy
b. Hypertrophic cardiomyopathy
c. Restrictive cardiomyopathy
d. Arrhythmogenic right ventricular cardiomyopathy
e. Myocarditis

66. A 20-year-old student sees his GP for blurred vision. On further questioning, he reports he had a 'lens problem' a year ago. On examination he also has pectus excavatum, a high arched palate and signs of hypermobility. Which of the following cardiac disorders is often associated with this patient's condition?

a. Aortic valve stenosis
b. Coarctation of the aorta
c. Mitral valve prolapse
d. Ventricular septal defect
e. Ebstein anomaly

67. A 27-year-old footballer presents with laboured breathing and chest pain. An ECG shows evidence of left ventricular hypertrophy. What is the most likely diagnosis?

a. Dilated cardiomyopathy
b. Hypertrophic cardiomyopathy
c. Restrictive cardiomyopathy
d. Arrhythmogenic right ventricular cardiomyopathy
e. Myocarditis

68. A 42-year-old woman presents with chest pain. She comments that the pain is worse on inspiration but is relieved by leaning forward. Her past medical history includes breast carcinoma. What is the most likely diagnosis?

a. Acute pericarditis
b. Pericardial effusion

c. Pericardial tamponade
d. Constrictive pericarditis
e. Myocarditis

69. A 65-year-old man sees his GP with worsening
central chest pain and breathlessness following
exertion for 3 months. These symptoms usually
resolve with rest. Lately he has also been feeling
dizzy. On examination a systolic murmur is heard.
ECG shows large R waves in leads I, aVL and V4–6,
and large R waves in leads V1–3. What is the most
likely diagnosis?
a. Myocardial infarction
b. Unstable angina
c. Stable angina
d. Aortic stenosis
e. Hypertrophic cardiomyopathy

70. A 43-year-old obese woman with known breast
cancer complains of shortness of breath. On
examination you note soft HSs and obscuration of
the apex beat. Which investigation is most likely to
lead to a diagnosis?
a. CXR
b. Echocardiogram
c. ECG
d. Arterial blood gas
e. Coronary angiography

71. A 63-year-old retired doctor presents with
nausea and headaches. His past medical history
includes type II diabetes mellitus. On examination
you note his blood pressure is 165/76 mmHg.
What is the next most appropriate step in
management?
a. Beta-blockers
b. Calcium channel antagonists
c. ACE inhibitors
d. Diuretics
e. Alpha-blockers

72. A previously fit and well 45-year-old man presents
to A&E with fevers and malaise. On examination
he has multiple splinter haemorrhages and
a systolic murmur. A diagnosis of infective
endocarditis is suspected. Dukes criteria is used
to help with the diagnosis of the condition. Which
of the following statements is INCORRECT in
Dukes criteria?
a. Presence of Osler nodes is a minor
criterion
b. Positive blood for rheumatoid factor is a minor
criterion
c. Echocardiographic evidence of prosthetic valve
dehiscence is a major criterion

d. Serological evidence of active infection with an
organism consistent with infective endocarditis (IE)
e. Definite diagnosis can be made with three minor
criteria

73. A 65-year-old hypertensive patient is reviewed in the
outpatient clinic complaining of visual disturbances.
On examination you note flame-shaped
haemorrhages. What is the most likely diagnosis?
a. Grade 1 retinal disease
b. Grade 2 retinal disease
c. Grade 3 retinal disease
d. Grade 4 retinal disease
e. Grade 5 retinal disease

74. A 45-year-old teacher with known mitral valve
prolapse presents to his GP with a 2-week history
of fevers, rigors, chest pain and breathlessness. He
recently underwent a tooth extraction. On examination
he is febrile with multiple splinter haemorrhages.
A systolic murmur is heard and appears to have
increased in intensity since his last GP visit. What is
the most likely causative agent in this case?
a. *Candida albicans*
b. *Staphylococcus aureus*
c. *Pseudomonas aeruginosa*
d. *Streptococcus viridans*
e. *Enterococcus*

75. A 64-year-old female comes to your surgery with
a past medical history of hypertension. She is on
an ACE inhibitor as well as on a range of other
medications. Which one of the following would be
most likely to blunt the antihypertensive effects of an
ACE inhibitor?
a. Chlorpromazine
b. Allopurinol
c. Ibuprofen
d. Spironolactone
e. Paracetamol

EXTENDED-MATCHING QUESTIONS (EMQs)

Cardiac murmurs and added sounds
Each answer can be used once, more than once or not
at all.
a. Aortic regurgitation
b. Aortic stenosis
c. Bicuspid aortic valve
d. Mitral regurgitation
e. Mitral stenosis
f. Patent ductus arteriosus

g. Transposition of the great vessels
h. Tricuspid regurgitation
i. Ventricular septal defect

For each scenario below, choose the most likely corresponding option from the list given above.

1. A 60-year-old man presents with heart failure. On examination he has a collapsing pulse, an early diastolic murmur and a displaced apex beat.
2. A 56-year-old man gives a history of rheumatic fever. He has flushed cheeks, an irregularly irregular pulse and a mid-diastolic murmur.
3. A 75-year-old woman presents to A&E following a drop attack. Her ECG shows left ventricular hypertrophy. On examination, a harsh systolic murmur is heard over both carotid arteries.
4. Three days following his MI, Mr Thompson has a sudden deterioration, developing left ventricular failure. He has a new pansystolic murmur radiating from the apex to the axilla.
5. A baby who is cyanotic at birth with a loud long systolic murmur in whom tetralogy of Fallot is suspected.

Chest pain

Each answer can be used once, more than once or not at all.

a. Angina pectoris
b. Pericarditis
c. Myocardial infarction
d. Aortic dissection
e. Reflux oesophagitis
f. Pulmonary infarct
g. Pneumonia
h. Costochondritis
i. Pneumothorax
j. Pulmonary embolus

For each scenario below, choose the most likely corresponding option from the list given above.

1. A middle-aged man presenting with a central crushing chest pain on exercise but relieved by rest.
2. Associated with central crushing chest pain which occurs at rest and may radiate to the jaw or arms.
3. Severe tearing chest pain which may radiate to the back.
4. Central chest discomfort which is sharp in nature with a tender area on palpation.
5. Sharp chest pain aggravated by movement, respiration and changes in posture.

Drugs

Each answer can be used once, more than once or not at all.

a. Propranolol
b. Nicorandil
c. Aspirin
d. Nifedipine
e. Captopril
f. Digoxin
g. Bisoprolol
h. Bendrofluazide
i. Clopidogrel
j. Simvastatin

For each scenario below, choose the most likely corresponding option from the list given above.

1. Used in the treatment of cardiac failure. Known to cause a persistent cough.
2. Contraindicated in renal artery stenosis.
3. Associated with bradycardia, headaches and fluid retention.
4. First-line management in acute coronary syndrome.
5. Specifically contraindicated in asthmatics and individuals with peripheral vascular disease.

Clinical features of cardiac disease

Each answer can be used once, more than once or not at all.

a. Aortic stenosis
b. Aortic regurgitation
c. Mitral stenosis
d. Mitral regurgitation
e. Infective endocarditis
f. Rheumatic fever
g. Tricuspid stenosis
h. Tricuspid regurgitation
i. Pulmonary hypertension
j. Pulmonary embolism

For each scenario below, choose the most likely corresponding option from the list given above.

1. A pansystolic murmur auscultated at the apex and radiating into the axilla.
2. Associated with erythematous macules on the palms and haemorrhages under the nails.
3. Associated with pink-coloured rings on the trunk and subcutaneous nodules over the joints.
4. Associated with a slow rising carotid pulse and ejection systolic murmur at the right upper sternal border.
5. Known to cause a right parasternal heave and a loud pulmonary second sound.

Murmurs

Each answer can be used once, more than once or not at all.

- a. Aortic regurgitation
- b. Aortic stenosis
- c. Austin–Flint murmur
- d. Flow murmur
- e. Graham Steell murmur
- f. Mitral regurgitation
- g. Mitral stenosis
- h. Tricuspid regurgitation
- i. Tricuspid stenosis
- j. Ventricular septal defect

For each scenario below, choose the most likely corresponding option from the list given above.

1. A 60-year-old Egyptian man with a pansystolic murmur loudest at the right sternal edge, a raised JVP and a pulsatile liver.
2. A 70-year-old woman in atrial fibrillation, an apex beat palpable in the mid-axillary line and a loud pansystolic murmur which is heard all over the heart.
3. A 14-year-old girl with a flat occiput, single palmar crease and a pansystolic murmur. She has a chromosomal abnormality affecting chromosome 21.
4. An elderly gentleman with a collapsing pulse and an early diastolic murmur which is loudest when sitting forward.
5. A diastolic murmur which is early and continues past mid-diastole.

Symptoms of heart failure

Each answer can be used once, more than once or not at all.

- a. Ankle swelling
- b. Cough
- c. Hepatomegaly
- d. Orthopnoea
- e. Paroxysmal nocturnal dyspnoea
- f. Pink frothy sputum
- g. Pulmonary fibrosis
- h. Pulmonary oedema
- i. Shortness of breath

For each scenario below, choose the most likely corresponding option from the list given above.

1. A patient has been on a cardiology ward for 3 weeks with a diagnosis of pulmonary oedema. He is receiving large doses of furosemide. His systolic blood pressure is 74mmHg and increases on being placed head down in bed. On auscultation he has fine crackles throughout both lung fields.

2. A patient complains of waking in the middle of the night and racing out of bed to the window, gasping for breath.
3. A patient sleeps on four pillows at night so he can catch his breath.
4. A patient with a diagnosis of heart failure complains of this symptom several weeks after starting an ACE inhibitor.
5. Congestion due to right heart failure can cause a nutmeg appearance and this symptom.

Electrocardiograph findings

Each answer can be used once, more than once or not at all.

- a. Anterior myocardial infarction
- b. Atrial fibrillation
- c. Atrial flutter with 2:1 block
- d. Digitalis effect
- e. Inferior myocardial infarction
- f. Pericarditis
- g. Posterior myocardial infarction
- h. Sick sinus syndrome
- i. Third-degree heart block
- j. Ventricular tachycardia

For each scenario below, choose the most likely corresponding option from the list given above.

1. ST depression in V1–3 and tall R wave in V1 and V2.
2. ST elevation that is present in all leads and is saddle shaped.
3. ST elevation of 3mm in leads II, III and aVF.
4. Broad complex QRS with a rate of 45 beats/min; P waves are present.
5. No P waves, narrow complex QRS rate of 150 beats/min with sawtooth baseline.

Heart disease

Each answer can be used once, more than once or not at all.

- a. Acute myocardial infarction
- b. Aortic stenosis
- c. Atrial myxoma
- d. Complete heart block
- e. Cor pulmonale
- f. Dilated cardiomyopathy
- g. Fibrinous pericarditis
- h. Infective endocarditis
- i. Mitral valve stenosis
- j. Tricuspid incompetence

For each scenario below, choose the most likely corresponding option from the list given above.

1. A 58-year-old woman with known asymptomatic aortic stenosis presents with fever and feeling

generally unwell. She has just had three fillings performed by her dentist.

2. A 49-year-old man presents to his GP with shortness of breath on walking up hills. He also experiences central chest pain which is relieved by resting, as well as occasional dizziness. He has a loud systolic murmur.

3. On the second day post-MI, a 71-year-old man develops pleuritic sounding chest pain. This is relieved by ibuprofen. The ECG demonstrates saddle-shaped ST changes.

4. A 63-year-old man presents to A&E with shortness of breath. He has a loud pansystolic murmur and a displaced apex beat. CXR demonstrates a straight left heart border and cardiothoracic ratio of >50%. He admits to previous excess alcohol intake.

5. A 44-year-old woman attends her respiratory clinic appointment. She has known chronic obstructive pulmonary disease and is a previous heavy smoker. Her most recent symptoms are ankle swelling and an exercise tolerance of 15 yards.

Chest pain

Each answer can be used once, more than once or not at all.

  a. Myocardial infarct
  b. Pulmonary embolus
  c. Pericarditis
  d. Left lower lobe pneumonia
  e. Rib fracture
  f. Oesophageal reflux disease
  g. Aortic dissection
  h. Costochondritis
  i. Angina pectoris
  j. Herpes zoster

For each scenario below, choose the most likely corresponding option from the list given above.

1. A 48-year-old housewife is admitted with left-sided chest discomfort, sharp in nature, which is worse on coughing. She has no sputum. She takes the oral contraceptive pill and propranolol hydrochloride (Half-Inderal LA). Her father and uncle died in their 60s from 'heart attacks'. She smokes 30 cigarettes a day. ECG: sinus tachycardia and right bundle-branch block. D-dimer 0.71 mg/L, troponin I 0.01 mg/L. CXR: no active disease (NAD).

2. A 58-year-old insulin-dependent diabetic is admitted at the request of his GP. He has been complaining of intermittent central chest pain for the past month. He is a poor historian but claims he has not noticed any relationship to the pain. He has suffered from AF and hypertension for 6 years. He currently takes digoxin, atenolol, diclofenac and simvastatin. O/E: body mass index 31 kg/m^2, no chest wall tenderness, HS I + II + ejection systolic murmur in aortic area. No clinical evidence of deep vein thrombosis. HbA1C 10.5%, random glucose 13.2 mmol/L, digoxin level 1.3 mmol/L. ECG: 1-mm depression in leads V1–V6. CXR: NAD.

3. A 45-year-old Moroccan man (working in the local chicken factory) attended A&E with central chest discomfort. His English is broken, but you establish that this has been a problem for the past week and that it is sharp in nature ('like a knife, doctor'). He has no recent trauma. Examination is unremarkable. CXR: scarring of right apex and calcified hilar nodes. You return to the patient and he confirms previously being treated for tuberculosis back in Morocco.

4. A 36-year-old man is admitted via A&E with right-sided chest pain associated with shortness of breath. There is no fever. O/E: Thin gentleman, smells of tobacco and alcohol. He is uncooperative to examination. Reduced breath sounds on the right side. Tender over the anterior chest wall. CXR: peripheral area of decreased lung markings on the right side.

5. A 56-year-old insulin-dependent diabetic is admitted at the request of a concerned relative (a local doctor). He has been complaining of niggling chest pain for the past 2 days, with an associated feeling of shortness of breath. O/E: apyrexial, no chest wall tenderness. Nil adventitious sounds. HS I + II + 0. CXR: NAD. ECG: ST elevation 3-mm leads V4–V6 with T-wave inversion. Troponin 6.5 mg/L.

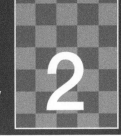

SINGLE BEST ANSWER (SBA) QUESTIONS

1. A 56-year-old man presents to the general practitioner (GP) complaining of weight loss of 2 kg over 3 months and lethargy. On further questioning he reveals that his stools are paler than normal, and his urine dark in colour. He denies being in any pain. On examination his sclerae look yellow. What is the most likely diagnosis?
   a. Gallstones
   b. Acute pancreatitis
   c. Autoimmune hepatitis
   d. Pancreatic cancer
   e. Hepatocellular carcinoma

2. A 40-year-old gentleman has been suffering from reflux symptoms for 1 year. He drinks approximately 40 units of alcohol a week and has recently managed to give up smoking. His GP sends him for an upper gastrointestinal (GI) endoscopy for further investigation. This looked suspicious for Barrett oesophagus, so a biopsy was taken. What would you expect the histology to show?
   a. Columnar cells
   b. Squamous cells
   c. Glandular cells
   d. Transitional cells
   e. Connective tissue cells

3. A 52-year-old female attended her local walk-in centre complaining of tiredness. On further questioning she had pruritus. A full panel of blood tests were sent off, and she was informed later in the week that one of the tests had come back positive for mitochondrial autoantibodies. What is the diagnosis?
   a. Primary biliary cirrhosis (PBC)
   b. Secondary biliary cirrhosis
   c. Primary sclerosing cholangitis
   d. Autoimmune hepatitis
   e. Wilson disease

4. A 58-year-old male went to the GP complaining of feeling more tired than usual. He also felt that he had become more 'tanned' throughout the winter months. On examination he had hepatomegaly. What is the diagnosis?
   a. Wilson disease
   b. Secondary biliary cirrhosis
   c. Iron-deficient anaemia

   d. Vitamin B_{12} deficiency
   e. Haemochromatosis

5. A 57-year-old alcohol-dependant lady presented for the first time to the accident and emergency department with abdominal pain and a distended abdomen. Examination of the abdomen reveals the presence of spider naevi and shifting dullness evident. She is treated for decompensated alcoholic liver disease. What vitamin should she be given intravenously?
   a. Vitamin A
   b. Vitamin B_1
   c. Vitamin B_{12}
   d. Vitamin C
   e. Vitamin D

6. A 32-year-old lady with type 1 diabetes went to see her GP complaining of a 10-day history of pain when swallowing both solids and liquids. She had recently completed a course of antibiotics for a urinary tract infection. She has been referred for an upper GI endoscopy. What is this most likely to show?
   a. Scleroderma
   b. Oesophageal carcinoma
   c. Achalasia
   d. Oesophageal candidiasis
   e. Benign oesophageal stricture

7. A 50-year-old male attended accident and emergency with a large-volume haematemesis. On examination he has gynaecomastia and spider naevi. Rectal (PR) examination revealed black stool. What is the most likely cause of his upper GI bleed?
   a. Oesophageal varices
   b. Oesophagitis
   c. Mallory–Weiss tear
   d. Duodenal ulcer
   e. Gastric carcinoma

8. A patient is brought into hospital after having a witnessed seizure lasting 2 minutes. He is known to have hepatic cirrhosis and has become confused and disorientated over the past few days. On examination he has a coarse flap with outstretched hands. What is the most likely diagnosis?
   a. Hyponatraemia
   b. Hepatic encephalopathy
   c. Carbon dioxide retention
   d. Epilepsy
   e. Illicit drug use

9. A 21-year-old male, who had been feeling unwell with flu-like symptoms for the past week, went to see the GP as his eyes looked yellow. Routine bloods showed a bilirubin of 68 µmol/L; however, the rest of his liver function tests (LFTs) were normal. What is the most likely diagnosis?
   a. Viral hepatitis
   b. Rotor syndrome
   c. Gilbert syndrome
   d. Dubin–Johnson syndrome
   e. Gallstones

10. A 23-year-old medical student organizes her elective in India. Whilst there, she develops fever, diarrhoea and abdominal cramps. The symptoms persist for a week before she visits a doctor for some advice. What is the most likely cause?
    a. Giardiasis
    b. Hepatitis A
    c. Salmonellosis
    d. Yersiniosis
    e. Rotavirus

11. A 51-year-old male was diagnosed last year with chronic respiratory disease, which was fairly severe and affected his mobility. This had come as a shock as he had never previously smoked. His LFTs had previously been mildly deranged. He went to see his GP as he looked more yellow than normal. What is the most likely cause?
    a. Gilbert syndrome
    b. Mirizzi syndrome
    c. Haemochromatosis
    d. α_1-Antitrypsin deficiency
    e. Alcoholic hepatitis

12. A 67-year-old lady presents with weight loss of 3 kg over 4 months and intermittent abdominal pain. Examination is unremarkable apart from an enlarged supraclavicular lymph node on the left side of the body. What is the most likely diagnosis?
    a. Cholangiocarcinoma
    b. Pancreatic cancer
    c. Sigmoid cancer
    d. Hepatocellular carcinoma
    e. Gastric cancer

13. A 71-year-old male presents to the GP with weight loss, lethargy and decreased appetite over the past 6 months. The GP organizes for blood samples to be taken and requests tumour markers. Alpha-fetoprotein (AFP) comes back elevated at 58 g/L. What is this suggestive of?
    a. Hepatocellular carcinoma
    b. Cholangiocarcinoma
    c. Ampullary adenoma

d. Colorectal cancer
e. Pancreatic cancer

14. A 21-year-old female presented to the accident and emergency department complaining of vomiting blood. She had been out the previous night and drank copious amounts of alcohol, and had been vomiting several times throughout the day. Examination was unremarkable, and there was no evidence of black stools. A nurse witnessed a vomit and reported that there were just small amounts of red streaks in it. What is the most likely diagnosis?
    a. Alcoholic hepatitis
    b. Acute gastritis
    c. Gastric ulcer
    d. Oesophageal varices
    e. Mallory–Weiss tear

15. A 23-year-old university student presented with general flu-like symptoms for 2 weeks including a sore throat. On examination she has enlarged cervical lymph nodes. Routine blood tests show the following measurements: bilirubin, 27 µmol/L; alanine transaminase (ALT), 494 IU/L; gamma-glutamyl transpeptidase, 62 IU/L; white cell count (WCC), 13.3; lymphocytes, 6.0. What is the likely cause of the raised liver enzymes?
    a. Gilbert syndrome
    b. Gallstone
    c. Viral illness
    d. Autoimmune hepatitis
    e. Acute pancreatitis

16. A 50-year-old male was being treated on a surgical assessment ward for acute pancreatitis. His initial GLASGOW score was 3. On ward round, 7 days after admission, the consultant requested an investigation to look for any evidence of pancreatic necrosis. What is the imaging used normally?
    a. Magnetic resonance imaging (MRI) abdomen
    b. Ultrasound scan (USS) abdomen
    c. Abdominal X-ray (AXR)
    d. Computed tomography (CT) abdomen
    e. Endoscopic ultrasound scan (EUS)

17. A 47-year-old female presents with severe intermittent abdominal pain over the last 2 months. She has had multiple previous admissions with acute pancreatitis. Her most recent CT scan showed calcified deposits in the pancreas. She denies any alcohol intake for the past 6 months. What is the most likely diagnosis?
    a. Acute pancreatitis
    b. Chronic pancreatitis
    c. Mesenteric ischaemia
    d. Pancreatic cancer
    e. Gastric ulcer

18. A 24-year-old male was referred for a colonoscopy to investigate his symptoms of weight loss and diarrhoea. The endoscopist thought that they could view skip lesions in the terminal ileum and took several biopsies. What is the histology most likely to show?
    a. Ulcerative colitis
    b. Coeliac disease
    c. Irritable bowel syndrome
    d. Crohn disease
    e. Bacterial enterocolitis

19. A 16-year-old female attends the GP surgery to ask for some advice. She suffers from severe travel sickness. The GP prescribes an antiemetic. Which one is likely to be the most effective?
    a. Levomepromazine
    b. Ondansetron
    c. Metoclopramide
    d. Domperidone
    e. Cyclizine

20. A 32-year-old male presented with abdominal pain and vomiting. He described the pain as a sudden onset, severe pain which radiates through to his back. He had an ultrasound earlier this year which showed gallstones. You suspect acute pancreatitis. What investigation is used to confirm this?
    a. Arterial blood gases
    b. Urea and electrolytes test results (U&Es)
    c. Serum amylase
    d. AXR
    e. CT abdomen

21. A 38-year-old male visits his GP complaining of intermittent abdominal pain. This is epigastric in nature and radiates through to the back. It is more severe before meal times and relieved by eating. A ^{14}C urea breath test is arranged which comes back positive. What is the most likely diagnosis?
    a. Duodenal ulcer
    b. Gastro-oesophageal reflux disease (GORD)
    c. Barrett oesophagus
    d. Achalasia
    e. Gastric ulcer

22. A patient had been in hospital for several weeks following a car crash. Whilst there, he developed offensive-smelling diarrhoea, passing at least six motions a day. He had a stool sample sent off which confirmed *Clostridium difficile*. Which of the following antibiotics is considered high risk for developing pseudomembranous colitis?
    a. Cefotaxime
    b. Vancomycin
    c. Flucloxacillin

    d. Doxycycline
    e. Ciprofloxacin

23. A 32-year-old male of Asian origin presents with weight loss, diarrhoea and stools that are difficult to flush away. He had a colonoscopy, and a biopsy later confirmed villous atrophy. He was started on a gluten-free diet; however, his symptoms failed to improve. What is the most likely diagnosis?
    a. Tropical sprue
    b. Coeliac disease
    c. Chronic pancreatitis
    d. Crohn disease
    e. Irritable bowel syndrome

24. A 70-year-old male has pancreatic cancer. He has recently been started on strong opioids to control his pain. He is visited by the palliative care nurses and complains of difficulty in opening his bowels, stating that his stools are much harder than they used to be. What is the most appropriate laxative to put him on?
    a. Lactulose
    b. Sodium docusate
    c. Fybogel
    d. MOVICOL
    e. Senna

25. A 42-year-old alcoholic presents with heartburn. He comments that it is aggravated by bending and lying down but relieved by drinking milk. What is the next most appropriate initial investigation?
    a. 24-hour oesophageal pH monitoring
    b. Barium swallow
    c. Upper GI endoscopy
    d. Chest X-ray
    e. AXR

26. A 40-year-old obese city worker presents with heartburn. He comments that he tried 'Gaviscon', which barely relieved the pain. Which management plan would you instigate first?
    a. H$_2$ receptor antagonists
    b. Domperidone
    c. Nissen fundoplication
    d. Proton-pump inhibitors
    e. Metoclopramide

27. A 35-year-old woman complains of difficulty in swallowing and weight loss. She comments that she is unable to swallow both liquid and solid food. A barium swallow demonstrates a tapered lower end of her oesophagus. What is the most likely diagnosis?
    a. Achalasia
    b. Systemic sclerosis

c. Diffuse oesophageal spasm

d. Hiatus hernia

e. Oesophageal carcinoma

28. A 65-year-old Chinese man presents complaining of swallowing difficulties and weight loss of approximately 2 stone over a 1-month period. An upper GI endoscopy is arranged which demonstrates evidence of a tumour mass. The following are all risk factors for squamous cell oesophageal carcinoma EXCEPT?

a. Pickled vegetables

b. Salted fish

c. Smoking

d. Alcohol

e. GORD

29. A middle-aged man presents complaining of swallowing difficulties and chest pain. A barium swallow is arranged which demonstrates a 'corkscrew'-like appearance. What is the most likely diagnosis?

a. Achalasia

b. Systemic sclerosis

c. Diffuse oesophageal spasm

d. Hiatus hernia

e. Oesophageal carcinoma

30. A 42-year-old man presents with pain in his stomach after meals. An endoscopy is performed which shows evidence of gastritis and infection with *Helicobacter pylori*. What is the next most appropriate step in management?

a. Metoclopramide, omeprazole and amoxicillin

b. Omeprazole, metronidazole and cimetidine

c. Omeprazole, metronidazole and clarithromycin

d. Omeprazole, ranitidine and amoxicillin

e. Domperidone, omeprazole and amoxicillin

31. A 56-year-old man presents with epigastric pain, vomiting and weight loss. He is a heavy drinker and admits to consuming half a bottle of vodka each day over a 10-year period. On examination you note a purple-coloured peri-orbital skin rash. What is the next most appropriate initial investigation?

a. Abdominal CT scan

b. Abdominal MRI scan

c. AXR

d. Upper GI endoscopy

e. EUS

32. A 42-year-old man presents with a 1-day history of haematemesis. On closer questioning he commented that when he opens his bowels his motion looks like tar. What is the most likely aetiological cause for his symptoms?

a. Mallory–Weiss tear

b. Reflux oesophagitis

c. Gastric varices

d. Oesophageal varices

e. Peptic ulcer

33. A 21-year-old rugby player presents to the accident and emergency with a 1-day history of haematemesis. He had recently been on a drinking binge following his team winning the local final. He comments that the bleeding began after an episode of severe vomiting. An endoscopy is performed. What is the most likely diagnosis?

a. Mallory–Weiss tear

b. Reflux oesophagitis

c. Gastric varices

d. Oesophageal varices

e. Peptic ulcer

34. A 75-year-old woman presents with a 1-day history of haematemesis. She comments she has been suffering from back pain for the past month for which she has been taking diclofenac as prescribed by her GP. What is the most likely aetiological cause for her symptoms?

a. Mallory–Weiss tear

b. Reflux oesophagitis

c. Peptic ulcer

d. Gastric varices

e. Oesophageal varices

35. While on call you are asked to see a patient who has just passed melaena. On examination you note he is drowsy with a pulse of 124 beats/min and blood pressure of 75/44 mmHg. Which management plan would you instigate first?

a. Upper GI endoscopy

b. Colonoscopy

c. Blood samples for group and save and cross-match

d. Intravenous (IV) access and fluid resuscitation

e. Laparotomy

36. A 45-year-old man presents with shortness of breath and fatigue. Routine blood investigations reveal a haemoglobin of 102 g/L, a mean corpuscular volume (MCV) of 75 fL and a serum ferritin of 10 µg/L. What is the next most appropriate initial investigation?

a. Upper GI endoscopy

b. Colonoscopy

c. Upper GI endoscopy and colonoscopy

d. Barium meal and follow through

e. Mesenteric angiography

37. A 14-year-old girl presents with abdominal pain and diarrhoea. She is found to be iron and folate deficient on initial investigation. What is the most likely diagnosis?
    a. Crohn disease
    b. Ulcerative colitis
    c. Whipple disease
    d. Irritable bowel syndrome
    e. Coeliac disease

38. A 19-year-old woman presents with abdominal pain and diarrhoea. She comments that there is a strong family history of coeliac disease. Which investigation is most likely to lead to a diagnosis?
    a. Upper GI endoscopy and distal duodenal biopsy
    b. Full blood count
    c. Small-bowel barium follow-through
    d. Immunoglobulin A (IgA) and tissue transglutaminase (tTG) serology
    e. Antireticulin antibodies

39. A 55-year-old man has recently undergone complicated small bowel surgery. He complains of producing loose stools which he describes as being offensive and difficult to flush. Which investigation is most likely to lead to a diagnosis?
    a. Upper GI endoscopy
    b. Rectal examination
    c. Hydrogen breath test
    d. Barium meal
    e. Abdominal CT scan

40. A middle-aged man with ulcerative colitis is referred to accident and emergency by his GP with an acute flare, opening his bowels eight times per day. Routine blood investigations reveal a platelet count of 576×10^9/L and C-reactive protein (CRP) of 156 mg/L. What is the next most appropriate step in management?
    a. Oral steroids
    b. IV steroids
    c. Ciclosporin
    d. Mesalazine
    e. Azathioprine

41. A patient with Crohn disease comes to see his GP. He is currently on mesalazine but has been experiencing an increase in bowel frequency and gradual onset of abdominal pain. What is the next most appropriate step in management?
    a. Steroids
    b. Ciclosporin
    c. Azathioprine
    d. Metronidazole
    e. Methotrexate

42. A 55-year-old woman presents with abdominal pain and diarrhoea. She notices fresh red blood in the toilet pan when she opens her bowels. She has smoked 25 cigarettes a day since the age of 30 and drinks 8 units of alcohol a week. Her mother was diagnosed with bowel cancer at 40 years of age. She enjoys eating steak but admits she does not have a taste for fruit or vegetables. You arrange a barium study which confirms the presence of a colonic tumour. What is the most likely aetiological cause for her tumour?
    a. Poor diet
    b. Smoking
    c. Alcohol
    d. Family history
    e. Age

43. A 32-year-old woman with severe Crohn disease underwent a subtotal colectomy with ileostomy formation. She comes to the GP complaining of increased stoma output. She comments that she is emptying her bag up to six times per day and that the contents are loose and watery. What is the next most appropriate initial investigation?
    a. Ileoscopy
    b. Barium meal and follow-through
    c. Hydrogen breath test
    d. Abdominal CT scan
    e. Stool culture

44. A 65-year-old woman is on long-term total parenteral nutrition (TPN) via a Hickman line following a small bowel resection. While on call you are asked to review the patient as she has a temperature of 38.5°C. What is the next most appropriate step in management?
    a. Peripheral blood cultures and continue TPN
    b. Hickman line blood cultures and continue TPN
    c. Peripheral and Hickman line blood cultures and continue TPN
    d. Peripheral and Hickman line blood cultures and stop TPN
    e. Paracetamol as required and recheck temperature in 30 minutes.

45. A 65-year-old man presents with right-sided abdominal pain. On examination you note a moderately enlarged liver and a yellow discoloration of his skin and eyes. What is the next most appropriate initial investigation?
    a. Abdominal USS
    b. Endoscopic retrograde cholangiopancreatography (ERCP)
    c. Viral markers
    d. Liver biopsy
    e. Magnetic resonance cholangiopancreatography (MRCP)

46. A 23-year-old South American man presents with abdominal pain and diarrhoea over a 3-day period followed by jaundice. He comments that his urine appears darker than usual but says he is drinking plenty of water. He has recently travelled to Lima to see his family. What is the most likely diagnosis?
    a. Hepatitis D
    b. Hepatitis A
    c. Hepatitis B
    d. Hepatitis C
    e. Hepatitis E

47. A 56-year-old Egyptian woman presents with fatigue and nausea. She complains that her skin feels itchy and that she has noticed blood when she passes urine. On examination you note a yellow tinge to her skin and sclera. What is the most likely diagnosis?
    a. Hepatitis A
    b. Hepatitis D
    c. Hepatitis B
    d. Hepatitis E
    e. Hepatitis C

48. A 32-year-old man presents with abdominal pain, diarrhoea and jaundice. He has recently been to Dubai with his wife. He comments that the best thing about Dubai is the seafood. What is the next most appropriate step in management?
    a. Alpha-interferon
    b. Lamivudine
    c. Ribavirin
    d. Watchful waiting
    e. Pegylated alpha-interferon

49. A 32-year-old man presents to accident and emergency following a paracetamol overdose. Routine blood investigations reveal an ALT of 1800 U/L and a prothrombin time of 42 seconds. On examination he appears drowsy and is not communicative. What is his grade of encephalopathy?
    a. Grade 1 encephalopathy
    b. Grade 2 encephalopathy
    c. Grade 3 encephalopathy
    d. Grade 4 encephalopathy
    e. Grade 5 encephalopathy

50. A middle-aged woman with autoimmune thyroiditis presents with nausea and fatigue. On examination you note jaundice and spider naevi. Which investigation is most likely to lead to a diagnosis?
    a. Abdominal USS
    b. Antinuclear antibodies
    c. Serum ferritin levels

    d. Hepatitis B testing
    e. IgM levels

51. A 43-year-old man with a long-standing history of alcohol abuse presents to accident and emergency with haematemesis. On examination you note a liver flap and evidence of moderate hepatomegaly. You suspect a diagnosis of cirrhosis. Which investigation is most likely to assess the patient's liver function?
    a. Liver biochemistry
    b. Serum electrolytes
    c. Serum AFP
    d. Prothrombin time
    e. Hepatitis serology

52. A 25-year-old city worker presents with a 2-day history of haematemesis following a weekend of binge drinking. Which management plan would you instigate first?
    a. Upper GI endoscopy
    b. IV terlipressin
    c. Laparotomy
    d. Transjugular intrahepatic portosystemic shunting (TIPS)
    e. Sucralfate

53. A middle-aged man is diagnosed with liver cirrhosis secondary to chronic alcohol abuse. On examination you note dullness in his flanks. Which management plan would you instigate first?
    a. Paracentesis
    b. Sodium restriction alone
    c. Sodium restriction and diuretics
    d. Transjugular intrahepatic portosystemic shunting (TIPS)
    e. Albumin infusion

54. A 35-year-old man with alcoholic cirrhosis complains of abdominal discomfort. On examination you note the presence of ascites and notable peritonism. Routine blood investigations reveal a WCC of 23×10^9/L and CRP of 107 mg/L. What is the most likely aetiological cause for his symptoms?
    a. *Staphylococcus aureus*
    b. *Escherichia coli*
    c. *Enterococcus faecalis*
    d. *Proteus mirabilis*
    e. *Staphylococcus epidermidis*

55. A middle-aged man presents to the accident and emergency with confusion. His wife comments that he does not appear to be his usual self and that he has been drinking excessively for many years. On examination you note a liver flap and a sweet smell on his breath. How would you usually make the diagnosis leading to his confusion?

a. Electroencephalography (EEG)
b. Head CT scan
c. Abdominal CT scan
d. Abdominal USS
e. Clinical assessment

56. A 47-year-old woman complains that her skin is feeling itchy and her stools are difficult to flush. On examination she has moderate hepatomegaly and investigations demonstrate a raised serum alkaline phosphatase. Which investigation is most likely to lead to a diagnosis?
a. Serum IgM
b. Serum aspartate aminotransferase (AST)
c. Serum bilirubin
d. Serum antimitochondrial antibodies (AMAs)
e. Antinuclear factor

57. A middle-aged man complains of malaise and arthropathy. He is a newly diagnosed diabetic and on examination has evidence of hepatomegaly. Which investigation is most likely to lead to a diagnosis?
a. Serum AST
b. Serum bilirubin
c. Serum albumin
d. INR
e. Serum ferritin

58. A middle-aged woman with suspected alcoholic liver disease is referred for a liver biopsy. The histology report states that there is necrosis of the liver cells and infiltration of leucocytes with the presence of Mallory bodies within the hepatocytes. What is the next most appropriate step in management?
a. Liver transplant
b. Steroids
c. Stop alcohol completely
d. Continue alcohol in moderation
e. Multivitamins and nutritional support

59. A 65-year-old man presents with weight loss and abdominal pain. On examination you note evidence of ascites. Routine blood investigations reveal a markedly raised AFP level and deranged LFTs. What is the next most appropriate initial investigation?
a. AXR
b. Abdominal MRI scan
c. Liver biopsy
d. USS
e. Hepatic angiogram

60. A middle-aged woman with chronic alcohol dependency presents with abdominal pain and weight loss. She comments that her stools are difficult to flush. What is the next most appropriate initial investigation?
a. Erect chest X-ray
b. AXR
c. ERCP
d. Abdominal CT scan
e. MRCP

61. An 85-year-old frail woman presents with abdominal pain and weight loss of over 2 stone in a 1-month period. An abdominal USS is performed which confirms the diagnosis as pancreatic cancer with liver metastases. What is the next most appropriate step in management?
a. Surgery
b. Palliative therapy
c. Radiotherapy
d. Chemotherapy
e. Surgery and chemotherapy

EXTENDED-MATCHING QUESTIONS (EMQs)

Liver problems

Each answer can be used once, more than once or not at all.
a. Alcoholic liver disease
b. Biliary atresia
c. Gallstones
d. Hepatitis A
e. Hepatitis B
f. Hepatitis C
g. Metastatic liver disease
h. Physiological jaundice
i. PBC
j. Wilson disease

For each scenario below, choose the most likely corresponding option from the list given above.

1. An obese 60-year-old man presents to the medical admissions unit following haematemesis with unsteadiness, a flapping tremor and erythematous palms.
2. Two years after major abdominal surgery, a 75-year-old woman presents to her GP with weight loss and jaundice. On examination she has an enlarged knobbly liver.
3. A 4-week-old baby girl is taken to see the GP by a concerned breastfeeding mother. The baby is deeply jaundiced.
4. A 20-year-old soldier returning from the Gulf has abdominal pain, vomiting and pale stools with jaundice. His liver edge is just palpable, smooth and slightly tender.

5. An overweight 45-year-old woman presents with right upper quadrant pain associated with meals. On examination she is slightly tender in the right upper quadrant on deep inspiration.

Hepatobiliary disorders
Each answer can be used once, more than once or not at all.
a. Wilson disease
b. α_1-Antitrypsin deficiency
c. Hepatitis A
d. Cirrhosis
e. Hepatitis E
f. Primary sclerosing cholangitis
g. Haemochromatosis
h. Hepatocellular carcinoma
i. Hepatitis C
j. PBC

For each scenario below, choose the most likely corresponding option from the list given above.

1. An autosomal recessive disorder associated with the C282Y mutation on chromosome 6.
2. An autosomal recessive disorder associated with cirrhotic changes and the presence of periodic acid–Schiff-positive staining globules within hepatocytes.
3. A condition known to primarily affect middle-aged women resulting in pruritus, jaundice, xanthomas and bone disease.
4. An autosomal recessive disorder known to cause basal ganglia damage and renal failure best managed by trientene.
5. A condition associated with abdominal pain, jaundice and cirrhosis seen in individuals with inflammatory bowel disease (IBD).

Gastrointestinal bleeding
Each answer can be used once, more than once or not at all.
a. Mallory–Weiss tear
b. Angiodysplasia
c. Haemorrhoids
d. Colon cancer
e. Duodenal ulcer
f. Oesophageal varices
g. Reflux oesophagitis
h. Gastritis
i. Gastric erosions
j. Anal fissure

For each scenario below, choose the most likely corresponding option from the list given above.

1. A 30-year-old female presenting with spots of bright red blood on the toilet paper after passing stool.

2. An 18-year-old university student presenting with haematemesis following a period of vigorous vomiting.
3. A cause of iron-deficiency anaemia affecting the colon, caecum or terminal ileum in individuals with aortic stenosis.
4. A 58-year-old bank manager comes to you with symptoms of heartburn and odynophagia.
5. A 67-year-old male has symptoms associated with epigastric discomfort which is typically relieved by food. The diagnosis was confirmed by a gram-negative bacterium seen on a biopsy slide.

Drugs
Each answer can be used once, more than once or not at all.
a. Omeprazole
b. Aspirin
c. Penicillamine
d. Acamprosate
e. Mesalazine
f. Steroids
g. Nifedipine
h. Cisapride
i. Chlordiazepoxide
j. Alpha interferon

For each scenario below, choose the most likely corresponding option from the list given above.

1. A 45-year-old male chronic alcohol user who has had three recent admissions to hospital following an alcoholic 'binge'. He is demanding medication to help prevent him drink again.
2. A 34-year-old patient with known ulcerative colitis admitted to accident and emergency following an acute flare.
3. A 65-year-old man with a history of stroke presenting with an episode of haematemesis.
4. A middle-aged obese man presenting with indigestion following consumption of spicy foods.
5. A 23-year-old female presenting with abdominal discomfort and diarrhoea. A colonoscopy and subsequent biopsies demonstrate evidence of transmural inflammation with noncaseating granulomas.

Dysphagia
Each answer can be used once, more than once or not at all.
a. Achalasia
b. Oesophageal carcinoma
c. Benign oesophageal stricture
d. Oesophagitis
e. Pharyngeal pouch

f. Oesophageal pouch
g. Oesophageal web
h. Foreign body
i. *Candida*
j. Cytomegalovirus

For each scenario below, choose the most likely corresponding option from the list given above.

1. A patient presenting with swallowing difficulties and oral discomfort following a recent renal transplant.
2. Associated with swallowing difficulties, persistent coughing and iron-deficiency anaemia.
3. Associated with regurgitation of food as a result of abnormal motility of the cricopharyngeus muscle and inferior constrictor.
4. A middle-aged man presenting with swallowing difficulties of both liquid and solid food following recent sclerotherapy of oesophageal varices.
5. Associated with intermittent dysphagia of both liquid and solid food. A chest radiograph demonstrates evidence of a fluid level behind the heart.

Gastroenteritis

Each answer can be used once, more than once or not at all.

a. *Clostridium perfringens*
b. *Campylobacter*
c. *Bacillus cereus*
d. *Vibrio cholerae*
e. *Escherichia coli*
f. *Yersinia enterocolitica*
g. *Salmonella*
h. *Staphylococcus aureus*
i. *Vibrio parahaemolyticus*
j. Norwalk virus

For each scenario below, choose the most likely corresponding option from the list given above.

1. Known to cause nausea, vomiting and diarrhoea approximately 1 to 6 hours following ingestion of contaminated dairy products or cold meat.
2. Associated with vomiting and later diarrhoea following consumption of reheated rice.
3. Associated with abdominal pain, diarrhoea and rectal bleeding following consumption of contaminated poultry.
4. Known to cause bloody diarrhoea within 1 to 2 days of consuming contaminated meat. The use of antibiotics is specifically contraindicated.
5. Associated with diarrhoea, abdominal pain and bloody stools following contact with infected animals or ice cream.

Pancreatitis

Each answer can be used once, more than once or not at all.

a. Alcohol
b. ERCP
c. Gallstones
d. Grey-Turner sign
e. Hyperlipidaemia
f. Pancreatic divisum
g. Pancreatic necrosectomy
h. Saponification
i. Scorpion venom
j. Trauma

For each scenario below, choose the most likely corresponding option from the list given above.

1. A 45-year-old care home assistant presents with acute onset of upper abdominal pain. His abdomen is guarded, with bowel sounds. He denies any alcohol consumption in the past 4 years. His serum amylase is 800 mmol/L; his serum sodium is 118 mmol/L. The laboratory technician calls to inform you of the low sodium, and you notice a milky flashback from the cannula in the man's hand.
2. A 23-year-old woman is involved in a traffic collision. Her motorcycle is hit from the side by a careless driver and she is found unconscious, lying on her back, by the ambulance crew. On admission, during the secondary survey, you notice she has bruising over her flanks.
3. A 47-year-old man presents with recurrent pancreatitis. He claims that he is abstinent from alcohol. At ERCP, the sphincter of Oddi cannot be cannulated, and the diagnosis is confirmed by MRCP.
4. A 25-year-old man presents to hospital with severe abdominal pain having returned from holiday in Gran Canaria (Spain). His serum amylase and lipase are significantly elevated. He denies having had a drink since his return 2 days ago.
5. A 40-year-old woman is admitted to hospital for treatment of acute pancreatitis. She describes a recent history of sharp right upper quadrant pain that would last for 2 hours at a time.

Diarrhoea

Each answer can be used once, more than once or not at all.

a. Angiotensin-converting enzyme inhibitor
b. Amoebic dysentery
c. Beta-blocker
d. Cancer of the colon
e. Diverticular disease
f. Giardiasis

g. Irritable bowel syndrome
h. Metformin
i. Ulcerative colitis
j. Zollinger–Ellison syndrome

For each scenario below, choose the most likely corresponding option from the list given above.

1. A 23-year-old man with type A personality presents with a change in bowel habit. He has alternating constipation with pellet-like stool and diarrhoea. He occasionally passes mucus but never any blood.
2. A 55-year-old man with newly diagnosed diabetes complains of diarrhoea after his last consultation with you.
3. A 68-year-old man presents with diarrhoea alternating with constipation and passage of blood per rectum. He has no weight loss or tenesmus. Colonoscopy demonstrates no masses but makes the diagnosis.
4. A 25-year-old woman presents with profuse diarrhoea with passage of blood and mucus. She describes cramping abdominal pains. Examination reveals left iliac fossa tenderness. She has also lost weight.
5. A 45-year-old man presents with diarrhoea in association with acid reflux. Gastroscopy reveals multiple duodenal ulcers, and serum gastrin levels are 10 times the upper limit of normal.

Altered bowel habit

Each answer can be used once, more than once or not at all.

a. Ulcerative colitis
b. Crohn disease
c. Colorectal carcinoma
d. Irritable bowel syndrome
e. Large bowel obstruction
f. Gastroenteritis
g. Diverticulitis
h. Scleroderma
i. Ischaemic colitis

For each scenario below, choose the most likely corresponding option from the list given above.

1. A 65-year-old retired policeman consults his GP with a 3-month history of diarrhoea associated with bloating sensations. His weight and appetite are stable. He admits to a variable diet over the years. He has been stressed lately following the death of his wife. O/E: Unremarkable. PR: normal. Proctoscopy: normal. Hb 96 g/dL, WCC 13.5 × 10^9/L, carcinoembryonic antigen (CEA) 3.4 ng/mL.
2. A 23-year-old university student attends the University Health Service with altered bowel

habit in the run up to her final examinations. Her weight and appetite are stable, but she admits to intermittent crampy abdominal pains. Her periods are regular. O/E: Unremarkable. CRP, WCC and alpha-1-glycoprotein are normal. Barium enema was normal at outpatients.

3. A 26-year-old accountant attends surgical outpatients complaining of ongoing diarrhoea with the occasional bloody stool. He has weight loss of 6 kg and a reduced appetite over the past 2 months. He is currently on ibuprofen for joint pains but is otherwise well. In the past 3 months he has taken 9 days of sick leave. O/E: His lips are swollen. The left iliac fossa (LIF) is mildly tender. No masses palpable. Proctoscopy: normal. Alpha-1-glycoprotein 3.6 kU/L. He is currently awaiting a barium enema and small bowel series.
4. A 45-year-old postman attends outpatients with a 3-month history of altered bowel habit, reduced appetite and occasional PR bleeding. He drinks 38 units of alcohol a week. His younger brother in Australia attends the hospital for a 'bowel problem'. O/E: Tender LIF with a fullness in the same area. 2-cm Hepar. Flexible sigmoidoscopy reveals an erythematous rectosigmoid. Barium enema: no focal lesion seen.
5. A 59-year-old man is admitted from the clinic with a 2-month history of tenesmus and a 4-kg weight loss over the past month. Admission blood test results: Hb 96 g/L, WCC 9.1 × 10^9/L, MCV 69.2 fL, K 3.2 mmol/L, Na 137 mmol/L, urea 6.0 mmol/L and creatinine 79 mmol/L. O/E PR: tender, blood on glove and impacted stool (poor cooperation from the patient). CEA 7.6 ng/mL. Barium enema: 'apple core stricture'.

Jaundice

Each answer can be used once, more than once or not at all.

a. Cholangiocarcinoma
b. Hepatic metastases
c. Hepatocellular carcinoma
d. Pancreatic carcinoma
e. Gallbladder carcinoma
f. Biliary colic
g. Alcoholic hepatitis
h. Hepatic cirrhosis
i. Chronic pancreatitis
j. Liver abscess

For each scenario below, choose the most likely corresponding option from the list given above.

1. A 64-year-old former miner is admitted with painless jaundice and a distended abdomen.

He admits to 10-kg weight loss over the past 2 months. His admission LFTs showed an obstructive picture. CA 19-9: 686 U/mL. He drinks 20 units of alcohol per week and is an ex-smoker of 3 years.

2. A 56-year-old lady is admitted with jaundice but is otherwise well. She has a history of hepatitis C acquired whilst a missionary in Africa 30 years ago. O/E: 2-cm firm hepar. No ascites or splenomegaly. USS: multiple focal lesions within the liver, confirmed on CT.

3. A 48-year-old salesman is admitted with severe epigastric pain of 2 days' duration. He admits to smoking 30 cigarettes a day and being a 'moderate drinker'. He is not aware of any change in the colour of his stools or urine. He has no past medical history and claims to have never been in hospital before. O/E: Mildly icteric with central abdominal discomfort. His amylase is 560 U/L. Your colleague informs you that she had problems controlling this patient's analgesic demands overnight. AXR: spiculated calcification on the left side extending over the midline.

4. A 71-year-old woman is transferred from a peripheral hospital following a 10-day admission with jaundice. An ERCP was performed which demonstrated mild extrahepatic duct dilatation. Her LFTs were of a mixed picture. You note that previous imaging investigations were performed 7 years ago whilst an inpatient in your hospital. An old AXR report commented: 'No obstruction or extraluminal gas. Porcelain gallbladder'.

5. A 49-year-old woman is admitted on the acute surgical 'take-in' with a 3-day history of jaundice, fever and lethargy. O/E: Overweight, icteric with right upper quadrant tenderness. No abdominal masses are palpable. Her chart shows a pyrexia of above 38°C with temperature spikes. She admits to avoiding fatty foods since her last admission 4 months ago when she underwent 'tests'. Old notes reveal these to be USS abdomen and ERCP. WCC 18.7 × 10^9/L, CRP 176 10^9 mg/L.

Dysphagia

Each answer can be used once, more than once or not at all.

a. Achalasia
b. Motor neurone disease
c. Oesophageal carcinoma
d. Pharyngeal pouch
e. Corrosive stricture
f. Barrett oesophagus
g. Hiatus hernia
h. Oesophageal varices
i. Retrosternal thyroid
j. Oesophageal web

For each scenario below, choose the most likely corresponding option from the list given above.

1. A 68-year-old man attends outpatients with a 4-month history of increasing dysphagia and halitosis. His weight is stable as is his appetite, although he complains of bringing up undigested food at times. He also complains of the feeling of food getting stuck in his throat. He is a teetotaller and nonsmoker. He is otherwise well. Examination is unremarkable.

2. A 52-year-old lady consults her GP with a 2-month history of increasing difficulty in swallowing. Her appetite is stable, although she is tired, but this has been ongoing for years. She has a history of microcytic anaemia and is on ferrous fumarate. She is a nonsmoker and teetotaller. She has never taken proton-pump inhibitors or H$_2$ receptor antagonists.

3. A 71-year-old former train driver is admitted to hospital with 2 stone in weight loss of unknown origin. On systematic questioning he admits to increasing difficulty with swallowing his favourite Sunday lunch and for the past 3 weeks has eaten only soup. He was previously a heavy drinker with 100 pack-years of smoking. O/E: 4 cm hard, irregular hepatomegaly. Barium swallow demonstrated a stricture in the lower third of the oesophagus.

4. A 65-year-old nun attends outpatients following a complaint to her GP of increasing difficulty swallowing. While awaiting this appointment, she tells you that she was admitted to hospital with a 'really bad' pneumonia on the right side of her chest for which she was given IV antibiotics. She is a teetotaller and nonsmoker. She has no medical history and on systemic review reveals no respiratory or neurological findings. O/E: no active disease (NAD). CXR: widening of the mediastinum with an air fluid level and a resolving right basal pneumonia.

5. A 36-year-old medical secretary visits surgical outpatients with a 2-month history of increasing difficulty swallowing and 1 stone in weight loss. She admits to poor sleep and occasional diarrhoea of late. O/E: Systolic flow murmur, weakness of the girdle muscles. No superficial neck swelling. CXR: superior mediastinal mass with mild tracheal shift. You are awaiting the results of full blood count/U&E/thyroid function tests and acetylcholine receptor antibodies.

Biliary disease

Each answer can be used once, more than once or not at all.

a. Acute cholecystitis
b. Acute pancreatitis
c. Biliary colic
d. Biliary peritonitis
e. Cholangiocarcinoma
f. Cholangitis
g. Empyema of the gallbladder
h. Gallbladder carcinoma
i. Gallstone in common bile duct
j. Mucocoele of the gallbladder

For each scenario below, choose the most likely corresponding option from the list given above.

1. A 70-year-old diabetic man with known ischaemic heart disease and gallstones presents with a history of right hypochondrial pain for 24 hours, which suddenly becomes severe and generalized. On examination, he is sweaty, but afebrile, has a tachycardia and generalized abdominal tenderness, especially on the right side, with absent bowel sounds.

2. A 57-year-old woman complains of a 6-month history of epigastric and right upper quadrant pain, which occurs once or twice a week and lasts for 1–5 hours. There are no significant abnormal findings on physical examination.

3. A 42-year-old woman with a history of biliary colic and intermittent jaundice is admitted as an emergency with a 2-day history of more severe abdominal pain radiating into her back, associated with profuse vomiting. On examination, she is morbidly obese, is dehydrated, has a tachycardia and generalized vague abdominal tenderness.

4. A 65-year-old man is admitted as an emergency with a 6-week history of intermittent abdominal pain. In the last few days, the pain has become more severe and he has felt 'fluish'. He has a swinging fever, is not clinically jaundiced, but has a right upper quadrant mass.

5. An 80-year-old man is admitted as an emergency with a 3-week history of progressive, painless jaundice. On examination, he is confused, deeply jaundiced, but afebrile. Abdominal examination is normal.

Respiratory 3

SINGLE BEST ANSWER (SBA) QUESTIONS

1. A 65-year-old lifelong smoker presents with a wheeze, breathlessness and cough with sputum production. On examination you note reduced chest expansion bilaterally. He has lived in central London since the age of 10. Which of the following is most likely to be causing his symptoms?
   a. Interstitial lung disease
   b. Asthma
   c. α_1-antitrypsin deficiency
   d. Chronic obstructive pulmonary disease (COPD)
   e. None of the above

2. A 60-year-old man with severe COPD is admitted with an acute exacerbation. What is the most appropriate initial investigation?
   a. Computed tomography (CT) chest scan
   b. Spirometry
   c. Arterial blood gas
   d. Peak flow
   e. Pulmonary function tests (PFTs)

3. A 68-year-old woman is admitted under your care with increasing breathlessness, wheeze and sputum production. She has COPD. What is the next most appropriate step in management?
   a. 60% oxygen
   b. 24% oxygen
   c. Oral steroids
   d. Noninvasive positive-pressure ventilation
   e. Antibiotics

4. An overweight middle-aged man presents to the general practitioner (GP) after his wife complains about his loud snoring. He tends to drink large amounts of alcohol in the evenings before going to bed. Which of the following features is he most likely to complain of?
   a. Morning headaches
   b. Nocturnal choking
   c. Reduced libido
   d. Daytime sleepiness
   e. Personality changes

5. A child is admitted with a cough and sputum production, which is thick, foul smelling and green in colour. The mother notes episodes of him coughing up blood. On examination he has notable finger clubbing with coarse crackles in both lung bases on auscultation. What is the most likely cause of his symptoms?
   a. Cystic fibrosis
   b. Inhaled foreign body
   c. Measles
   d. *Klebsiella*
   e. Whooping cough

6. You suspect bronchiectasis in a young patient. Which of the following investigations is most likely to confirm the diagnosis?
   a. Sputum culture
   b. Sweat test
   c. Bronchoscopy
   d. Chest X-ray (CXR)
   e. High-resolution CT

7. A child recently diagnosed with cystic fibrosis is admitted following an exacerbation of his symptoms. What is the next most appropriate step in management?
   a. Prednisolone
   b. *N*-acetylcysteine
   c. Sodium reabsorption blockers
   d. Antibiotics
   e. Aminophylline

8. A teenager presents to the GP with symptoms indicative of cystic fibrosis. A sweat test is performed. Which of the following is diagnostic?
   a. A chloride value between 40 and 60 mmol/L
   b. A chloride value less than 40 mmol/L
   c. A sodium value of less than 60 mmol/L
   d. A sodium value above 60 mmol/L
   e. A sodium value between 40 and 60 mmol/L

9. A 35-year-old farmer presents with acute wheeze, cough and shortness of breath (SOB). He has smoked 10 cigarettes a day for 6 months. He likes to keep fit by running marathons. His grandfather had asthma as a child. He has lived in central London for the past year. Which of the following is the most likely cause of his condition?
   a. Asthma
   b. COPD
   c. Occupation
   d. Exercise
   e. Air pollution

10. A known asthmatic presents to the GP complaining of gradually worsening of her symptoms. She is already taking a regular β_2 agonist inhaler. What is the next most appropriate step in management?
    a. Long-acting β_2 agonist inhaler
    b. Low-dose inhaled steroid
    c. High-dose inhaled steroid
    d. Oral prednisolone
    e. Intravenous hydrocortisone

11. A woman is admitted to hospital with acute severe asthma. Her respiratory rate is greater than 25 breaths/min and peak flow is less than 50% of her predicted value. What is the next most appropriate step in management?
    a. Noninvasive ventilation
    b. Antibiotic therapy
    c. Intravenous magnesium
    d. Intravenous aminophylline
    e. Nebulized salbutamol

12. A middle-aged woman is admitted to hospital with a cough, sputum production, fever and dyspnoea. A diagnosis of pneumonia is made. Which of the following organisms is most likely to account for her symptoms?
    a. Streptococcus pneumoniae
    b. Haemophilus influenzae
    c. Legionella pneumophila
    d. Staphylococcus aureus
    e. Aspergillus fumigatus

13. An elderly woman is admitted to hospital with pneumonia. The following are all risk factors used in predicting mortality in community-acquired pneumonia EXCEPT?
    a. Urea greater than 7 mmol/L
    b. Age of 65 years
    c. Respiratory rate of 20 breaths/min or more
    d. Systolic blood pressure less than 90 mmHg
    e. Confusion

14. A middle-aged man presents with a cough, sputum production, fever and dyspnoea. Red-coloured papules are noted on the back of his hands. Routine blood investigations demonstrate that he is anaemic. Which of the following organisms is most likely to account for his condition?
    a. Chlamydia pneumoniae
    b. Haemophilus influenzae
    c. Staphylococcus aureus
    d. Mycoplasma pneumoniae
    e. Legionella pneumophila

15. A 42-year-old man presents to the GP with symptoms suggestive of pneumonia. He also complains of generalized muscular pains. He has many pets at home and mentions he recently bought two parrots. Which of the following organisms would account for his condition?
    a. Chlamydia psittaci
    b. Haemophilus influenzae
    c. Staphylococcus aureus
    d. Mycoplasma pneumoniae
    e. Legionella pneumophila

16. A 23-year-old known intravenous drug abuser is admitted with a fever, productive cough and dyspnoea. Which of the following organisms is most likely to account for his condition?
    a. Chlamydia pneumoniae
    b. Haemophilus influenzae
    c. Staphylococcus aureus
    d. Mycoplasma pneumoniae
    e. Legionella pneumophila

17. A 32-year-old man presents to the GP with a fever, productive cough and chest pain. He has recently been abroad to Dubai and stayed at a newly built hotel. He mentioned that he had bouts of diarrhoea in the last few days of his trip, which he put down to the foreign food. Which of the following organisms is most likely to account for his condition?
    a. Chlamydia pneumoniae
    b. Haemophilus influenzae
    c. Staphylococcus aureus
    d. Mycoplasma pneumoniae
    e. Legionella pneumophila

18. A 40-year-old man is diagnosed with a mild pneumonia. He has no known drug allergies. What is the most appropriate treatment?
    a. Amoxicillin
    b. Metronidazole
    c. Azithromycin
    d. Cefuroxime
    e. Flucloxacillin

19. You suspect pneumonia in a 35-year-old woman. Which of the following investigations is most likely to confirm the diagnosis?
    a. Blood culture
    b. Sputum culture
    c. White cell count
    d. CXR
    e. Arterial blood gas

20. An Asian man presents with a 2-month history of fever and a cough productive of blood-tinged sputum. He has recently moved to the United

Kingdom from abroad. What is the most likely causative organism?

a. *Mycoplasma pneumoniae*
b. *Streptococcus pneumoniae*
c. *Mycobacterium avium-intracellulare*
d. *Mycobacterium tuberculosis*
e. *Pneumocystis jiroveci*

21. A West Indian immigrant has recently been diagnosed with tuberculosis (TB). Which of the following cells are solely responsible for engulfing bacilli and forming granulomatous lesions?

a. Neutrophils
b. Macrophages
c. Langhans giant cells
d. Epithelioid cells
e. T lymphocytes

22. An Asian immigrant presents with a fever and a cough productive of blood-tinged sputum. On examination you note an enlarged liver and enlarged cervical lymph nodes. A CXR shows patchy shadowing in the upper zones. You suspect TB. What is the next most appropriate investigation you would order to confirm your suspicion?

a. Bronchoscopy
b. Sputum smear
c. Mantoux test
d. Lymph node biopsy
e. CT chest scan

23. A middle-aged man is diagnosed with TB. He has no known drug allergies. Which is the least likely drug to be included in the initial treatment?

a. Ethambutol
b. Pyrazinamide
c. Streptomycin
d. Rifampicin
e. Isoniazid

24. A 55-year-old man has recently been diagnosed with TB. He has been started on quadruple therapy and complains of a colour change in his urine. What drug is most likely to be responsible for this?

a. Rifampicin
b. Isoniazid
c. Ethambutol
d. Pyrazinamide
e. Streptomycin

25. An Afro-Caribbean man presents with increasing dyspnoea. A CXR shows bilateral hilar lymphadenopathy. Routine blood investigations demonstrate a raised serum calcium. Which of the following is also likely to be affected?

a. Heart
b. Central nervous system
c. Bones and joints
d. Liver
e. Eyes

26. You suspect sarcoidosis in an Afro-Caribbean man who presents with a cough and evidence of lymphadenopathy. Which of the following investigations is likely to be most useful in confirming a diagnosis?

a. CXR
b. Lung function tests
c. CT chest
d. Serum angiotensin-converting enzyme (ACE)
e. Lymph node biopsy

27. A middle-aged man presents with exertional dyspnoea and a nonproductive cough. On examination he has finger clubbing and fine inspiratory crackles are noted bibasally on auscultation. What is the most likely diagnosis?

a. Silicosis
b. Pneumoconiosis
c. TB
d. Cryptogenic fibrosing alveolitis
e. Allergic bronchopulmonary aspergillosis

28. Which of the following is the most common cause of extrinsic allergic alveolitis?

a. Forking mouldy hay
b. Handling pigeons
c. Turning germinating barley
d. Turning mushroom compost
e. Contaminated humidifier systems in air conditioners

29. A shipbuilding yard worker presents with breathlessness. A CT chest scan is ordered, and a diagnosis of asbestos-induced lung damage is made. He is distraught with the diagnosis and wants to know if he is eligible for industrial injury benefits. Which of the following findings would allow him to pursue a claim?

a. Pleural plaques
b. Asbestosis
c. Mesothelioma
d. Bilateral diffuse pleural thickening
e. All of the above

30. A 65-year-old woman presents with breathlessness and haemoptysis. She is diagnosed with squamous cell carcinoma (SCC) of the lung. She has been a smoker for as long as she can remember. She has lived in central London for almost 30 years now and she worked in a shipbuilding yard for most of

her working life. Both her father and mother died of lung cancer. Which of the following is the most likely cause of her cancer?
a. Smoking
b. Gender
c. Family history
d. Occupation
e. City living

31. A middle-aged man is diagnosed with lung cancer. He worked in a shipbuilding yard for most of his life. He is distraught with the diagnosis as he says he has never smoked in his life. Which of the following types of lung cancer is he most likely to suffer from?
a. Squamous
b. Large cell
c. Adenocarcinoma
d. Alveolar cell
e. Small cell

32. A 53-year-old woman is diagnosed with lung cancer. Her main symptoms on presentation included breathlessness and haemoptysis. She complained of stretch marks on her abdomen and that her skin bruised easily. On examination you note purple abdominal striae. Which of the following types of lung cancer is she most likely to suffer from?
a. Squamous
b. Large cell
c. Adenocarcinoma
d. Alveolar cell
e. Small cell

33. A 63-year-old man is diagnosed with lung cancer. Which of the following extrapulmonary manifestations is he most likely to suffer from?
a. Clubbing
b. Dermatomyositis
c. Lambert–Eaton myasthenic syndrome (LEMS)
d. Hypercalcaemia
e. Thrombophlebitis migrans

34. With regard to pleural fluid, which of the following is most important in determining whether an effusion is a transudate or exudate?
a. Bacterial count
b. Amylase levels
c. Malignant cells
d. Glucose levels
e. Protein levels

35. Which of the following typically causes a transudative pleural effusion?
a. Heart failure
b. Pneumonia
c. Bronchial carcinoma

d. Pancreatitis
e. Connective tissue disease

36. A 45-year-old woman presents with SOB and chest pain. She comments that she has recently travelled to Australia. An electrocardiogram demonstrates evidence of right heart strain. You suspect a pulmonary embolus. Which investigation is most likely to lead to a diagnosis?
a. CT pulmonary angiogram (CTPA)
b. D dimers
c. Ventilation perfusion scan
d. CXR
e. Arterial blood gas

37. You are called to review a 70-year-old man admitted for treatment of pneumococcal pneumonia, who has become more unwell with swinging fevers, worsening breathlessness and pleuritic chest pain. His inflammatory markers are rising and a repeat CXR shows a new right-sided pleural effusion. What is the next most appropriate diagnostic investigation?
a. CT scan
b. Bronchoscopy
c. Ultrasound-guided diagnostic pleural tap
d. PFTs
e. Recheck the sputum for resistant organisms

38. A 76-year-old man with COPD was admitted to accident and emergency department with acute on chronic SOB. He has a chest drain inserted for a pneumothorax. Which of the following is true of chest drain management?
a. He should have his drain clamped if he has to travel to the radiology department without a medical escort.
b. The drain should only be removed when it has stopped bubbling.
c. The drain may be clamped if it only bubbles on coughing.
d. The drain should only be removed when it has stopped swinging.
e. Pain relief is usually not necessary in the first few days after insertion.

39. A 76-year-old man is admitted to intensive care unit (ICU) for potassium replacement. A central venous line is inserted via the subclavian vein. During the procedure he becomes acutely breathless with decreasing oxygen saturation. What is the most likely diagnosis?
a. The wire has threaded into the left ventricle
b. His chronic obstructive airways disease has been exacerbated
c. A pneumothorax has been created
d. A myocardial infarction has been induced
e. Air embolism has occurred

40. A 58-year-old man with longstanding emphysema presents to the emergency department with sudden onset of breathlessness and left-sided pleuritic chest pain. On arrival, he is hypoxic, tachypnoeic, hypotensive and tachycardic. His trachea is deviated to the right and breath sounds are markedly reduced on the left side of his chest. What is the next step in the management of this patient?
    a. CXR
    b. Insert large bore cannula into the left second intercostal space
    c. Insert chest drain with negative suction on the left side
    d. 1-L saline bolus
    e. Oxygen via nasal cannulae

41. A 40-year-old nonsmoker presents to the emergency department with sudden-onset breathlessness and left-sided chest pain. On examination, he is unable to complete sentences and has low oxygen saturation levels. He has diminished breath sounds on the left side with tracheal deviation towards the right. Heart sounds are normal. What is the most likely explanation for these findings?
    a. Pneumonia
    b. Asthma
    c. Congestive heart failure
    d. Pneumothorax
    e. Pulmonary embolism

42. A 66-year-old woman with history of weight loss presents to the respiratory clinic with an 8-week history of nonproductive cough and chronic clearing of throat. She has a 52-pack year smoking history and quit 25 years ago. She was subsequently diagnosed with carcinoma of the lung. Which of the following is NOT a complication of carcinoma of the lung?
    a. Adrenal metastases
    b. Hypertrophic pulmonary osteoarthropathy
    c. Hypocalcaemia
    d. Hyponatraemia
    e. Ptosis

43. A 65-year-old factory worker presents with a dry cough, right-sided chest pain and finger clubbing. He has lost 4 kg in weight in the last 2 weeks. He has a 30-year smoking history. On examination the right lung is dull to percussion with reduced chest expansion. What is the most likely diagnosis?
    a. Asbestosis
    b. Bronchioalveolar lung cancer
    c. Mesothelioma
    d. Coal worker's pneumoconiosis
    e. Small cell lung cancer (SCLC)

44. A 50-year-old heavy smoker of 30 pack years presents to his GP with weight loss of 8 kg over 4 months and a chronic cough with two episodes of haemoptysis. He denies any history of fever. Chest radiograph shows a rounded lesion measuring 5 cm in diameter in the right upper lobe. What is the most likely diagnosis?
    a. Cytomegalovirus infections
    b. Granulomatous inflammation
    c. *Pneumocystis carinii (jirovecii)* pneumonia
    d. Bronchial carcinoma
    e. Mesothelioma

45. An outbreak of pneumonia involving over 20 cases, some fatal, has occurred in one town and most of the sufferers have stayed in the same hotel. Features of the illness were high fever, rigors, confusion, myalgia, abdominal pain, vomiting and diarrhoea. Chest radiograph showed bilateral shadowing. The clinical diagnosis was confirmed by a fluorescent antibody titre, which showed a significant rise in paired sera taken a month apart. What is the most likely pathogen?
    a. *Haemophilus influenzae*
    b. *Legionella pneumophilia*
    c. *Mycoplasma pneumoniae*
    d. *Staphylococcus aureus*
    e. *Streptococcal pneumoniae*

46. You see a 55-year-old female for the first time. She has a 2-year history of chronic daily cough; thick, malodorous sputum and occasional haemoptysis. She has been treated with antibiotics for recurrent respiratory infections, but is frustrated with her continued symptoms. She has never smoked. Her forced expiratory volume in 1 second:forced vital capacity (FEV_1:FVC) ratio is 60% and a CT scan shows bronchial wall thickening and luminal dilatation. Which of the following is the most likely diagnosis?
    a. Asthma
    b. Bronchiectasis
    c. COPD
    d. Bronchiolitis
    e. Emphysema

47. A 67-year-old obese man presents with loud chronic snoring and gasping episodes during sleep. His wife has witnessed episodes where it appears as if he has stopped breathing. He reports unrefreshing sleep, multiple awakenings from sleep and morning headaches. He has excessive daytime sleepiness, which is interfering with his daily activities. He has been treated for hypertension, gastro-oesophageal reflux and type 2 diabetes. For adults with

obstructive sleep apnoea, which one of the following is the most effective treatment?
a. Continuous positive airway pressure (CPAP)
b. Mandible-positioning oral appliances
c. Modafinil
d. Uvulopalatal surgery
e. Weight reduction to achieve a body mass index <30 kg/m^2

48. A 35-year-old man who has recently been treated for Hodgkin lymphoma presents to you with a nonproductive cough. His CXR shows shadowing in one of the upper zones. His oxygen saturation is 95% on air. What is the most likely diagnosis?
a. Bleomycin toxicity
b. *Pneumocystis carinii* pneumonia
c. Pulmonary lymphoma
d. Radiation pneumonitis
e. TB

49. A 56-year-old female is seen in the respiratory clinic with a 1-year history of breathlessness. Physical examination shows tachypnoea, widespread crackles and finger clubbing. Spirometry shows a low vital capacity and total lung capacity associated with a relatively well-preserved peak flow rate. Arterial blood gases reveal hypoxaemia. What is the most likely diagnosis?
a. Emphysema
b. Bronchial asthma
c. Pulmonary fibrosis
d. Bilateral pleural effusions
e. Bronchitis

50. A 65-year-old retired rock miner sees his GP with worsening breathlessness, decreased exercise tolerance, dry cough and weight loss. He reports no past medical history. On examination he appears slightly tachypnoeic at rest. Fine inspiratory crackles are heard in the upper zones. Subsequent chest radiograph reveals multiple round opacities in the upper lobes with calcified hilar lymphadenopathy. What is the most likely diagnosis?
a. Asbestosis
b. Silicosis
c. Cystic fibrosis
d. Aspergillosis
e. TB

51. A 60-year-old nonsmoker presents to his GP with worsening breathlessness for several months, mainly on exertion. He has also developed a nonproductive cough and nonpainful deformities of his fingernails. He worked in the building industry for 30 years before his retirement this year. On examination, there are bibasal fine end-inspiratory crackles and evidence of finger clubbing. A subsequent plain chest radiograph shows evidence of lower lobe fibrotic changes. What is the most likely cause in this patient's condition?
a. Smoking
b. Silicosis
c. Asbestosis
d. Chronic bronchitis
e. Hypersensitivity pneumonitis

52. A 30-year-old woman known to have asthma presents to the emergency department with a 2-day history of worsening breathlessness and chest tightness despite regular salbutamol inhalers. She has been suffering from an upper respiratory tract infection for the past few days. Which of the following findings on clinical examination would be an ominous sign for an impending respiratory failure in this patient?
a. Tachycardia
b. Tachypnoea
c. Silent chest
d. Increased wheezing
e. All of the above

53. A 36-year-old woman with a history of moderate persistent asthma presents to the emergency department with progressive worsening of SOB, wheezing and cough over 3 days. She has been compliant with her maintenance asthma regimen, which consists of an inhaled corticosteroid and a leukotriene receptor antagonist for maintenance therapy and salbutamol as rescue therapy. Which one of the following is most consistent with a diagnosis of asthma?
a. Reduced FEV$_1$ and reduced FEV$_1$:FVC ratio
b. Reduced FEV$_1$ and normal FEV$_1$:FVC ratio
c. Reduced FEV$_1$ and increased FEV$_1$:FVC ratio
d. Reduced FVC$_1$ and normal FEV$_1$:FVC ratio
e. Reduced FVC$_1$ and increased FEV$_1$:FVC ratio

EXTENDED-MATCHING QUESTIONS (EMQs)

Pneumonia

Each answer can be used once, more than once or not at all.

a. *Mycoplasma pneumoniae*
b. *Chlamydia psittaci*
c. *Staphylococcus aureus*
d. *Legionella pneumophila*

e. *Haemophilus influenzae*
f. Aspiration pneumonia
g. *Pseudomonas aeruginosa*
h. *Pneumocystis jiroveci*
i. *Streptococcus pneumoniae*
j. *Mycobacterium avium intracellulare*

For each scenario below, choose the most likely corresponding option from the list given above.

1. A 32-year-old man presenting with SOB and feeling generally unwell. He has a known history of cystic fibrosis.
2. A common cause of pneumonia in patients with COPD.
3. A middle-aged man presenting with a cough and generalized muscular pains. He is known to be a keen collector of rare birds.
4. An intravenous drug abuser presenting with SOB and a fever.
5. A middle-aged woman having recently returned from Las Vegas presenting with a nonproductive cough, fever and diarrhoea.

Respiratory drugs

Each answer can be used once, more than once or not at all.

a. Ethambutol
b. Pyrazinamide
c. Isoniazid
d. Rifampicin
e. Metronidazole
f. Erythromycin
g. Clarithromycin
h. Flucloxacillin
i. Tobramycin
j. Ticarcillin

For each scenario below, choose the most likely corresponding option from the list given above.

1. Associated with induction of liver enzymes.
2. Associated with blurred vision and colour blindness.
3. An intravenous drug abuser diagnosed with pneumonia associated with patchy areas of consolidation on his CXR.
4. Known to cause liver inflammation and gout.
5. A middle-aged woman recently diagnosed with a stroke aspirates when given some water.

Lung cancer

Each answer can be used once, more than once or not at all.

a. Lambert–Eaton myasthenic syndrome (LEMS)

b. Dermatomyositis
c. Herpes zoster
d. Acanthosis nigricans
e. Hypertrophic pulmonary osteoarthropathy
f. Horner syndrome
g. Pancoast tumour
h. Cushing syndrome
i. Thrombophlebitis migrans
j. Clubbing

For each scenario below, choose the most likely corresponding option from the list given above.

1. A 75-year-old man recently diagnosed with lung cancer complaining of painful wrists and ankles.
2. A middle-aged man recently presenting with haemoptysis and shoulder pain.
3. A 65-year-old woman presenting with breathlessness, haemoptysis and pigmented skin in her axillae.
4. A middle-aged woman with known lung cancer presenting with dropping of her upper eyelid, pupillary constriction and a sunken eye on the right side.
5. A patient recently diagnosed with lung cancer presenting with lower limb weakness and difficulty in climbing stairs.

Diseases of the respiratory tract

Each answer can be used once, more than once or not at all.

a. Bronchiectasis
b. Sinusitis
c. Rhinitis
d. Pharyngitis
e. Laryngotracheobronchitis
f. Influenza
g. Emphysema
h. Acute bronchitis
i. Asthma
j. Obstructive sleep apnoea

For each scenario below, choose the most likely corresponding option from the list given above.

1. Dilatation and destruction of lung tissue distal to terminal bronchioles.
2. A 23-year-old man presenting with sudden-onset cough, fever and muscular aches.
3. Associated with a hoarse voice and barking cough.
4. An 18-year-old woman with cystic fibrosis presenting with a persistent cough productive of yellow/green-coloured sputum.
5. A middle-aged man presenting with cough, chest tightness and wheeze.

Investigative findings

Each answer can be used once, more than once or not at all.

    a. COPD
    b. Obstructive sleep apnoea
    c. Sarcoidosis
    d. Wegener granulomatosis
    e. Bronchiectasis
    f. Cystic fibrosis
    g. Extrinsic allergic alveolitis
    h. Asthma
    i. Cryptogenic fibrosing alveolitis
    j. Pneumonia

For each scenario below, choose the most likely corresponding option from the list given above.

    1. A middle-aged woman with SOB and a ground-glass appearance on her CXR.
    2. A 55-year-old farmer presenting with a cough and SOB. His CXR demonstrates fluffy nodular shadowing.
    3. A lifelong smoker with an FEV_1:FVC ratio of 62% with an increase in FEV_1 of 12% following use of salbutamol.
    4. A 23-year-old woman presenting with a fever, cough and SOB. Routine blood investigations reveal a white cell count of 23×10^9/L. A CXR demonstrates evidence of patchy consolidation.
    5. A 45-year-old man presenting with haemoptysis. A CXR reveals evidence of cavitation and routine blood investigations demonstrate increased levels of antineutrophil cytoplasmic antibodies.

Lung diseases

Each answer can be used once, more than once or not at all.

    a. Asbestosis
    b. Asthma
    c. Bird fancier's lung
    d. COPD
    e. Cor pulmonale
    f. Pleural effusion
    g. Pneumoconiosis
    h. Pulmonary embolus
    i. Rheumatoid lung
    j. Pneumothorax

For each scenario below, choose the most likely corresponding option from the list given above.

    1. A 65-year-old woman with tar-stained fingers, central cyanosis and a widespread wheeze.
    2. A 30-year-old man who was involved in a road traffic accident has an area of bruising over his chest, has a respiratory rate of 30 breaths/min and has absent breath sounds on the right side of his chest.
    3. A 60-year-old man who has been a lifelong smoker and has been losing weight presents with acute SOB, absent breath sounds and dullness to percussion on the left side.
    4. A 58-year-old woman who has painful, swollen hands, a hump at the top of her spine and fine bibasal inspiratory crackles.
    5. A 70-year-old man who worked in the steel industry, presenting with swollen ankles, a raised jugular venous pressure and fine inspiratory bibasal lung crackles.

Shortness of breath

Each answer can be used once, more than once or not at all.

    a. Pulmonary embolus
    b. Aortic stenosis
    c. Congestive cardiac failure
    d. Asthma
    e. Cryptogenic fibrosing alveolitis
    f. Pleural effusion
    g. Bronchial carcinoma
    h. COPD
    i. Right middle lobe pneumonia
    j. Pneumothorax

For each scenario below, choose the most likely corresponding option from the list given above.

    1. A 55-year-old baker is admitted with increasing SOB over the past 6 weeks along with chest tightness and two syncopal episodes whilst at work. He suffered from asthma as a child. He admits to 20 pack years of smoking. Admission blood test results, including D-dimer, are unremarkable. CXR: No active disease (NAD). Peak expiratory flow rate 450 L/min.
    2. A 32-year-old woman of childbearing age recently returned from a 2-month sabbatical in Thailand. She has been short of breath for the past week. O/E: Reduced air entry at the right middle and lower zones. No calf swelling. Oxygen saturations 92% (right atrial (RA)). D-dimer 0.45 mg/L, white cell count (WCC) 13.6×109 /L. CXR: indistinct right heart border.
    3. A 61-year-old retired plumber is admitted with increasing SOB over the past 2 months. He smokes 20 cigarettes a day. SOB is associated with mild pleuritic chest pain. O/E: Reduced breath sounds at the left lower zone and decreased vocal resonance. CXR: loss of the left hemidiaphragm silhouette. Hb 12.6 g/dL, WCC 8.4×10^9/L.

4. A 24-year-old male master's student is admitted to a district general hospital acutely SOB for the past day. He recalls a similar incident during his first year at university. He returned from a summer tour of Australasia 1 week ago. O/E: Oxygen saturations 93% (RA). Haemodynamically stable. Reduced breath sounds on left side and asymmetrical chest expansion. A medical student informs you 'the lungs look different' on the CXR.

5. A 73-year-old former mill worker is admitted dyspnoeic with mild haemoptysis mixed with her sputum. She has had three previous admissions in the last 5 months with similar presentations. O/E: Thin, grade 2 finger clubbing. Increased anteroposterior chest diameter with scattered wheeze and a few bibasal crepitations, right more than left. Arterial blood gas (on 28% oxygen): partial pressure of oxygen (PO_2) 13.6 kPa, partial pressure of carbon dioxide (PCO_2) 5.6 kPa. CXR: borderline cardiomegaly, blunted right costophrenic angle. Chronic inflammatory changes throughout and a bulky left hilum.

Respiratory infections
Each answer can be used once, more than once or not at all.

a. Cytomegalovirus
b. *Staphylococcus aureus*
c. *Pseudomonas aeruginosa*
d. *Escherichia coli*
e. *Legionella pneumophila*
f. *Streptococcus pneumoniae*
g. *Candida albicans*
h. *Mycobacterium tuberculosis*
i. *Coxiella burnetii*
j. *Mycoplasma pneumoniae*

For each scenario below, choose the most likely corresponding option from the list given above.

1. The patient has been ventilated on the intensive therapy unit (ITU) for a week following a complicated laparotomy and now has lung infiltrates and mucopurulent secretions coming up the endotracheal tube.

2. A young, previously fit man presents acutely unwell with pneumonia and his chest radiograph shows numerous small abscesses.

3. A middle-aged man is admitted to ITU with a severe, acute pneumonia. He is the second ITU admission and the third case of pneumonia occurring in workers at the same factory in town.

4. A 71-year-old woman develops a chest infection 3 days after an uncomplicated operation to remove a Duke's A colonic carcinoma.

5. A 36-year-old woman has a 3-day history of fever, cough and pleuritic pain. She has coughed up a bit of blood in some purulent sputum. She has a pleural rub and her chest radiograph shows segmental consolidation in the left upper lobe.

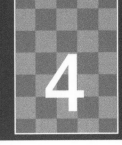

SINGLE BEST ANSWER (SBA) QUESTIONS

1. A 45-year-old man complains of breathlessness and feeling tired for the past week. He also remarks that he has not been passing as much urine as usual. On clinical examination he is not dehydrated. He has a serum creatinine of 500 μmol/L. Urine analysis reveals a urine osmolality of 650 mOsm/kg and a urine sodium of 15 mmol/L. You diagnose acute kidney injury (AKI). What is the least likely cause of his renal failure?
   a. Decreased cardiac output
   b. Severe liver failure
   c. Hypovolaemia
   d. Renal artery obstruction
   e. Acute tubular necrosis

2. A middle-aged woman presents with breathlessness for the last week. She also comments that she has been feeling more tired than usual and that she has been passing urine infrequently. On examination you note that her skin is pale and pigmented with several small bruises. What is the most appropriate initial investigation?
   a. Urea and electrolytes
   b. Urine Stix testing and microscopy
   c. Serum calcium, phosphate and uric acid
   d. Full blood count
   e. Renal ultrasound

3. A 51-year-old man is diagnosed with AKI. He has recently been suffering from diarrhoea and vomiting and has lost his appetite. He takes captopril for his high blood pressure. He is oliguric with a urine output of less than 300 mL/day. Routine blood tests reveal a potassium of 6.5 mmol/L. What is the first most appropriate step in his management?
   a. Treat his high potassium
   b. Fluid replacement
   c. Diuretics
   d. Withdraw captopril
   e. Nutrition replacement

4. A patient with AKI is referred for dialysis. The following are all indications for dialysis EXCEPT?
   a. Severe metabolic acidosis
   b. Uncontrollable hyperkalaemia
   c. Pulmonary oedema
   d. Pericarditis
   e. Anaemia

5. A 56-year-old man is diagnosed with AKI. The cause of this was attributed to interstitial nephritis. The following drugs all cause interstitial nephritis EXCEPT?
   a. Nonsteroid antiinflammatory drugs (NSAIDs)
   b. Angiotensin-converting enzyme (ACE) inhibitors
   c. Allopurinol
   d. Penicillin
   e. Cimetidine

6. A 65-year-old man complains of waking up in the night to pass urine for the past 3 weeks. He feels generally quite tired and complains of muscle weakness. Routine blood tests reveal a serum calcium of 1.76 mmol/L, a serum phosphate of 3.4 mmol/L, a low vitamin D level and a raised parathyroid hormone level. You diagnose renal osteodystrophy. Which of the following radiological signs is least likely?
   a. Bamboo spine
   b. Subperiosteal erosions
   c. Salt and pepper skull
   d. Brown tumours
   e. Pseudofractures

7. A 67-year-old diabetic patient complains of bone and muscle pain for the last 4 weeks. She remarks that she feels more tired than usual and is constantly itching. Routine blood investigations reveal an estimated glomerular filtration rate 28 mL/min per 1.73 m² and a haemoglobin of 8.7 g/dL. In addition, her vitamin D level is low. What is the most appropriate step in her management?
   a. Review of diabetic medication
   b. Reduction of protein intake
   c. Erythropoietin injections
   d. Referral for dialysis
   e. Vitamin D analogues

8. A 68-year-old man with chronic renal failure is referred for peritoneal dialysis. What is the most likely complication of this form of dialysis?
   a. Cardiovascular disease
   b. Peritonitis
   c. Amyloidosis
   d. Shoulder pain
   e. Carpal tunnel syndrome

9. A 51-year-old man complains of pain in his loins and passing blood in his urine for the past 2 weeks. There is a strong family history of polycystic kidney disease (PKD). On examination his blood pressure is recorded

as 160/95 mmHg. What investigation is most likely to confirm the diagnosis of PKD?
a. 24 Hour ambulatory blood pressure monitoring
b. Urea and electrolytes
c. Urine Stix testing and microscopy
d. Renal ultrasound
e. Excretion urography

10. A 67-year-old man complains of loin pain and passing blood in his urine for the past week. On examination you note the presence of large irregular kidneys. You are concerned about the possibility of PKD. What is the most common mode of inheritance of this condition?
a. Autosomal recessive
b. X-linked recessive
c. Autosomal dominant
d. X-linked dominant
e. Y linked

11. A 57-year-old man presents with haematuria, loin pain and a solid mass in his right flank. Excretion urography demonstrates the presence of a space-occupying lesion. What is the most appropriate step in his management?
a. Medroxyprogesterone acetate
b. Surgery
c. Interleukin 2
d. Alpha-interferon
e. Radiotherapy

12. A 70-year-old man complains of waking up in the night to pass urine, nonspecific bone pain and weight loss. He mentions that there is often a delay in initiating urination and a sense of incomplete voiding. What is the most appropriate initial investigation after a digital rectal examination?
a. Urea and electrolytes
b. Serum prostate-specific antigen (PSA)
c. Renal ultrasound
d. Transrectal ultrasound
e. Excretion urography

13. A 30-year-old man complains of a painless swelling in his right testicle. Routine blood tests reveal a beta-human chorionic gonadotropin (beta-hCG) level that is higher than normal. Surgical exploration and subsequent histological examination of the testis reveal the presence of cystic spaces. What is the most likely diagnosis?
a. Seminoma
b. Teratoma
c. Sertoli cell adenoma
d. Leydig cell adenoma
e. Testicular torsion

14. A 31-year-old man complains of a painless swelling in his left testicle. Routine blood tests reveal a beta-hCG level that is higher than normal. In addition, his AFP level is markedly raised. What is the most likely diagnosis?
a. Seminoma
b. Teratoma
c. Sertoli cell adenoma
d. Leydig cell adenoma
e. Testicular torsion

15. A 29-year-old man presents with a painless swelling in his left testicle. He complains of a cough and shortness of breath. Ultrasound scanning reveals the presence of a testicular tumour. Surgical exploration and subsequent histological examination reveal no cystic spaces. In addition to an orchidectomy, what is the next most appropriate step in management?
a. Chemotherapy
b. Radiotherapy
c. Watchful waiting
d. Goserelin
e. Cyproterone acetate

16. A 35-year-old woman complains of accidentally passing urine when she coughs or laughs. She has given birth to three children. Urine Stix testing reveals a trace of protein. What is the most likely diagnosis?
a. Functional incontinence
b. Urge incontinence
c. Stress incontinence
d. Overflow incontinence
e. Urinary tract infection (UTI)

17. A 61-year-old man complains of hesitancy, a poor stream and terminal dribbling when passing urine. On examination you note the presence of a distended bladder palpable suprapubically. Which investigation is most likely to lead to a diagnosis?
a. Radionuclide studies
b. Urodynamic study
c. Abdominal ultrasound
d. Bladder scan
e. Cystoscopy

18. A 43-year-old man with gout complains of severe intermittent loin pain and microscopic haematuria which has lasted for several hours. What is the initial most appropriate step in management?
a. Fluid replacement
b. Allopurinol
c. Pain relief
d. Shock wave lithotripsy
e. Nephrolithotomy

19. A 23-year-old marathon runner complains of severe intermittent loin pain and vomiting soon after a training session for her next marathon. On examination she is severely dehydrated. Which of the following investigations is most likely to lead to a diagnosis?
    a. Serum calcium levels
    b. Abdominal X-ray of kidneys, ureters and bladder (KUB)
    c. Urea and electrolytes
    d. Midstream specimen of urine for culture and sensitivity
    e. 24-Hour urine collection for calcium

20. A 24-year-old woman complains of urinary frequency and dysuria. What organism is the most likely cause of her symptoms?
    a. *Escherichia coli*
    b. *Proteus mirabilis*
    c. *Klebsiella aerogenes*
    d. Enterococci
    e. *Staphylococcus saprophyticus*

21. A 30-year-old man complains of urinary frequency, dysuria and suprapubic tenderness for the past week. What is the most appropriate initial investigation?
    a. Urine microscopy and culture
    b. Bladder scan
    c. Abdominal X-ray
    d. Urodynamic studies
    e. Cystoscopy

22. An elderly man is catheterized having failed to pass urine for the past 2 days. Soon after, he becomes significantly confused and complains of generalized loin pain. On examination he is pyrexial with a temperature of 39.5°C. What is the most appropriate step in his management?
    a. High fluid intake
    b. Trimethoprim
    c. Nitrofurantoin
    d. Amoxicillin
    e. Gentamicin

23. A 4-year-old boy presents with swelling of his ankles, genitals and abdomen. On examination you also note slight swelling of his arms. His jugular venous pressure is not raised. His mother mentions that his urine appears frothy. Which investigation is most likely to lead to a diagnosis?
    a. 24-Hour urinary protein and serum albumin measurement
    b. Urine microscopy and culture
    c. Plasma lipids measurement

    d. Urea and electrolytes
    e. Renal ultrasound

24. A 6-year-old boy is diagnosed with nephrotic syndrome. What is the most likely underlying cause of this condition?
    a. Amyloidosis
    b. Membranous nephropathy
    c. Minimal change disease
    d. Focal segmental glomerulosclerosis
    e. Systemic lupus erythematosus

25. A patient presents to accident and emergency (A&E) with bilateral pitting oedema, ascites and severe loin pain. His urine dipstick shows proteinuria, liver function tests show hypoalbuminaemia, and U&Es show an AKI. On examination his left kidney is palpable. Which of the following medications should be prescribed?
    a. Co-amoxiclav
    b. Dalteparin
    c. Diclofenac
    d. Prednisolone
    e. Warfarin

26. A patient known to have HIV presents to A&E with pitting oedema. He also describes his urine as being frothy. A urine dip on admission shows proteinuria, but no haematuria. A renal biopsy is taken and shows deposition of immunoglobulin M (IgM) and C3 in some of the glomeruli. What is the most likely underlying diagnosis?
    a. Berger disease
    b. Focal segmental glomerulosclerosis
    c. Goodpasture syndrome
    d. Mesangiocapillary glomerulonephritis type II
    e. Proliferative glomerulonephritis

27. A 67-year-old man with stage 5 CKD presents to A&E with sharp central chest pain. The pain is made worse on inspiration and when he lies down. The pain can be relieved slightly by sitting forwards. Which of the following treatment regimens should be started to treat this patient's underlying condition?
    a. Allopurinol
    b. Colchicine
    c. Diclofenac
    d. Haemodialysis
    e. Primary coronary angioplasty

28. A patient with PKD has reached end-stage renal failure, and is about to undergo his first dialysis session. Routine blood tests are taken. Which of the following is most likely to be within the normal range in this patient?

a. Haemoglobin
b. Parathyroid hormone
c. Serum creatinine
d. Serum phosphate
e. Serum urate

29. A patient with ongoing membranous nephropathy has developed hypoalbuminaemia as a result of proteinuria. Which of the following drugs would reduce the loss of albumin via the kidneys?
    a. Amiloride
    b. Bumetanide
    c. Ramipril
    d. Indapamide
    e. Human albumin solution

30. A 32-year-old male is brought into hospital after passing dark brown urine following an accident at work where he was pinned against a wall by a loader. Which of the following treatments should be initiated immediately?
    a. IV 0.9% saline
    b. IV sodium bicarbonate
    c. IV insulin and 50% dextrose
    d. IV dexamethasone
    e. Haemodialysis

31. A 43-year-old female presents to A&E with shortness of breath, cough and haemoptysis. She also reports haematuria. Initial blood tests show a raised white cell count (eosinophilia), raised urea, erythrocyte sedimentation rate, C-reactive protein and perinuclear antineutrophil cytoplasmic antibodies (P-ANCA). Which of the following is the most likely underlying diagnosis?
    a. Churg–Strauss syndrome
    b. Goodpasture syndrome
    c. Kawasaki disease
    d. Microscopic polyangiitis
    e. Wegener granulomatosis

32. A 62-year-old male was started on ramipril by his general practitioner (GP) to treat his high blood pressure. Three days later, he presented to A&E with a cough, dyspnoea and wheeze, which is made worse by lying down. On examination he was found to have bilateral fine inspiratory crackles throughout both lungs. His arterial blood gas showed a type 1 respiratory failure. Which of the following conditions is this patient likely to have, which has resulted in his symptoms?
    a. Acquired angioedema
    b. Asthma
    c. Bilateral renal artery stenosis

d. Congestive cardiac failure
e. Pulmonary fibrosis

33. A 69-year-old female is referred to the renal clinic for worsening kidney function. Her GP noticed a gradual increase in creatinine over the past few years. On examination there were two large ballotable masses on both flanks, as well as a nontender suprapubic mass, which is dulled to percussion. Which of following is the most likely cause of the decline in renal function?
    a. Amyloidosis
    b. Bilateral renal artery stenosis
    c. Hydronephrosis
    d. PKD
    e. Metastatic lung cancer

34. A 60-year-old woman with end-stage renal failure on haemodialysis is found unconscious at home by her husband. Her husband reports that she has missed two dialysis sessions this past week. Electrocardiogram (ECG) shows evidence of hyperkalaemia. Which of the following ECG findings is associated with hyperkalaemia?
    a. Short PR interval
    b. ST-segment depression
    c. T-wave inversion
    d. U waves
    e. Tall T waves

35. A 38-year-old man was referred to the nephrology department by his GP following abnormal findings on urinalysis. Which of the following is NOT true in patients with nephrotic syndrome?
    a. Massive proteinuria
    b. Hypoalbuminemia
    c. Periorbital oedema
    d. Hyperlipidemia
    e. Prolonged bleeding time

36. A 65-year-old man known to have end-stage renal failure secondary to diabetes mellitus, who has been on haemodialysis for 8 years, presents to his GP with a 2-month history of numbness and tingling of his left hand. Clinical examination shows atrophy of thenar prominence. What is his most likely diagnosis?
    a. Carpal tunnel syndrome
    b. Cervical root impingement
    c. Thoracic outlet syndrome
    d. Myocardial infarction
    e. Pronator teres syndrome

EXTENDED-MATCHING QUESTIONS (EMQs)

Renal disease

Each answer can be used once, more than once or not at all.

a. Acute nephritic syndrome
b. Nephrotic syndrome
c. UTI
d. Tubulointerstitial nephritis
e. Renal stone disease
f. Urinary tract obstruction
g. PKD
h. Medullary sponge kidney
i. Renal carcinoma
j. Renal hypertension

For each scenario below, choose the most likely corresponding option from the list given above.

1. An uncommon condition associated with dilatation of the collecting ducts in the papillae and cyst formation.
2. An autosomal dominant condition associated with cyst formation and mutations in the *PKD1* gene.
3. A 7-year-old boy presenting with haematuria and proteinuria following a sore throat.
4. A condition associated with proteinuria, oedema and hypoalbuminaemia.
5. A middle-aged man presenting with polyuria and nocturia. He is known to suffer from rheumatoid arthritis for which he takes NSAIDs.

Complications of renal failure

Each answer can be used once, more than once or not at all.

a. Anaemia
b. Osteomalacia
c. Osteoporosis
d. Osteosclerosis
e. Amyloidosis
f. Autonomic neuropathy
g. Cardiomyopathy
h. Peptic ulceration
i. Acute pancreatitis
j. Gout

For each scenario below, choose the most likely corresponding option from the list given above.

1. Associated with an increase in trabeculae typically in cancellous bone.

2. Associated with the deposition of insoluble fibrillar protein and diagnosed by Congo Red staining of tissues.
3. A multifactorial pathogenesis associated with depressed bone marrow activity and decreased erythropoietin formation.
4. A 65-year-old man with known renal failure presenting with postural hypotension, nausea and vomiting.
5. A condition characterized by incomplete mineralization of osteoid tissue.

Clinical features of renal disease

Each answer can be used once, more than once or not at all.

a. Acute nephritic syndrome
b. Nephrotic syndrome
c. Acute renal failure
d. Tubulointerstitial nephritis
e. Renal stone disease
f. Urinary tract obstruction
g. Chronic renal failure
h. Medullary sponge kidney
i. Renal carcinoma
j. Renal hypertension

For each scenario below, choose the most likely corresponding option from the list given above.

1. Typical features include swelling of the ankles, genitals and abdomen.
2. Associated with shortness of breath, generalized lethargy and bone pain.
3. Typical features include haematuria, loin pain and a mass in the flank.
4. May be associated with pain and swelling of the big toe.
5. Typical features include haematuria, proteinuria and oedema in children following a sore throat.

Investigations

Each answer can be used once, more than once or not at all.

a. Urea and electrolytes
b. PSA
c. Urine microscopy and culture
d. Magnetic resonance angiography
e. X-ray of the kidneys, ureters and bladder
f. Renal ultrasound
g. Renal biopsy
h. Serum albumin
i. Cystoscopy
j. Urodynamics

For each scenario below, choose the most likely corresponding option from the list given above.

1. A patient with known ischaemic heart disease taking ACE inhibitors who subsequently develops renal failure.
2. A 24-year-old long-distance runner presenting with severe right-sided groin pain and vomiting.
3. A 65-year-old man presenting with a poor urinary stream, terminal dribbling and hesitancy.
4. A 75-year-old woman presenting with confusion, pain on passing urine and fever.
5. A 35-year-old woman presenting with urinary incontinence following coughing or standing.

Management of renal disease

Each answer can be used once, more than once or not at all.

a. Haemodialysis
b. Peritoneal dialysis
c. Surgery
d. Alpha-blockers
e. Amoxicillin
f. Analgesia
g. Prednisolone
h. Haemofiltration
i. Transplantation
j. Antihypertensives

For each scenario below, choose the most likely corresponding option from the list given above.

1. A 60-year-old gentleman presenting with frequency, nocturia and postvoid dribbling.
2. A 22-year-old marathon runner presenting with severe left-sided loin pain.
3. An elderly gentleman presenting with fever, confusion and dysuria.
4. A condition associated with proteinuria and hypoalbuminaemia.
5. The mainstay form of treatment in individuals presenting with haematuria, loin pain and a mass in the flank.

Diseases of the tubules and interstitium

Each answer can be used once, more than once or not at all.

a. Toxic acute tubular necrosis
b. Amyloidosis
c. PKD
d. Urate nephropathy
e. UTI
f. Sickle-cell disease nephropathy
g. Chronic pyelonephritis
h. Drug-induced tubulointerstitial nephritis
i. Goodpasture syndrome
j. Ischaemic acute tubular necrosis
k. Acute pyelonephritis

For each scenario below, choose the most likely corresponding option from the list given above.

1. A 26-year-old woman who is 26 weeks pregnant presents with a 2-day history of dysuria and increased frequency of micturition. On inspection of the urine sample, you notice it is cloudy.
2. A 63-year-old man who has vesicoureteric reflux presents to the GP's surgery with a 3-day history of fever, general malaise and loin pain. He says he had also noticed that he suddenly needs to go to the toilet without warning.
3. A 28-year-old male dies from a motorcycle accident in which he lost a lot of blood following trauma to his abdomen. Histological examination of the kidneys reveals infiltration of inflammatory cells and tubular cells, flattened and vacuolated tubular cells and interstitial oedema.
4. A 33-year-old woman undergoing chemotherapy for leukaemia goes into AKI.
5. A 30-year-old woman is found to have severe hypertension. Her mother reports that she had bouts of 'undiagnosed' fever as a young child and wet the bed until age 12 following which she has always had nocturia. Urinalysis reveals the presence of protein.

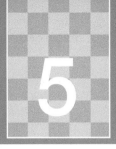
SINGLE BEST ANSWER (SBA) QUESTIONS

1. A 35-year-old woman complains of generalized facial weakness along with difficulties in chewing. On examination you note ptosis and a slow downward drift of her outstretched arms. In addition, you observe that her speech appears slower than normal. What is the most appropriate initial investigation?
   a. Acetylcholine receptor antibodies
   b. Electromyography (EMG)
   c. Muscle biopsy
   d. Creatine kinase levels
   e. Head computed tomography (CT) scan

2. A 45-year-old lawyer complains of difficulty in releasing his grasp after shaking peoples' hands. What term most appropriately describes this?
   a. Myositis
   b. Muscular dystrophy
   c. Myasthenia
   d. Myopathy
   e. Myotonia

3. A 7-year-old boy presents with difficulty in running and in rising to an erect position from the floor. His mother mentions that to become upright he often uses his hands to climb up his legs. What is the most likely diagnosis?
   a. Limb girdle dystrophy
   b. Facioscapulohumeral dystrophy
   c. Duchenne muscular dystrophy
   d. Becker muscular dystrophy
   e. Myotonia congenita

4. A 32-year-old alcoholic complains of numbness and tingling sensation in his hands. On general examination you note nystagmus. What is the most likely diagnosis?
   a. Vitamin B_6 deficiency
   b. Vitamin B_1 deficiency
   c. Vitamin B_{12} deficiency
   d. Vitamin A deficiency
   e. Vitamin C deficiency

5. A 45-year-old man presents with a 1-week history of progressive weakness and numbness in his distal limbs. On examination you note areflexia and muscle weakness but with normal sensation. Nerve conduction studies demonstrate slowing of motor conduction with segmental demyelination. You decide to perform a lumbar puncture (LP). What is the most likely finding on cerebrospinal fluid (CSF) analysis?
   a. Normal protein, normal glucose, normal cell count
   b. Low protein, raised glucose, raised cell count
   c. Low protein, low glucose, low cell count
   d. Raised protein, normal glucose, raised cell count
   e. Raised protein, normal glucose, normal cell count

6. A 54-year-old woman with diabetes presents with pain and tingling in her right hand. On examination you note wasting of her thenar muscles. Which nerve is most likely to be affected?
   a. Radial
   b. Ulnar
   c. Median
   d. Brachial
   e. Musculocutaneous

7. A 65-year-old man presents with weakness in his hands and arms. On examination you note significant wasting and fasciculation. You suspect the possibility of motor neurone disease. Which investigation is most likely to lead to a diagnosis?
   a. EMG
   b. Muscle biopsy
   c. Creatine kinase levels
   d. Head CT scan
   e. None of the above

8. A 32-year-old man presents with ataxia, dysarthria and visual disturbance. On examination you note absent lower limb tendon reflexes and an upgoing plantar response. You also note absence of joint position and vibration sense in his lower limbs. A visual examination demonstrates nystagmus and pale-coloured optic discs. What is the most likely diagnosis?
   a. Cauda equina lesion
   b. Friedreich ataxia
   c. Syringomyelia
   d. Syringobulbia
   e. Spinal cord compression

9. A 40-year-old woman presents with difficulty in walking. Neurological examination reveals significant weakness in her legs, as well as notable spasticity. In addition, you note a loss of sensation to pain and

temperature in her upper limbs. Which investigation is most likely to lead to a diagnosis?
a. Spinal magnetic resonance imaging (MRI) scan
b. Spinal X-ray
c. Spinal CT scan
d. Muscle biopsy
e. EMG

10. A 54-year-old woman presents with back pain and weakness in her legs. On examination you note significant spasticity in her legs. Appropriate imaging demonstrates the presence of a vertebral lesion. What is the most appropriate step in management?
a. Dexamethasone
b. Surgical decompression
c. Physiotherapy
d. Neck brace
e. Baclofen

11. A 38-year-old man complains of headaches that typically last for 4 weeks followed by a period of remission. He describes the headache as being quite severe and located primarily around his right eye. During such episodes he suffers from watering of his eye, as well as significant redness. What is the most likely diagnosis?
a. Trigeminal neuralgia
b. Giant-cell arteritis
c. Cluster headache
d. Migraine
e. Tension headache

12. A 65-year-old woman complains of a headache and scalp tenderness when she combs her hair. She also suffers from jaw pain while eating and has noticed that her vision is intermittently poor. What is the most likely diagnosis?
a. Trigeminal neuralgia
b. Giant-cell arteritis
c. Cluster headache
d. Migraine
e. Tension headache

13. A 60-year-old woman complains of a headache and scalp tenderness when she combs her hair. On examination you note her temporal arteries are tender, firm and pulseless. What is the next most appropriate step in management?
a. Paracetamol
b. Triptans
c. Ergotamine
d. Pizotifen
e. Steroids

14. A 61-year-old woman complains of a headache and scalp tenderness when she combs her hair. She presents as an emergency due to sudden loss of vision in her right eye. Routine blood investigations reveal an erythrocyte sedimentation rate (ESR) of 65 mm/h. You perform a routine fundoscopy assessment. What is most likely to be seen on fundoscopy?
a. Cherry-red spot
b. Flame-shaped haemorrhages
c. Cotton wool spots
d. Silver wiring
e. Papilloedema

15. A 28-year-old woman complains of a throbbing headache accompanied by nausea, vomiting and difficulty looking at bright lights. Prior to her headache, she recalls seeing flashes and jagged lines. What is the most likely diagnosis?
a. Trigeminal neuralgia
b. Giant-cell arteritis
c. Cluster headache
d. Migraine
e. Tension headache

16. A 30-year-old man complains of a throbbing headache and visual loss. He mentions that the headache comes on after eating chocolate biscuits which he is very fond of. What is the most likely aetiological cause for his headache?
a. Serotonin
b. Adrenaline
c. Noradrenaline
d. Dopamine
e. Acetylcholine

17. A 35-year-old man complains of a 2-day history of headaches. During the consultation, he begins to experience a headache which he describes as throbbing in nature. He also mentions he feels nauseous and his vision is deteriorating. His past medical history includes ischaemic heart disease. What is the next most appropriate step in management?
a. Sumatriptan
b. Ergotamine
c. Methysergide
d. Paracetamol and metoclopramide
e. Pizotifen

18. A 63-year-old man accompanied by his wife presents with headaches and vomiting. His wife is keen to mention that he has become generally slow and that his personality is not what it used to be. She is worried as he is beginning to show

little interest in his usual hobbies. He is referred for a CT head scan which reveals the presence of a tumour. What is the most likely site of his tumour?
a. Temporal lobe
b. Parietal lobe
c. Frontal lobe
d. Occipital lobe
e. Cerebellum

19. A 55-year-old man presents with headache, vomiting and papilloedema. He describes the headache as getting worse when he coughs but decreasing when he stands up. A CT head scan reveals the presence of a tumour. What additional findings may there be on neurological examination?
a. Cranial nerve (CN) II nerve palsy
b. CN III nerve palsy
c. CN IV nerve palsy
d. CN V nerve palsy
e. CN VII nerve palsy

20. A 55-year-old woman complains of a sudden-onset severe headache and an intolerance of bright lights. On examination you note neck stiffness. Routine observations reveal a temperature of 38.5°C. You suspect meningitis. What is the most likely organism responsible for her symptoms?
a. *Neisseria meningitidis*
b. *Staphylococcus aureus*
c. Group B streptococci
d. *Listeria monocytogenes*
e. Enterovirus

21. A 10-year-old boy presents with a headache and difficulty when looking at bright lights. On examination you note neck stiffness and a nonblanching rash on his abdomen. He is pyrexial with a temperature of 39°C. There is no known history of drug allergies. What is the next most appropriate step in management?
a. Paracetamol
b. Cefotaxime
c. Ampicillin
d. Benzylpenicillin
e. Chloramphenicol

22. A 19-year-old university student complains of a headache and a stiff neck. He also mentions that he finds it difficult to look at bright lights. Observations reveal a temperature of 39°C. What is the most appropriate initial investigation?
a. Blood culture
b. LP
c. Viral serology

d. Head CT scan
e. Syphilis serology

23. A 23-year-old university student is diagnosed with meningitis of bacterial aetiology. The cause has been assigned as bacterial. What is the most likely finding on CSF analysis?
a. Lymphocytes, increased protein, normal glucose
b. Lymphocytes, decreased protein, increased glucose
c. Lymphocytes, normal protein, normal glucose
d. Polymorphs, normal protein, normal glucose
e. Polymorphs, increased protein, decreased glucose

24. A 35-year-old man presents with blurred vision and right-sided eye pain. In addition, he mentions he experiences a 'pins and needles'-like sensation on occasions. The following are all sites which may be affected in his condition EXCEPT?
a. Optic nerve
b. Periventricular white matter
c. Spinal cord
d. Cerebellum
e. Peripheral nerves

25. A 32-year-old man presents with blurred vision and right-sided eye pain. In addition, he complains of numbness and weakness in his legs. What is the most appropriate initial investigation?
a. MRI brain scan
b. Electrophysiology
c. LP
d. Brain CT scan
e. Cerebral angiography

26. A 31-year-old woman is diagnosed with MS following investigations which include an LP. What is the most likely finding on CSF analysis?
a. Decreased polymorphs
b. Monoclonal bands
c. Increased glucose
d. Decreased protein
e. Oligoclonal bands

27. A 32-year-old man complains of a tremor when he holds a glass or spoon. He notices it improves when he drinks alcohol. What is the most likely diagnosis?
a. Chorea
b. Hemiballismus
c. Myoclonus
d. Benign essential tremor
e. Tic

28. A 45-year-old man with Parkinson disease complains of a jerky movement which spreads from one part of his body to the other ever since he was started on treatment for his condition. What is the most likely diagnosis?
   a. Chorea
   b. Hemiballismus
   c. Myoclonus
   d. Benign essential tremor
   e. Tic

29. A 35-year-old woman with epilepsy was witnessed as having a sudden jerking movement of her right arm while she fell asleep. What is the most likely diagnosis?
   a. Chorea
   b. Hemiballismus
   c. Myoclonus
   d. Benign essential tremor
   e. Tic

30. A 30-year-old man complains of prolonged spasms of muscle contraction. He is now receiving botulinum toxin which has improved his symptoms dramatically. What is the most likely diagnosis?
   a. Chorea
   b. Hemiballismus
   c. Myoclonus
   d. Dystonia
   e. Tic

31. A 65-year-old woman presents with a hand tremor. She has slowed considerably in day to day activities and now requires support for activities of daily living. On examination you note an expressionless face, slowness of movements and marked rigidity in her upper limbs. What is the initial most appropriate step in management?
   a. Bromocriptine
   b. Selegiline
   c. Amantadine
   d. Benzhexol
   e. Levodopa

32. A 62-year-old man presents with a shuffling gait and reduced arm swing. On examination you note a resting tremor. Which neurotransmitter is he most likely to be lacking?
   a. Dopamine
   b. Serotonin
   c. Noradrenaline
   d. Adrenaline
   e. Acetylcholine

33. A 53-year-old schizophrenic presents with a resting hand tremor. On examination you note slowness of movements, marked rigidity in his upper limbs and an inability to move his eyes vertically. What is the most likely diagnosis?
   a. Drug-induced parkinsonism
   b. Idiopathic parkinsonism
   c. Parkinsonism plus
   d. Methylphenyltetrahydropyridine-induced parkinsonism
   e. Postencephalitic parkinsonism

34. A 28-year-old man presents to accident and emergency (A&E) following a fitting episode. His girlfriend witnessed the event and described it as a jerking action of his entire body. She mentioned that the event did not last long. After the episode, the gentleman remembers feeling drowsy and that his tongue was sore. What is the most likely diagnosis?
   a. Tonic-clonic seizure
   b. Absence seizure
   c. Simple partial seizure
   d. Complex partial seizure
   e. Myoclonic seizure

35. A 7-year-old girl was witnessed by her father as having episodes where she suddenly stopped what she was doing, stared and then regained normal activity. What is the most likely diagnosis?
   a. Tonic-clonic seizure
   b. Absence seizure
   c. Simple partial seizure
   d. Complex partial seizure
   e. Myoclonic seizure

36. A 45-year-old man presents following a fitting episode. He described it as a jerking-like movement which began in his right hand and spread to the left side of his body. Following the episode, he mentioned his upper limbs felt weak. What is the most likely diagnosis?
   a. Tonic-clonic seizure
   b. Absence seizure
   c. Focal motor seizure
   d. Complex partial seizure
   e. Myoclonic seizure

37. A 39-year-old woman presents following a fitting episode. She recalls experiencing the smell of burning rubber during the event. What is the most likely diagnosis?
   a. Tonic-clonic seizure
   b. Absence seizure
   c. Simple partial seizure
   d. Complex partial seizure
   e. Myoclonic seizure

38. A 32-year-old man is diagnosed with grand mal epilepsy. He is started on appropriate

treatment. After 4 weeks, he complains of hair loss. Routine blood investigations reveal an alanine aminotransferase of 55 U/L, an aspartate aminotransferase of 55 U/L, an alkaline phosphatase of 140 U/L and a bilirubin of 3 mg/dL. Which drug is most likely to be responsible for these findings?
a. Phenytoin
b. Carbamazepine
c. Ethosuximide
d. Sodium valproate
e. Vigabatrin

39. A 36-year-old man is diagnosed with grand mal epilepsy. He is started on appropriate treatment. During a routine review with his general practitioner (GP), blood investigations reveal a folate of 1.8 µg/L and a low vitamin D level. Which drug is most likely to be responsible for these findings?
a. Phenytoin
b. Carbamazepine
c. Ethosuximide
d. Sodium valproate
e. Vigabatrin

40. A 34-year-old man is diagnosed with epilepsy. He is started on appropriate treatment. He goes to see his GP complaining of a generalized skin rash and 'night terrors'. Which drug is most likely to be responsible for this?
a. Phenytoin
b. Carbamazepine
c. Ethosuximide
d. Sodium valproate
e. Vigabatrin

41. A known epileptic is admitted to A&E following two consecutive seizures. Since the episode, he has failed to regain consciousness. He has a history of poor compliance with medication. As the house officer on call you attempt to obtain intravenous access but fail. What is the next most appropriate step in management?
a. Phenytoin
b. Enobarbital
c. Clonazepam
d. Lorazepam
e. Diazepam

42. A known epileptic is admitted to A&E following two consecutive seizures. Since the episode he has failed to regain consciousness. He is known to drink heavily. What is the most appropriate initial investigation?
a. Serum electrolytes
b. Head CT scan
c. LP

d. Blood glucose
e. Blood cultures

43. A 55-year-old man presents with a sudden-onset severe headache. On examination you note neck stiffness and that his right eye is abducted and looking down. Fundoscopy assessment reveals papilloedema. What is the most appropriate initial investigation?
a. Head CT scan
b. Head MRI scan
c. LP
d. Cerebral angiography
e. Visual field assessment by perimetry

44. A 54-year-old man presents with a sudden-onset severe headache. On examination you note neck stiffness. An LP is performed which reveals a yellow-coloured supernatant after centrifugation of the CSF. What is the most likely diagnosis?
a. Intracerebral haemorrhage
b. Subarachnoid haemorrhage
c. Subdural haematoma
d. Extradural haematoma
e. None of the above

45. A 38-year-old alcoholic presents following a serious fall. He complains of a severe headache. On examination he appears drowsy and confused. What is the most likely diagnosis?
a. Intracerebral haemorrhage
b. Subarachnoid haemorrhage
c. Subdural haematoma
d. Extradural haematoma
e. None of the above

46. A 35-year-old man was found unconscious following a boxing match. He regains consciousness while in A&E. During neurological assessment, he rapidly deteriorates and becomes less aware of his surroundings. Which artery is most likely to have been ruptured?
a. Anterior cerebral
b. Middle cerebral
c. Posterior cerebral
d. Vertebral
e. Middle meningeal

47. A 62-year-old man presents with weakness on his right side. His symptoms, however, dramatically improve within 24 hours. What is the most likely diagnosis?
a. Stroke
b. Stroke in evolution
c. Minor stroke
d. Transient ischaemic attack (TIA)
e. Completed stroke

48. A 60-year-old woman is diagnosed as having had a TIA arising from emboli in her internal carotid artery. She is likely to display all of the following features EXCEPT?
    a. Amaurosis fugax
    b. Aphasia
    c. Hemiparesis
    d. Hemisensory loss
    e. Transient global amnesia

49. A 45-year-old obese man presents with right-sided weakness, loss of sensation and visual disturbances. On examination you note increased tone, brisk reflexes and an upgoing plantar response. Which artery is most likely to be occluded?
    a. Anterior cerebral
    b. Middle cerebral
    c. Posterior cerebral
    d. Vertebral
    e. Middle meningeal

50. A 53-year-old man presents with sudden-onset vomiting and vertigo. On examination you note left-sided facial numbness and a diminished gag reflex. There is also reduced sensitivity to pain and temperature on the right side and evidence of a broad-based ataxic gait. Which artery is most likely to be occluded?
    a. Anterior cerebral
    b. Middle cerebral
    c. Posterior cerebral
    d. Posterior inferior cerebellar artery (PICA)
    e. Middle meningeal

51. A diabetic lifelong smoker presents with weakness on his right side. On examination you note an audible bruit in his internal carotid artery. What is the most appropriate initial investigation?
    a. Head CT scan
    b. Plasma glucose
    c. Carotid Doppler
    d. Urea and electrolytes
    e. Magnetic resonance angiography

52. An obese lifelong smoker presents with a 12-hour history of right-sided weakness, loss of sensation and visual disturbances. On examination you note increased tone, brisk reflexes and an upgoing plantar response. His blood pressure is 145/95 mmHg. A head CT scan reveals the presence of a cerebral infarct. What is the next most appropriate step in management?
    a. Antihypertensives
    b. Thrombolysis
    c. Heparin
    d. Warfarin
    e. Aspirin

53. A 32-year-old alcoholic presents to A&E. On examination his speech is notably confused. His eyes open spontaneously and he withdraws to pain. What is his Glasgow Coma Scale (GCS) Score?
    a. 9
    b. 10
    c. 11
    d. 12
    e. 13

54. A 35-year-old man presents with visual disturbance. He is later diagnosed with MS. What is the most likely type of his visual loss?
    a. Scotoma
    b. Bitemporal hemianopia
    c. Homonymous hemianopia
    d. Homonymous quadrantanopia
    e. None of the above

55. A 32-year-old man is found unconscious at his home. He is immediately transferred to A&E. On examination he is noted to have bilateral pupillary constriction. The following are all causes of pupil constriction EXCEPT?
    a. CN III nerve palsy
    b. Horner syndrome
    c. Argyll Robertson pupil
    d. Opiate addiction
    e. Lesion at the pons

56. A 31-year-old woman presents with ptosis of her right eye. On examination you note that her right eye is abducted, pointing down and fixed to light. Which artery is most likely to be affected in this presentation?
    a. Anterior cerebral
    b. Middle cerebral
    c. Posterior cerebral
    d. Posterior communicating
    e. Middle meningeal

57. A 56-year-old woman presents with left-sided facial weakness. On examination you note dribbling from the corner of her mouth and that she is unable to close her eyes. She complains of hearing disturbance and you observe the presence of vesicles in her left ear. What is the most likely diagnosis?
    a. Otitis media
    b. Bell palsy
    c. Ramsay Hunt syndrome
    d. Guillain–Barré syndrome
    e. Otitis externa

58. A middle-aged man complains of a sensation whereby his surroundings are revolving around him.

He was recently prescribed gentamicin following a severe episode of pneumonia. What structure is most likely to be affected in his condition?

a. Labyrinth
b. CN VIII
c. Brainstem
d. Cerebellum
e. Basal ganglia

59. A middle-aged man is diagnosed with a pseudobulbar palsy. The following are all findings of such a condition EXCEPT?

a. Dysarthria
b. Dysphagia
c. Nasal regurgitation
d. Exaggerated jaw jerk
e. Tongue fasciculations

60. A middle-aged man with MS presents with an ataxic broad-based gait. He is likely to demonstrate the following signs EXCEPT?

a. Intention tremor
b. Vertical nystagmus
c. Dysarthria
d. Pendular reflexes
e. Decreased tone

61. A 40-year old man suffered a femoral shaft fracture following a road traffic accident. Forty-eight hours later, he became increasingly drowsy with a rash on his chest and abdomen and died soon after. A postmortem examination shows multiple petechial haemorrhages in the corpus callosum and centrum semiovale of the brain region. What is the most likely diagnosis?

a. Diffuse axonal injury
b. Fat embolism
c. Watershed infarction
d. Septic embolism
e. Pulmonary embolism

62. A 55-year old woman presents to her GP with a 3-month history of progressive cognitive impairment, urinary incontinence and unsteady gait leading to falls noticed by her son. Other than suffering from subarachnoid haemorrhage in her youth, she has no other medical history. What is the most likely diagnosis?

a. Hereditary spinocerebellar ataxia
b. Wilson disease
c. Normal pressure hydrocephalus (NPH)
d. Huntington disease
e. Pseudotumour cerebri

63. A previously fit and well 55-year old woman is brought to the emergency department by her husband. She initially complained of epigastric fullness, which was followed by a period of unresponsiveness where she looked 'blank'. Shortly afterwards, she started to smack her lips. She appeared confused and disorientated for a short period afterwards. She could not remember the events. Clinical examination is unremarkable. What is the most likely diagnosis?

a. Simple partial seizure
b. Cocaine overdose
c. Complex partial seizure
d. Tonic-clonic seizure
e. Absence seizure

64. A 24-year old man presents to his GP with a change in personality. His girlfriend reports that he has become aggressive, irrational and labile in mood in the last 2 months, which is 'not his usual self at all'. Subsequent brain CT shows evidence of a brain tumour. Which part of his brain is most likely to be affected?

a. Temporal lobe
b. Parietal lobe
c. Pituitary gland
d. Occipital lobe
e. Frontal lobe

65. A 62-year old man presents to his GP with severe progressive memory loss, initially noticed by his wife. She has also noticed speech disturbance, unsteadiness on walking, uncontrollable trembling and tendency to fall asleep during the day. On examination he has an ataxic gait. The patient reports no family history of psychiatric or neurological diseases. What is the most likely diagnosis?

a. Creutzfeldt–Jakob disease (CJD)
b. Fatal familial insomnia
c. Kuru
d. Gerstmann–Straussler–Scheinker syndrome
e. Normal old age phenomenon

66. An 80-year old man is accompanied to the GP surgery by his daughter. She expresses concerns that her father may be suffering from Alzheimer disease (AD) and would like a formal assessment. Which of the following is not characteristic of AD?

a. Aphasia
b. Apraxia
c. Agnosia
d. Sudden cognitive decline
e. Repetitive statements

67. A 30-year-old teacher presents to her GP with a 2-year history of recurrent severe headaches.

The headaches occur two to three times per year, with each episode lasting 3–4 hours. They are unilateral and usually associated with vomiting and photophobia. She has tried various analgesics but with minimal effect. Neurological examination is unremarkable. What is the most likely diagnosis?

a. Migraine
b. Tension headache
c. Cluster headache
d. Temporal arteritis
e. Analgesia-related headache

68. A 35-year old woman presents to the emergency department with severe right-sided headaches. She tells you that these 'attacks' happen every few months, and are associated with watering of her right eye and nasal congestion. Each episode can last for up to 2 hours. She is completely well in between these episodes. Which of the following management is most likely to provide relief for this patient?

a. Oxygen inhalation
b. Corticosteroids
c. Nonsteroidal antiinflammatory drugs
d. Amitriptyline
e. Verapamil

69. A 34-year-old woman presents to her GP with sudden-onset severe dizziness and vomiting but no other symptoms. On examination she has a horizontal nystagmus with the fast phase to the right. What is the most likely explanation for these findings?

a. Acoustic neuroma on the right side
b. Horizontal nystagmus probably indicates a central cause
c. Tertiary syphilis
d. Otitis externa
e. Viral labyrinthitis

70. A 25-year old man sees his GP for muscle weakness. He underwent a left-sided lymph node biopsy recently to investigate a painless lump found in the posterior triangle of his neck. Since then, he has been complaining of difficulty shrugging his left shoulder and tilting his head to the left side. On examination his left scapula is more prominent than the right, especially on left shoulder abduction, and his left shoulder appears more drooped than the right. Which one of the following nerves is most likely to be injured?

a. Long thoracic nerve
b. Suprascapular nerve
c. Accessory nerve

d. Musculocutaneous nerve
e. Dorsal scapular nerve

71. A 20-year old man presents to the emergency department with weakness in his left wrist, following a party the night before where he drank heavily and slept uncomfortably on a chair overnight. On examination there is no obvious injury, but he has a left-sided wrist drop. What is the most likely causative agent in this case?

a. Injury to median nerve
b. Injury to ulnar nerve
c. Injury to radial nerve
d. Fracture of the distal radius
e. Carpal tunnel syndrome

72. A secondary school rugby player reports a history of progressive inability to participate in the sport over the last month. Initially, he had double vision following a practice session. He was better the following morning, but his symptoms recurred the day after. Now he has double vision most of the time, except right after sleeping. He says his strength and agility are declining, and his coach thinks he is playing too poorly to remain on the team. On examination he has mild ptosis, which increases if he tries to maintain an upward gaze. His arm strength is initially 5/5, but he tires very rapidly. After a few minutes of isotonic exertion, he cannot lift his arms against gravity. His deep tendon reflexes are normal. Which of the following is the most likely diagnosis?

a. Guillain–Barré syndrome
b. Psychophysiologic weakness
c. Postconcussion syndrome
d. Myasthenia gravis (MG)
e. Myotonic dystrophy

73. A 40-year-old woman presents to her GP with a 1-month history of fatigue and weakness. She reports that her eyes feel droopy as the day progresses. She also has difficulty in swallowing and food tends to be left in her mouth after an attempt to swallow. She is otherwise well with no known medical history. Clinical examination is unremarkable except for the presence of mild bilateral ptosis. Which of the following radiological finding is most likely to be associated with this patient's condition?

a. A widened mediastinum on chest X-ray
b. Air–fluid level on chest X-ray
c. Dilated bowel loops on abdominal plain X-ray
d. Multiple lesions in liver on abdominal CT
e. Solitary pulmonary nodule on chest X-ray

EXTENDED-MATCHING QUESTIONS (EMQs)

Delirium
Each answer can be used once, more than once or not at all.

a. Concussion
b. Diabetic ketoacidosis
c. Encephalitis
d. Hepatic encephalopathy
e. Hypercalcaemia
f. Hypercapnia
g. Hyperosmolar, nonketotic state
h. Hyponatraemia
i. Opiate analgesia
j. Subarachnoid haemorrhage
k. Subdural haematoma

For each scenario below, choose the most likely corresponding option from the list given above.

1. A previously fit and well 13-year-old boy presents to A&E with a 24-hour history of increasing confusion. On examination he is unwell, smells of ketones and is dehydrated.
2. A 70-year-old lifelong smoker who is attending the oncologist presents to the medical admission unit with a 48-hour history of increasing confusion and vomiting. His blood gases are normal, but he is dehydrated.
3. A 60-year-old smoker with a 75-pack year history presents with a productive cough and feeling short of breath. He is drowsy but rousable. He has a bounding pulse and a flapping tremor.
4. An 82-year-old lady with a history of dementia and falls presents with increasing confusion and more frequent falls. She is drowsy with a mental test score of 2/10. She has a right-sided weakness and upgoing plantars.
5. A previously fit 25-year-old man presents to A&E with a severe headache and increasing confusion. While you are examining him, he starts to fit. While applying the oxygen mask, you notice a cold sore.

Cranial nerve lesions
Each answer can be used once, more than once or not at all.

a. I
b. II
c. III
d. IV
e. V
f. VI
g. VII
h. VIII
i. IX
j. X

For each scenario below, choose the most likely corresponding option from the list given above.

1. Associated with unilateral ptosis and a 'down and out' pupil.
2. Known to cause loss of taste on the anterior two-thirds of the tongue.
3. Associated with diplopia when looking down and away from the affected side.
4. Associated with unilateral visual loss in the form of an area of depressed vision within the visual field.
5. Associated with unilateral sensory loss on the face and tongue.

Diseases of the peripheral nerves
Each answer can be used once, more than once or not at all.

a. Vitamin B$_6$ deficiency
b. Vitamin B$_1$ deficiency
c. Vitamin B$_{12}$ deficiency
d. Charcot–Marie–Tooth disease
e. Guillain–Barré syndrome
f. Carpal tunnel syndrome
g. Mononeuritis multiplex
h. Amyloidosis
i. HIV associated neuropathy
j. Autonomic neuropathy

For each scenario below, choose the most likely corresponding option from the list given above.

1. A diabetic patient presenting with pain and numbness in her hands, in addition to wasting of her thenar muscles.
2. Associated with distal limb wasting and weakness. In advanced cases, the legs may resemble inverted champagne bottles.
3. Associated with weakness and complaints of numbness in the distal limbs. Additional features include respiratory muscle weakness and postural hypotension.
4. Seen commonly in individuals with a long-standing history of alcohol abuse.
5. A sensory neuropathy seen occasionally in individuals on isoniazid therapy.

Diseases of the muscle
Each answer can be used once, more than once or not at all.

a. Limb girdle dystrophy
b. Facioscapulohumeral dystrophy

c. Myasthenia gravis
d. Dystrophia myotonica
e. Myotonia congenita
f. Cushing syndrome
g. Hypothyroidism
h. Hyperthyroidism
i. Osteomalacia
j. Duchenne muscular dystrophy

For each scenario below, choose the most likely corresponding option from the list given above.

1. Presents in early childhood with weakness in the proximal leg muscles.
2. Fatigability of proximal limb muscles in association with immunoglobulin G (IgG) acetylcholine receptor antibodies.
3. An autosomal dominant condition characterized by distal muscle weakness and myotonia.
4. An autosomal dominant condition characterized by myotonia in childhood.
5. An autosomal recessive disorder associated with abnormal muscle function of the shoulder and pelvic girdle.

Epilepsy

Each answer can be used once, more than once or not at all.

a. Grand mal
b. Petit mal
c. Myoclonic seizure
d. Jacksonian motor seizure
e. Temporal lobe epilepsy
f. Status epilepticus
g. West syndrome
h. Juvenile myoclonic epilepsy
i. Frontal lobe epilepsy
j. Lennox–Gastaut syndrome

For each scenario below, choose the most likely corresponding option from the list given above.

1. A patient presenting with muscle jerking and incontinence of urine.
2. Commonly seen in childhood whereby the individual ceases activity and stares for a few seconds.
3. Associated with jerking movements beginning in the corner of the mouth and spreading to involve the limbs on the opposite side.
4. Phenytoin is the first-line treatment in this form of epilepsy.
5. Associated with feelings of unreality or undue familiarity.

Extrapyramidal diseases

Each answer can be used once, more than once or not at all.

a. Idiopathic Parkinson disease
b. Multiple sclerosis
c. Drug-induced Parkinson disease
d. Parkinsonism plus
e. Benign essential tremor
f. Chorea
g. Huntington disease
h. Hemiballismus
i. Myoclonus
j. Tics

For each scenario below, choose the most likely corresponding option from the list given above.

1. A condition associated with signs of parkinsonism and an inability to move the eyes vertically or laterally.
2. Associated with violent swinging movement of one side of the body.
3. An autosomal dominant condition associated with a defective gene on chromosome 4.
4. Brief repeated stereotypical movements involving the face and shoulders.
5. A condition typically presenting in adult life associated with perivenular plaques of demyelination.

Headache 1

Each answer can be used once, more than once or not at all.

a. Cervical spondylitis
b. Chronic sinusitis
c. Giant-cell arteritis
d. Malignancy
e. Meningitis
f. Ménière disease
g. Migraine
h. Subarachnoid haemorrhage
i. Subdural haematoma
j. Tension headache

For each scenario below, choose the most likely corresponding option from the list given above.

1. A fit and well 30-year-old man presents with a sudden-onset severe headache, confusion, photophobia and neck stiffness.
2. A 45-year-old woman presents with recurrent headaches for the last year. She has no focal neurological deficit and the headaches have not been worsening.
3. A 79-year-old with hypertension presents with worsening headaches over the sides of his head, and jaw ache on chewing.

4. An 18-year-old student who has just started university presents with a worsening headache and marked photophobia. Neck stiffness is not detectable.

Nerves of the upper limb

Each answer can be used once, more than once or not at all.

a. Axillary nerve
b. Long thoracic nerve of Bell
c. Lower brachial plexus
d. Medial cutaneous nerve of forearm
e. Median nerve
f. Musculocutaneous nerve
g. Nerve to coracobrachialis
h. Radial nerve
i. Ulnar nerve
j. Upper brachial plexus

For each scenario below, choose the most likely corresponding option from the list given above.

1. A 14-year-old boy presents with an inability to grip in his right arm after falling from a tree and catching himself on a low-lying branch.
2. A 30-year-old pregnant woman presents with numbness and reduced grip in her left hand, symptoms which are worse at night. On examination the numbness appears limited to the thumb, index and middle fingers. The thumb is particularly weak in flexion, opposition and abduction.
3. A 25-year-old man presents to A&E with a broken arm following an arm wrestling contest. X-ray demonstrates a fracture of the proximal third of the humerus. He has wrist drop and has a loss of sensation over the web space between the thumb and index finger.
4. The same gentleman as above, on further examination, has anaesthesia over the regimental patch and is unable to abduct his arm.
5. A 58-year-old woman presents having had a mastectomy and axillary node clearance. On asking her to press her hands against the wall in front of her, you notice that the scapula on the affected side is more prominent, with the medial border standing proud.

Headache 2

Each answer can be used once, more than once or not at all.

a. Bacterial meningitis
b. Benign intracranial hypertension
c. Cerebral abscess
d. Cerebral metastasis

e. Cluster headache
f. Giant-cell arteritis
g. Subarachnoid haemorrhage
h. Subdural haemorrhage
i. Temporomandibular joint disease
j. Tension headache

For each scenario below, choose the most likely corresponding option from the list given above.

1. A 22-year-old woman presents to her GP with frontal headaches, worse in the morning. She has no other symptoms. On examination she has a body mass index of $32 \, \text{kg/m}^2$ with nothing else to note. CT of the head and LP are normal. Her condition settles with dietary advice.
2. A 60-year-old man presents to his GP with severe headaches over the frontal region and shoulders. The examination is unremarkable except for a thick band palpable over the right temple. The ESR is 97 mm/h.
3. A 54-year-old woman presents with severe headaches; she is completely incapacitated by the pain which is present over her right eye. She often sees zig-zag lines before the headache and they are so severe that she presses over her eye to try and relieve the pain. These attacks last several hours and disappear as quickly as they start.
4. A 27-year-old man complains of headaches to his GP. They are temporal and are relieved by sleeping. He is anxious as his company is merging and he risks losing his job.
5. A 19-year-old medical student presents with headache and photophobia of 3 hours' duration. She is unable to touch her chest with her chin. There are no signs of raised intracranial pressure. The CSF shows reduced glucose and numerous polymorphs.

Strokes

Each answer can be used once, more than once or not at all.

a. Lacunar infarct
b. Partial anterior circulation infarct (PACI)
c. Partial anterior circulation syndrome (PACS)
d. Partial occipital circulation syndrome (POCS)
e. Pontine stroke
f. PICA occlusion
g. Total anterior circulation syndrome (TACS)
h. TIA
i. Vertebrobasilar insufficiency

For each scenario below, choose the most likely corresponding option from the list given above.

1. A 60-year-old hypertensive man with ischaemic heart disease presents to A&E with a 'funny turn'. On examination he has right hemiparesis, right inattention and a right homonymous hemianopia.
2. A 72-year-old diabetic woman with renal disease presents to A&E with a right hemiparesis affecting her right arm and leg; sensation is normal on the right and left.
3. A 55-year-old obese man is admitted to the ward following a stroke. On admission he was found to have loss of pain and temperature sensation on the left side of his body and the right side of his face, nystagmus to the right and a right Horner syndrome.
4. A 90-year-old woman attends her GP following an episode of weakness that affected her right side: she was unable to stand or use her arm. She is quite distressed, and worries that the symptoms may return. On questioning, the episode seems to have lasted around 4 hours.
5. A 78-year-old man is admitted with a stroke. CT demonstrates an infarct in the anterior circulation. On examination he has a right hemiparesis and a right homonymous hemianopia.

Headache 3

Each answer can be used once, more than once or not at all.

a. Subarachnoid haemorrhage
b. Migraine
c. Skull fracture
d. Tension headache
e. Subdural haematoma
f. Extradural haematoma
g. Intracerebral haemorrhage
h. Cerebral infarct
i. Cerebral sinus thrombosis
j. Idiopathic intracranial hypertension
k. Viral encephalitis

For each scenario below, choose the most likely corresponding option from the list given above.

1. An 18-year-old man was riding pillion on a motorbike without a helmet. At 50 mph (80.5 km/h) he was seen to fall from the bike onto the road. At the scene, he was found to have sustained multiple traumatic injuries to the thorax and limbs. His GCS score was 8. His left pupil had a sluggish reaction to light. Work-up imaging included CT brain which revealed an elliptical, roughly $3 \times 4\,cm^2$ area of high attenuation peripherally.
2. A 26-year-old postgraduate university student was admitted with headache and a 2-day history of recent alteration in her sense of smell. A mild pyrexia was noted by nursing staff. LP revealed a normal protein content, slightly raised leucocytes (lymphocytes predominant) and a normal plasma:CSF glucose ratio. CT brain was reported as normal. MRI brain (T2 weighted) revealed a slightly asymmetrical distribution of high signal within the temporal lobes bilaterally, more so on the right side.
3. A 28-year-old mother of two is seen at outpatient clinic with a short history of headache, which was worse in the mornings and on stooping to attend to her young children. She has no past medical history, although she is attending a dietitian-led weight loss clinic. Her only medication is the oral contraceptive pill as she does not wish for further children at present. O/E: Bilateral papilloedema. CT brain: normal.
4. A 73-year-old lady who lives alone was found by her neighbour to be behaving oddly of late and more unsteady on her feet over the past couple of weeks. She has a medical history that includes hypertension, atrial fibrillation, previous total hip replacement (THR) and Parkinson disease. O/E: She is disorientated in time and place. Her mood was fluctuant. CT brain: low attenuation crescenteric region adjacent to the right temporal bone.
5. A 28-year-old working mother reattended outpatient clinic complaining of a 9-month history of headache. They are now occurring around three times a week, mostly on weekdays, and were partially responsive to codeine-based analgesics. The headache is felt across the whole head, with no visual disturbance or nausea. Complete neurological examination was normal. Brain CT had been done at her second visit, largely on patient request for peace of mind and was reported as normal.
6. A 76-year-old lady was admitted to A&E following a collapse at home. She lives alone and was found by her daughter on the bedroom floor. Her past medical history included angina and peripheral vascular disease. Skull X-ray taken initially was normal. O/E: Right-sided weakness. Speech was normal. CT brain (at 24 hours): low attenuation area in the region of left internal capsule with adjacent oedema.

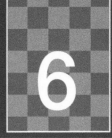

6

SINGLE BEST ANSWER (SBA) QUESTIONS

1. A 65-year-old man complains of pain and stiffness in his hands. On examination you note swelling of the distal interphalangeal (DIP) joints and first carpometacarpal joint. What is the most likely diagnosis?
   a. Rheumatoid arthritis
   b. Osteoarthritis
   c. Psoriatic arthritis
   d. Gout
   e. Pseudogout

2. A 70-year-old woman presents with pain, swelling and stiffness in her knees. The latter is for a short period (<30 minutes), worse early in the morning. Which investigation is most likely to lead to a diagnosis?
   a. Full blood count
   b. Erythrocyte sedimentation rate (ESR)
   c. Rheumatoid factor (RF)
   d. Knee X-ray
   e. C-reactive protein (CRP)

3. A 50-year-old man presents to his general practitioner (GP) with pain in his hands. The GP notes small swellings on his distal and proximal interphalangeal (PIP) joints. What is the next most appropriate step in management?
   a. Surgery
   b. Heat therapy
   c. Hydrotherapy
   d. Steroids
   e. Paracetamol

4. A 35-year-old woman presents with pain, swelling and stiffness in her hands. On examination you note swelling of the PIP joints as well as small nodules just below her elbows. Which investigation is most likely to lead to a diagnosis?
   a. Platelet count
   b. Haemoglobin levels
   c. RF
   d. Antinuclear factor
   e. ESR

5. A 45-year-old woman presents to the GP with marked ulnar deviation of her hands. You note an obvious swan neck deformity of her fingers. What extra manifestation is she most likely to suffer from?
   a. Anaemia
   b. Pleural effusion

   c. Pericarditis
   d. Felty syndrome
   e. Scleromalacia perforans

6. A 30-year-old man is diagnosed with rheumatoid arthritis. He mentions that the pain is difficult to cope with and has been ongoing for the last 4 months. What is the next most appropriate step in management?
   a. Nonsteroidal antiinflammatory drugs (NSAIDs)
   b. Cyclooxygenase-2 (COX-2) inhibitors
   c. Surgery
   d. Tumour necrosis factor-α blockers
   e. Methotrexate

7. A 23-year-old man presents with increasing pain, swelling and stiffness in his lower back. On examination you note a reduction in chest expansion and obvious kyphosis. What is the most likely diagnosis?
   a. Ankylosing spondylitis
   b. Psoriatic arthritis
   c. Osteoarthritis
   d. Reactive arthritis
   e. Enteropathic arthritis

8. A 20-year-old man returns from a trip to Amsterdam. He complains of pain in his knees as well as pain on passing urine. What is the most likely diagnosis?
   a. Ankylosing spondylitis
   b. Psoriatic arthritis
   c. Osteoarthritis
   d. Reactive arthritis
   e. Enteropathic arthritis

9. A 52-year-old man presents to his GP with pain in his hands. The GP notes swelling of his DIP joints as well as pitting of his nails. What is the most likely diagnosis?
   a. Ankylosing spondylitis
   b. Psoriatic arthritis
   c. Osteoarthritis
   d. Reactive arthritis
   e. Enteropathic arthritis

10. A 30-year-old woman is admitted with a painful right knee. On examination the knee is warm to touch. Joint aspiration confirms the presence of a gram-positive coccus. What is the most appropriate step in management?
    a. NSAIDs
    b. COX-2 inhibitors

c. Bed rest
d. Joint mobilization
e. Flucloxacillin and fusidic acid

11. A 25-year-old woman presents with a rash on her nose and cheeks, which she mentions gets worse in the sunlight. She also complains of joint pains in her hands. Which investigation is most likely to provide a diagnosis?
a. Full blood count
b. Antinuclear antibodies (ANAs)
c. Anticardiolipin antibodies
d. Complement levels
e. RF

12. A 45-year-old woman presents with pain in her hands. On examination you note thickening of her skin and tapering of her fingers. She also mentions that she has difficulty opening her mouth. Which investigation is most likely to support the diagnosis?
a. Full blood count
b. Hand X-ray
c. Anticentromere antibodies
d. Anti-Jo 1 antibodies
e. Anti-Ro antibodies

13. A 55-year-old man presents with weakness in his shoulders. He mentions that he has difficulty raising his hands above his head. On examination you note a purple-coloured rash on his face. What is the most likely diagnosis?
a. Dermatomyositis
b. Polymyositis
c. Polymyalgia
d. Overlap syndrome
e. Systemic lupus erythematosus (SLE)

14. A 60-year-old woman presents with weakness in her shoulders and lower limbs. She mentions that she has difficulty walking upstairs and getting up from sitting. You suspect a diagnosis of polymyositis. Which investigation is most likely to confirm the diagnosis?
a. Anti-Jo 1 antibodies
b. ESR
c. Electromyography (EMG)
d. Magnetic resonance imaging (MRI) of the spine
e. Muscle biopsy

15. A middle-aged woman presents with dry eyes and a dry mouth. She also mentions that her fingers feel colder than usual. Which antibody is usually present?
a. Anti-Ro and Anti-La antibodies
b. Anti-Jo 1 antibodies
c. Anticentromere antibodies

d. Anticardiolipin antibodies
e. Lupus anticoagulant

16. A child is taken to the GP by his mother. On examination the GP notes a rash on his legs and buttocks. The mother mentions that he has difficulty walking and is particularly worried as she has noticed blood in his urine. The child was recently treated for a chest infection. What is the most likely diagnosis?
a. Churg–Strauss syndrome
b. Henoch–Schönlein purpura
c. Microscopic polyangiitis
d. Polyarteritis nodosa
e. Juvenile arthritis

17. A 55-year-old man presents with severe pain and swelling of his right big toe. He is obese and a heavy drinker. What is the most appropriate step in management?
a. Allopurinol
b. Probenecid
c. Colchicine
d. NSAIDs
e. Steroids

18. An elderly woman who was diagnosed recently with haemochromatosis presents with pain and stiffness in her knees resembling osteoarthritis. Which of the following investigations is most likely to provide a diagnosis?
a. White cell count (WCC)
b. Knee X-ray
c. Serum calcium
d. Joint fluid microscopy
e. Uric acid levels

19. An Asian woman presents to the GP complaining of generalized muscle pains. She mentions that she is struggling to walk and has difficulty rising from her chair. What is the most likely abnormality on serum investigation?
a. High potassium
b. High calcium
c. Low sodium
d. Low vitamin D
e. Low magnesium

20. A 70-year-old woman has been diagnosed with osteoporosis. She is a heavy smoker and drinker. Her medical history includes a fractured distal radius. What is the most appropriate step in management?
a. Stop smoking
b. Stop alcohol
c. Hormone replacement therapy
d. Bisphosphonates
e. Raloxifene

21. A 75-year-old man presents with significant pain in his legs. On examination you note bowing of his tibia. You suspect a diagnosis of Paget disease. Which investigation is most likely to confirm your suspicion?
    a. Serum magnesium levels
    b. Serum alkaline phosphatase (ALP) levels
    c. Vitamin B_{12} levels
    d. Serum folate levels
    e. Serum sodium levels

EXTENDED-MATCHING QUESTIONS (EMQs)

Limp
Each answer can be used once, more than once or not at all.
a. Chondromalacia patellae
b. Compartment syndrome
c. Congenital dislocation of the hip
d. Fractured neck of femur
e. Gout
f. Osteoarthritis of hip
g. Osteoarthritis of knee
h. Perthes disease
i. Slipped upper femoral epiphysis
j. Trochanteric bursitis

For each scenario below, choose the most likely corresponding option from the list given above.

1. On a GP visit to a nursing home, you are asked to see an 85-year-old woman with dementia, recurrent falls and pain on mobilizing. She can now only walk with assistance. On examination, when lying supine, she has a shortened externally rotated left leg.
2. A 65-year-old man with high blood pressure and ischaemic heart disease presents with a hot, swollen and erythematous knee joint. His regular medications include a thiazide diuretic.
3. A 13-year-old boy presents with niggly pain in the hip that is much worse after being tackled at football.
4. A 25-year-old man presents in accident and emergency (A&E) with a limp and excruciating pain in the lateral aspect of his lower leg following training for a marathon.
5. A 58-year-old man presents to his GP with pain in his left knee of several months' duration. On examination he has a restricted range of movement in his left hip.

Finger clubbing
Each answer can be used once, more than once or not at all.
a. Alcoholic liver disease
b. Crohn disease
c. Emphysema
d. Familial clubbing
e. Fibrosing alveolitis
f. Infective endocarditis
g. Pulmonary abscess
h. Scleroderma
i. Squamous cell carcinoma

For each scenario below, choose the most likely corresponding option from the list given above.

1. A 40-year-old man with right-sided chest pain with weight loss of 3 months' duration and a grumbling pyrexia.
2. A 20-year-old man with intermittent lower abdominal pain on defecation associated with blood and mucus.
3. A 48-year-old woman presents with dyspnoea. On examination she has bilateral, fine, late inspiratory crackles.
4. An 18-year-old intravenous drug abuser who presents with fever and weight loss and who is short of breath.
5. A 15-year-old boy who presents to his GP surgery with asthma.

The painful joint
Each answer can be used once, more than once or not at all.
a. Ankylosing spondylitis
b. Fibromyalgia
c. Gout
d. Osteoarthritis
e. Pseudogout
f. Psoriatic arthritis
g. Reiter syndrome
h. Rheumatoid arthritis
i. Septic arthritis
j. SLE

For each scenario below, choose the most likely corresponding option from the list given above.

1. A 27-year-old man with low back pain and morning stiffness. He had an episode of iritis a year previously.
2. A 40-year-old woman with symmetrically painful fingers and wrists. There is little evidence of synovitis. Her ESR is raised and she has an erythematous rash over her nose and cheeks.

3. A 37-year-old man with gonococcal urethritis presents with pain in the hip and a limp.
4. An 82-year-old woman presents with a painful right hip and knee, worse on exercise. On examination she has a positive Trendelenburg test and walks with a limp.
5. A 75-year-old man with a painful great toe, 1 week after starting therapy for mild heart failure.

Arthritis

Each answer can be used once, more than once or not at all.

a. Enteropathic arthritis
b. Juvenile idiopathic arthritis
c. Tuberculous arthritis
d. Septic arthritis
e. Reactive arthritis
f. Osteoarthritis
g. Psoriatic arthritis
h. Rheumatoid arthritis
i. Gonococcal arthritis
j. *Salmonella* arthritis

For each scenario below, choose the most likely corresponding option from the list given above.

1. Involvement of the DIP joints and first carpometacarpal joint of the hands.
2. Involvement of the metacarpophalangeal joints (MCPs) and PIP joints of the hands.
3. Involvement of the MCPs and PIP joints of the hands with pitting of the nails.
4. Involvement of the knee joint with visual discomfort and pain on passing urine.
5. Involvement of the lower limb joints in a patient with ulcerative colitis.

Connective tissue disease

Each answer can be used once, more than once or not at all.

a. Antiphospholipid syndrome
b. Systemic sclerosis
c. SLE
d. Discoid lupus
e. Polymyositis
f. Dermatomyositis
g. Overlap syndrome
h. Sjögren syndrome
i. Polymyalgia
j. Eczema

For each scenario below, choose the most likely corresponding option from the list given above.

1. A woman presenting with a butterfly rash and joint discomfort.

2. A woman presenting with a scaly facial rash made worse by sunlight.
3. A 25-year-old woman with a history of three consecutive miscarriages.
4. A 55-year-old man with a purple-coloured rash around his eyes.
5. A 65-year-old woman presenting with difficulty in opening her mouth and palpable swellings in her fingers.

Vasculitis

Each answer can be used once, more than once or not at all.

a. Polymyalgia rheumatica
b. Temporal arteritis
c. Kawasaki disease
d. Wegener granulomatosis
e. Churg–Strauss syndrome
f. Henoch–Schönlein purpura
g. Essential cryoglobulinaemia
h. Polyarteritis nodosa
i. Behçet disease
j. Microscopic polyangiitis

For each scenario below, choose the most likely corresponding option from the list given above.

1. A 75-year-old man complaining of a history of stiffness and intense pain in his shoulder and back.
2. A 55-year-old woman complaining of a sudden-onset headache associated with a loss of pulsation in her temporal artery.
3. A middle-aged man with abdominal pain and deranged renal function. A renal biopsy confirms inflammation of medium-sized arteries.
4. A middle-aged man presenting with generalized abdominal pain and haematuria. Urine dipstick reveals the presence of blood and protein. An autoantibody screen reveals the presence of perinuclear antineutrophil cytoplasmic antibodies.
5. A 43-year-old woman presenting with mouth ulcers and red-coloured painful lumps on her thighs.

Drugs

Each answer can be used once, more than once or not at all.

a. Methotrexate
b. Penicillamine
c. Azathioprine
d. Sulfasalazine
e. Hydroxychloroquine
f. Auranofin
g. Sodium aurothiomalate
h. Diclofenac

i. Infliximab
j. Leflunomide

For each scenario below, choose the most likely corresponding option from the list given above.

1. Associated with mouth ulcers, proteinuria and thrombocytopenia.
2. Associated with headaches and visual disturbances.
3. A therapeutic agent associated with a blue-coloured skin discoloration in sunlight.
4. Associated with male infertility and hepatitis.
5. A therapeutic agent administered intramuscularly known to cause mouth ulcers and pulmonary fibrosis.

Back pain

Each answer can be used once, more than once or not at all.

a. Prolapsed intervertebral disc
b. Spondylolisthesis
c. Spinal stenosis
d. Ankylosing spondylitis
e. Bacterial osteomyelitis
f. Myeloma
g. Cauda equina syndrome
h. Tuberculosis osteomyelitis
i. Osteoporosis
j. Paget disease

For each scenario below, choose the most likely corresponding option from the list given above.

1. A middle-aged woman presenting with low back pain, groin numbness and urinary retention.
2. Associated with an aching pain in the lower back when walking with radiation into the lower limbs. The pain is eased by rest.
3. A 23-year-old man presenting with sudden-onset back pain after weightlifting, which is exacerbated by movement and coughing.
4. A 54-year-old man complaining of back stiffness and shooting pains down his legs that worsens throughout the day. On examination you note obvious lordosis and a waddling-like gait.
5. Pain and stiffness in the lower back known to affect late teens.

Joint pain

Each answer can be used once, more than once or not at all.

a. Rheumatoid arthritis
b. Psoriatic arthritis
c. Ankylosing spondylitis
d. Reactive arthritis
e. Pseudogout
f. Gout
g. Septic joint
h. Bone infarct
i. Pathological fracture
j. SLE

For each scenario below, choose the most likely corresponding option from the list given above.

1. A 65-year-old lady presented to her GP with an acutely swollen left knee. She had no chronic illnesses and is on no medication. On examination of her knee joint, there was evidence of an effusion. It was painful on palpation. All other joints were unremarkable. Her old notes reveal a similar problem in the past (an X-ray was taken previously). It reported chondrocalcinosis of the left knee.
2. A 9-year-old child presented to A&E with a 16-hour history of a red, hot, tender, right knee. On examination the right knee was warm to the touch and exquisitely painful. The knee was aspirated but no crystals were noted. WCC was elevated. Ultrasound demonstrated a large effusion. No bony erosion seen.
3. A 45-year-lady was seen at the outpatient clinic with a year-long history of pain in the small joints of hands, feet and the left wrist. She complained of stiffness on waking in the mornings. Her GP had undertaken a number of blood tests: ESR and CRP were elevated, ANA and RF were reported as within normal range. O/E: warmth and swelling over multiple MCP and PIP joints bilaterally in keeping with active synovitis. No rash or nodules noted. Radiographs of hands and feet: periarticular erosions at right third and fourth and left third MCP joints. Soft tissue swelling noted adjacent to multiple MCP and PIP joints in both hands.
4. A 39-year-old gentleman was referred by his GP with lower back and joint pains. He had not sustained any injury and gives an 8-month history of lower back pain and more recently discomfort of the wrists and several fingers in the left hand. O/E: swelling and tenderness of the second, third and fourth DIP joints in the left hand. Both wrists tender and reduced range of active movement. Inflammatory markers were raised. ANA and RF negative. Radiographs of hands reveal normal bone density. Erosions at the DIP joints correlate with clinical findings.
5. A 35-year-old lady is admitted to hospital with a number of symptoms, including painful joints, tiredness and a rash. This has caused her to be off work for the last 6 weeks. O/E: pale. Apyrexic. A number of small joints of both hands are tender to touch. Admission blood tests reveal

the following: ESR, 67 mm/h; CRP, 8 ng/L; Hb, 10.2 g/dL; WCC, 2.4×10^9/L. Radiographs and ultrasound of the joints were normal.

6. A 49-year-old man with a history of hypertrophic obstructive cardiomyopathy and grade 3 heart failure is admitted to the cardiology unit with acute pulmonary oedema. ECHO confirms preexisting disease and an estimated ejection fraction of 24%. He receives treatment in addition to his regular cardiac medications. On day 4 of his admission, he complains of a red, hot, swollen right elbow. A cannula is sited in his left forearm for intravenous medication administration. X-ray reveals soft tissue swelling.

7. A 47-year-old man is currently an inpatient in the hepatology unit, which he has attended on a number of occasions in the past 5 years. He has been a diabetic for the past 4 years. He develops an acutely sore right knee. It is hot, red and swollen, both subjectively and objectively. Ultrasound of the knee confirms an effusion. It is aspirated, the results of which shows no growth.

Endocrine and diabetes

SINGLE BEST ANSWER (SBA) QUESTIONS

1. A middle-aged man is diagnosed with a pituitary tumour following a magnetic resonance imaging (MRI) head scan. One of his complaints includes gradual loss of vision. With regard to his visual loss, which of the following features is he most likely to demonstrate?
   a. Paracentral scotoma
   b. Mononuclear field loss
   c. Bitemporal hemianopia
   d. Homonymous hemianopia
   e. Homonymous quadrantanopia

2. A 53-year-old woman is diagnosed with hypopituitarism. Which of the following hormones is most likely to be affected first?
   a. Follicle-stimulating hormone (FSH) and luteinizing hormone (LH)
   b. Thyroid-stimulating hormone (TSH)
   c. Adrenocorticotropic hormone (ACTH)
   d. Prolactin
   e. Growth hormone

3. A 65-year-old man is diagnosed with an underactive pituitary gland. Which of the following is the most common cause of hypopituitarism?
   a. Infection
   b. Vascular
   c. Immunological
   d. Trauma
   e. Neoplasm

4. A 41-year-old woman visits the general practitioner (GP) complaining of a sore mouth. On examination her tongue is very tender, and she feels that it has changed colour slightly. She was recently started on vitamin B_{12} injections for pernicious anaemia. What is the likely cause?
   a. Candidiasis
   b. Herpes simplex virus
   c. Glossitis
   d. Sialadenitis
   e. Carcinoma of the tongue

5. A 25-year-old woman is diagnosed with hypopituitarism. Which of the following hormones is essential to replace first when managing her condition?
   a. Thyroid hormone
   b. Oestrogen
   c. Growth hormone
   d. LH
   e. FSH

6. A 29-year-old man complains of headaches and visual disturbances. He also remarks that he can express milk from his breasts. What is the most appropriate initial investigation?
   a. MRI pituitary scan
   b. Visual field assessment by perimetry
   c. Thyroid function tests
   d. Serum prolactin level
   e. Serum testosterone level

7. A 42-year-old man complains of visual disturbances and headaches. He remarks his wedding ring feels tighter than usual. On examination you note a protruding jaw, interdental separation and spade like hands. Which investigation is most likely to confirm the diagnosis?
   a. Serum growth hormone
   b. Serum insulin-like growth factor 1 (IGF-1)
   c. Serum prolactin
   d. Fasting glucose
   e. Visual field assessment by perimetry

8. A 40-year-old Caucasian woman presents to her GP complaining of tiredness, weight gain and feeling unusually cold. On general examination the GP notes a slow relaxing ankle jerk. The GP diagnoses hypothyroidism. The patient enquires about the cause of her condition. Which of the following is the most likely cause of her hypothyroidism?
   a. Idiopathic
   b. Iodine deficiency
   c. Dyshormonogenesis
   d. Pituitary insufficiency
   e. Hashimoto thyroiditis

9. A 35-year-old man complains of weight gain and feeling cold. Thyroid function tests demonstrate a low T4 and a raised TSH. He is also notably anaemic with a haemoglobin of 10.2 g/dL. What is the most likely type of anaemia he will demonstrate?
   a. Aplastic anaemia
   b. Macrocytic
   c. Microcytic
   d. Autoimmune haemolytic anaemia
   e. Nonautoimmune haemolytic anaemia

10. A 55-year-old man with treated hypothyroidism presents with confusion. His hypothyroidism is due to an underactive pituitary gland. Blood tests reveal a sodium of 128 mmol/L and a glucose of 2.8 mmol/L. Routine observations reveal a temperature of 35°C. What is the most appropriate step in management?
    a. Sodium replacement
    b. Glucose replacement
    c. Intravenous (IV) T3 replacement
    d. IV hydrocortisone
    e. Warmed IV fluids

11. A 35-year-old woman is diagnosed with an overactive thyroid gland. What is the most likely aetiological cause of her thyrotoxicosis?
    a. Toxic multinodular goitre
    b. Solitary toxic nodule
    c. de Quervain thyroiditis
    d. Graves disease
    e. Thyroiditis factitia

12. A 40-year-old woman complains of weight loss and heat intolerance. Routine blood investigations confirm a diagnosis of Graves disease. Which of the following features are specific to this disease?
    a. Lid lag
    b. Tremor
    c. Proximal myopathy
    d. Atrial fibrillation
    e. Ophthalmoplegia

13. A 35-year-old man complains of weight loss and heat intolerance. On examination you note an obvious goitre and red-coloured lesions on his shins. You suspect Graves disease. Which investigation is most likely to lead to a diagnosis?
    a. TSH
    b. T4 and T3 levels
    c. Thyroid ultrasound
    d. TSH receptor antibodies
    e. Thyroglobulin antibodies

14. A 32-year-old woman complains of weight loss and heat intolerance. She mentions that her heart is always racing. A quick examination reveals marked exophthalmos. What is the next most appropriate step in management?
    a. Propranolol
    b. Carbimazole
    c. Radioactive iodine
    d. Surgery
    e. Propylthiouracil

15. A middle-aged woman is diagnosed with hyperthyroidism. Her GP commences carbimazole. Which of the following is the most likely side effect of this medication?
    a. Rash
    b. Nausea and vomiting
    c. Arthralgia
    d. Jaundice
    e. Agranulocytosis

16. A 29-year-old woman is diagnosed with hyperthyroidism. She is currently 28 weeks' pregnant. The following are all suitable treatments for hyperthyroidism EXCEPT?
    a. Carbimazole
    b. Propranolol
    c. Radioactive iodine
    d. Surgery
    e. Propylthiouracil

17. A 35-year-old woman has recently undergone radioactive iodine therapy for an overactive thyroid. Her condition deteriorates and she becomes notably restless and delirious. On examination she has a pulse rate of 120 beats/min and a temperature of 40°C. She is severely dehydrated. What is the first most appropriate step in her management?
    a. Dexamethasone
    b. Potassium iodide
    c. Propranolol
    d. Carbimazole
    e. IV fluids

18. A patient presents with exophthalmos and ophthalmoplegia. She has a known history of hyperthyroidism. Which of the following is the first most appropriate step in management?
    a. Steroids
    b. Orbit irradiation
    c. Watchful waiting
    d. Lateral tarsorrhaphy
    e. Normalization of thyroid status

19. A 36-year-old woman presents with a significantly enlarged goitre. She complains of a discomfort in her neck as well as breathing difficulties. On examination you note a solitary nodule. She is worried about the possibility of cancer. Which of the following investigations is most likely to reveal such a diagnosis?
    a. TSH
    b. T4 and T3 levels
    c. Chest radiography
    d. Fine-needle aspiration for cytology
    e. Thyroid scan (^{125}I)

20. A 40-year-old woman presents with a goitre. On examination you note a nodule that feels hard and irregular in size. You also note the presence of enlarged cervical lymph nodes. Fine-needle aspiration confirms the presence of malignant cells. Routine blood investigations reveal a calcium level of 3.67 mmol/L. Which one of the following is the most likely type of her thyroid cancer?
    a. Papillary
    b. Follicular
    c. Anaplastic
    d. Medullary cell
    e. Lymphoma

21. A 35-year-old woman is diagnosed with thyroid cancer. Histological assessment confirms the diagnosis as anaplastic with pulmonary metastases. What is the next most appropriate step in management?
    a. Palliative
    b. Radioactive iodine
    c. Subtotal thyroidectomy
    d. Total thyroidectomy
    e. Chemotherapy

22. A 43-year-old man is diagnosed with Cushing syndrome. Which one of the following is most likely to be decreased or inhibited in this condition?
    a. Protein catabolism
    b. Free water clearance
    c. Circulating neutrophils
    d. Uric acid production
    e. Circulating lymphocytes

23. A 35-year-old woman complains of lethargy, low mood and loss of weight. On examination you note increased pigmentation of her buccal mucosa and skin creases. Her blood pressure drops to 85/60 mmHg from 122/63 mmHg on standing. Which of the following investigations is most likely to confirm her diagnosis?
    a. Serum urea and electrolytes
    b. Adrenal antibodies
    c. Abdominal X-ray
    d. Tetracosactide (synacthen) short test
    e. Tetracosactide (synacthen) long test

24. A middle-aged man is diagnosed with adrenal gland insufficiency. What is the most likely aetiological cause for this condition?
    a. Autoimmune
    b. Adrenal gland tuberculosis
    c. Haemorrhage
    d. Pituitary disease
    e. Adrenal gland tumour

25. A middle-aged woman is admitted to the medical admissions unit with severe abdominal pain and weakness. On examination she has a pulse rate of 120 beats/min, a blood pressure of 95/65 mmHg and a urine output of less than 30 mL/h. Routine blood tests reveal a random plasma glucose of 3.0 mmol/L. You note deep pigmentation of her buccal mucosa and skin creases. Her GP referral letter comments that she has been feeling tired, low in mood and suffering weight loss for the past 1 month. What is the first most appropriate step in her management?
    a. Intramuscular hydrocortisone
    b. IV glucose
    c. IV hydrocortisone
    d. IV dextrose
    e. IV fludrocortisone

26. A 45-year-old gentleman is diagnosed with impaired adrenal function. He has been taking steroids on and off for the past 2 years for treatment of severe Crohn disease. Which of the following investigations is most likely to reveal the cause of his adrenal failure?
    a. Urea and electrolytes
    b. Adrenal antibodies
    c. Abdominal X-ray
    d. Tetracosactide (synacthen) short test
    e. Tetracosactide (synacthen) long test

27. A 53-year-old woman complains that she has put on a considerable amount of weight over the past 2 months. She also mentions that her skin feels thin and bruises easily. On examination you note a plethoric complexion and purple striae on her abdomen. A 24-hour urinary cortisol is three times the upper limit of normal. What is the most likely cause of her condition?
    a. Adrenal adenoma
    b. Adrenal carcinoma
    c. Adrenal hyperplasia
    d. Pituitary adenoma
    e. Carcinoid tumour

28. A 45-year-old woman is diagnosed with Cushing syndrome. Routine blood tests reveal a significantly raised ACTH level. High-dose dexamethasone suppresses plasma cortisol after 48 hours. What is the most likely cause of her condition?
    a. Adrenal adenoma
    b. Adrenal carcinoma
    c. Adrenal hyperplasia
    d. Pituitary adenoma
    e. Carcinoid tumour

29. A 50-year-old man complains of feeling low in mood. On examination his blood pressure is 140/85 mmHg. His body mass index (BMI) is 31 kg/m². He has purple streaks on his abdomen as well as pigmentation of skin creases. Investigations confirm Cushing syndrome secondary to a pituitary adenoma. What is the next most appropriate step in management?
    a. External beam irradiation
    b. Aminoglutethimide
    c. Ketoconazole
    d. Metyrapone
    e. Surgical excision of tumour

30. A 30-year-old woman is admitted to accident and emergency (A&E) complaining of nausea and headaches. She appears mildly confused and is unaware of her surroundings. On examination her blood pressure is 125/80 mmHg with no postural drop. Investigations show a serum sodium of 122 mmol/L, a low plasma osmolality, a urine osmolality, which is much higher than plasma, and a urinary sodium level, which is greater than 30 mmol/L. What is the most likely cause of her symptoms?
    a. Renal tubular acidosis
    b. Glucocorticoid deficiency
    c. Syndrome of inappropriate antidiuretic hormone (SIADH)
    d. Renal failure
    e. Salt-wasting nephropathy

31. What is the most appropriate management for the patient described above?
    a. Furosemide
    b. Hypertonic saline
    c. Hypotonic saline
    d. Dimethylchlorotetracycline
    e. Fluid restriction

32. A 32-year-old man with a recent diagnosis of mania is treated with lithium. Three weeks later he returns complaining of feeling thirsty and going to pass urine up to eight times a day. Which of the following investigations is most likely to confirm the diagnosis?
    a. Urine volume measurement
    b. Plasma sodium concentration
    c. Urine osmolality
    d. Plasma osmolality
    e. Water deprivation test

33. A 25-year-old woman complains of abdominal pain and nonspecific bone pain for the past 2 weeks. She also mentions that she has been feeling generally low in herself. Routine blood tests reveal a raised parathyroid hormone level and a low vitamin D level.

Her corrected serum calcium level is 2.01 mmol/L. What is the most likely diagnosis?
    a. Primary hyperparathyroidism
    b. Secondary hyperparathyroidism
    c. Tertiary hyperparathyroidism
    d. DiGeorge syndrome
    e. Pseudohypoparathyroidism

34. A 42-year-old woman with breast cancer complains of nonspecific bone pain, abdominal discomfort and not opening her bowels for the past 1 week. Her GP decides to admit her. Upon arrival, you note she is severely dehydrated and confused. Routine blood tests reveal a corrected serum calcium level of 4.0 mmol/L. What is the first most appropriate step in her management?
    a. Prednisolone
    b. IV fluid replacement
    c. Bisphosphonates
    d. Calcitonin
    e. Phosphate

35. A 35-year-old man complains of numbness around his mouth. On examination you note opposition of his thumb, extension of his interphalangeal joints and flexion of his metacarpophalangeal joints. His corrected serum calcium is 1.70 mmol/L. What is the most likely cause of his symptoms?
    a. Osteomalacia
    b. Pseudohypoparathyroidism
    c. DiGeorge syndrome
    d. Idiopathic hypoparathyroidism
    e. Renal failure

36. You suspect primary hyperaldosteronism in a 65-year-old man with hypertension. Which of the following investigations is most important in helping to confirm such a diagnosis?
    a. Plasma aldosterone-to-renin ratio
    b. Serum aldosterone
    c. Adrenal computed tomography (CT) scan
    d. Adrenal MRI scan
    e. Serum renin

37. A 45-year-old man complains of headaches, sweating and nausea. On examination his pulse rate is 135 beats/min and his blood pressure is 138/95 mmHg. Routine blood tests reveal a random plasma glucose of 10.2 mmol/L. You suspect the possibility of a catecholamine-producing tumour. Which of the following investigations is most likely to confirm the diagnosis?
    a. Clonidine suppression and glucagon stimulation test
    b. Abdominal CT scan
    c. Abdominal MRI scan

d. 24-Hour urinary collection of metanephrines

e. Metaiodobenzylguanidine CT scintigraphy

38. A 57-year-old man presents to the GP complaining of feeling thirsty, weight loss and passing urine up to nine times a day. His BMI is 32 kg/m^2. Routine blood tests reveal a random blood glucose of 12.2 mmol/L. What is the next most appropriate step in management?
a. Diet therapy
b. Glibenclamide
c. Insulin
d. Acarbose
e. Rosiglitazone

39. A 55-year-old man has been recently diagnosed with type II diabetes. His BMI is 35.5 kg/m^2. What is the most appropriate medical management?
a. Glibenclamide
b. Metformin
c. Acarbose
d. Repaglinide
e. Pioglitazone

40. A newly diagnosed diabetic is commenced on metformin. What is the most common side effect of this drug?
a. Lactic acidosis
b. Hypoglycaemia
c. Pruritis
d. Rash
e. Diarrhoea

41. A 17-year-old boy complains of feeling tired, thirsty and going to pass urine more frequently than normal. He has also developed abdominal pain and vomiting in the last 2 hours. His serum glucose level is 22 mmol/L and urinalysis shows ketonuria. What is the next most appropriate step in management?
a. Acarbose
b. Lifestyle modification alone
c. Insulin
d. Metformin
e. Pioglitazone

42. A diabetic patient on insulin is found unconscious at home. He is immediately transferred to hospital. Routine blood tests reveal a glucose level of 1.9 mmol/L. What is the next most appropriate step in management?
a. Intramuscular glucagon
b. Oral carbohydrate
c. IV dextrose
d. Diazoxide
e. Octreotide

43. A 32-year-old diabetic man on insulin is admitted to hospital having been found unconscious at home. He quickly regains consciousness on arrival. On examination his eyes are sunken and his tongue appears dry. His breathing is deep at a rate of 25 breaths/min. His blood pressure is 110/65 mmHg. Routine blood tests reveal a plasma glucose of 22 mmol/L. You perform an arterial blood gas, which demonstrates a pH of 7.10, a partial pressure of carbon dioxide (PCO$_2$) of 3.5 kPa and a bicarbonate of 19 mmol/L. What is the next most appropriate step in his management?
a. IV saline
b. IV insulin
c. Sodium bicarbonate infusion
d. IV colloids
e. Intramuscular glucagon

44. A 65-year-old diabetic man who is a poor clinic attendee presents to his GP complaining of blurred vision. Fundoscopy reveals the presence of yellow-coloured exudates as well as cotton wool spots. What is the most likely diagnosis?
a. Background retinopathy
b. Maculopathy
c. Preproliferative retinopathy
d. Proliferative retinopathy
e. Cataracts

45. A 55-year-old diabetic woman complains of numbness, tingling and pain in her toes and hands. She reports that she feels like she is 'walking on cotton'. Examination reveals bilateral loss of sensation on the palms and soles. What is the most likely diagnosis?
a. Autonomic neuropathy
b. Acute painful neuropathy
c. Diabetic mononeuropathy
d. Diabetic amyotrophy
e. Symmetrical sensory neuropathy

46. A 29-year-old diabetic woman is trying for a baby. She visits her GP to ask about whether her diabetes may affect her pregnancy. Diabetes may result in the following complications during pregnancy EXCEPT?
a. Macrosomia
b. Polyhydramnios
c. Respiratory distress syndrome
d. Preeclampsia
e. Neonatal hyperglycaemia

47. A 31-year-old man complains of sweating and palpitations. He remarks that he often sees double. Routine blood tests reveal a fasting plasma glucose of 2.2 mmol/L. He undergoes an abdominal CT scan which reveals the presence of a pancreatic

tumour. What is the next most appropriate step in management?

a. Surgical excision of tumour
b. Diazoxide
c. Octreotide
d. Chemotherapy
e. Radiotherapy

48. A 51-year-old man presents to A&E with nausea and vomiting. His wife, who attends with him, remarks that earlier in the day he had a terrible headache, which felt as if he had 'been hit on the head with a baseball bat'. She told him to get some rest and on his way to the door he walked into a coffee table. He has a medical history of hypertension. His current blood pressure is 82/46 mmHg. On inspection the patient appears confused, weak and sweaty. On examination he has a third-nerve palsy and bitemporal hemianopia. What is the most likely diagnosis?

a. Sheehan syndrome
b. Ruptured craniopharyngioma
c. Pituitary macroadenoma
d. Pituitary microadenoma
e. Pituitary apoplexy

49. A 35-year-old woman was referred to the hospital by her GP with polyuria, polydipsia and altered sensations in her limbs that has been progressively worsening over the last 3 weeks. The hospital rules out type 2 diabetes but investigations reveal she is hypertensive (154/80 mmHg), as well as hypokalaemic and alkalotic. The doctor diagnoses Conn syndrome. What is the cause of Conn syndrome?

a. Cortisol and aldosterone deficiency
b. ACTH-secreting tumour
c. Adrenaline-secreting tumour
d. Aldosterone-secreting tumour
e. Chronic excessive cortisol secretion

50. A 42-year-old male was admitted to the endocrinology ward with increasing weight, central obesity and depression. He also has been having erectile dysfunction for the last month. Cushing disease is the suspected cause and an overnight dexamethasone suppression test is ordered to confirm. What is the underlying cause of Cushing disease?

a. Adrenal adenoma
b. Pituitary adenoma
c. Iatrogenic (i.e., steroid treatment)
d. Ectopic ACTH
e. Primary hyperaldosteronism

51. A 25-year-old woman presents to her GP with a 2-month history of polydipsia, polyuria and malaise. On further questioning, the patient reveals that she has not lost any weight, she goes to the toilet approximately once every half an hour and passes large amounts of dilute urine. She has a past medical history of a brain injury that occurred 1 year ago when she was in a road traffic accident. What is the most likely diagnosis?

a. Type 1 diabetes
b. Type 2 diabetes
c. Nephrogenic diabetes insipidus
d. Neurogenic diabetes insipidus
e. Pituitary adenoma

52. A 40-year-old man who has been hospitalized with a subarachnoid haemorrhage becomes progressively more confused and agitated. His urinary output is low. Blood tests show hyponatraemia, low plasma osmolality and high urine osmolality. His blood pressure is 130/86 mmHg and he is euvolaemic. What is the most likely diagnosis?

a. Undiagnosed diabetes
b. Undiagnosed hypothyroidism
c. SIADH
d. Addison disease
e. Acute renal failure

53. A 67-year-old woman has a bone mineral density (BMD) of >2.5 standard deviations below the mean BMD. She has been advised to stop smoking and given calcium and vitamin D supplements. She has no independent clinical risk factors for fracture. What is the most appropriate pharmacological intervention?

a. Bisphosphonates
b. Teriparatide
c. Calcitonin
d. Strontium ranelate and raloxifene
e. No pharmacological intervention is required

54. A 45-year-old man was admitted to the emergency department after he was found confused by his family at home. His notes show that he has been complaining of headaches and blurred vision for the last 4 months, as well as polyuria. He is overweight and you suspect that he has undiagnosed diabetes mellitus type 2. What would be the most appropriate test to perform to confirm hyperglycaemia in this patient?

a. 2-Hour plasma glucose
b. Fasting glucose
c. Glycosylated haemoglobin (HbA1c)
d. Random blood glucose
e. Urine dipstick for glucose

55. A 29-year-old man is referred to the endocrinology clinic with a 5-week history of unexplained flushing in his face and upper chest. The man has also been

experiencing diarrhoea and vomiting that have worsened over time. The man has no family history of any relevant conditions. The doctor examines the patient and notes several murmurs on auscultation that were not previously noted by the man's GP. The doctor suspects cardiac damage secondary to carcinoid syndrome. If liver metastases are the source of the hormones, damage to which two valves in the heart is associated with carcinoid syndrome?

a. Pulmonary and aortic
b. Pulmonary and tricuspid
c. Aortic and mitral
d. Tricuspid and mitral
e. Pulmonary and mitral

56. A 19-year-old woman presents to her GP complaining that she has been unable to get pregnant despite trying for 2 years. The woman has also been having irregular periods since she started puberty. The woman has hirsutism and poorly controlled acne, and her hair has also been getting progressively thinner during the last few weeks. Her family history reveals that her mother is obese and suffers from type 2 diabetes. The patient is 135 cm tall and weighs 62 kg. The GP suspects polycystic ovary syndrome (PCOS) and refers the girl for tests at the hospital. Which of these hormones is raised in PCOS?

a. LH
b. FSH
c. Oestradiol
d. Human chorionic gonadotrophin
e. 17-Hydroxyprogesterone

57. A 75-year-old man with type 2 diabetes mellitus who normally takes long-acting insulin once daily is admitted to hospital with a urinary tract infection. He is hyperglycaemic, with ketones and glucose on urinalysis. He is orientated, alert and not vomiting. What is the most appropriate hypoglycaemic agent during his acute illness?

a. Increase in long-acting insulin
b. Soluble human insulin
c. Metformin
d. An oral sulphonylurea
e. A combination of metformin and a sulphonylurea

58. A 55-year-old man with type 2 diabetes mellitus complicated by diabetic retinopathy sees his GP regularly for blood pressure monitoring. What is the optimal blood pressure for patients with diabetes mellitus?

a. 130/90 mm/Hg
b. 130/80 mm/Hg
c. 140/80 mm/Hg
d. 150/70 mm/Hg
e. As low a blood pressure as the patient tolerates

59. A 56-year old patient presented with a month's history of nocturia and feeling dehydrated all the time. He was diagnosed with type 2 diabetes mellitus and was started on sulphonylureas (gliclazide). Which one of the followings is NOT true regarding this medication?

a. Evidence of long-term prevention of macrovascular complications of type 2 diabetes.
b. Hypoglycaemic effect of sulphonylureas is due to enhancement of insulin secretion by pancreatic beta cells.
c. Preferably used in nonobese diabetic patients.
d. Sulphonylureas reduce fasting plasma glucose by an average of 2–4 mmol/L and HbA1c by 1% to 2%.
e. The most common and most serious side effect of sulphonylureas is hypoglycaemia.

60. A 75-year-old man was brought to the GP by a neighbour who was worried that he was not eating and drinking properly since his wife had died. The examination was normal apart from what appeared clinically to be a folliculitis over his trunk and buttocks. He was treated with antibiotics. He returned 4 months later with marked bruising in the same distribution and now with gingival hypertrophy and bleeding aphthous ulcers. The full blood count and clotting screen were normal. What is the most likely diagnosis?

a. Chronic lymphocytic leukaemia
b. Gingivitis
c. Chronic myeloid leukaemia
d. Scurvy
e. Vitamin K deficiency

61. A previously fit and well 68-year-old retired nurse presents to her GP for routine health check. She does not drink or smoke, and is not taking any regular medications. Initial blood tests show Na 136 mmol/L, K 3.1 mmol/L, bicarbonate 34 mmol/L and chloride 94 mmol/L. A subsequent CT scan is performed due to an elevated aldosterone-to-renin ratio, which shows bilateral adrenal enlargement. Which of the following is the most appropriate treatment for this patient?

a. Amiloride
b. Amlodipine
c. Clonidine
d. Bendroflumethiazide
e. Spironolactone

62. A 50-year-old woman presents to the emergency department with a 3-day history of worsening nausea, lethargy, abdominal pain and bony pains. She is a chronic heavy smoker and has been recently diagnosed with lung cancer, and is awaiting treatment. Clinically she appears cachectic and dehydrated. Blood results show a serum calcium of 2.90 mmol/L (2.25–2.5 mmol/L). What is the most appropriate initial step in her management?
   a. Calcitonin
   b. Pamidronate
   c. Thiazide diuretic
   d. IV saline
   e. Prednisolone

63. A 23-year-old woman with cystic fibrosis complicated by chronic cholestasis presents to her GP with a 1-week history of muscle weakness and tremor in her hands. She admits that she has been noncompliant with her medications. Neurological examination reveals diminished tendon reflexes throughout. What is the most likely diagnosis?
   a. Hypoglycaemia
   b. Vitamin K deficiency
   c. Vitamin E deficiency
   d. Vitamin B deficiency
   e. Vitamin D deficiency

64. A 50-year-old woman is brought to the emergency department by ambulance after she was found on the floor unresponsive by her husband. She is severely hypoglycaemic on arrival, but regains consciousness following IV glucose. She reports no medical conditions and is not on any medications, but tells you that in the last 2 months she has had intermittent episodes of dizziness, sweating and tremors, which seem to improve after eating a chocolate bar or biscuit. Subsequent blood tests show raised insulin, C-peptide, proinsulin and glucagon levels. What is the most likely diagnosis?
   a. Insulinoma
   b. Glucagonoma
   c. Somatostatinoma
   d. Pancreatic adenocarcinoma
   e. Insulin administration

65. A 10-year-old boy presents to the emergency department with worsening fatigue, dizziness, muscle weakness, vomiting and diarrhoea. On arrival he appears dehydrated and hypotensive. Blood tests show sodium of 125 mmol/L, K 5.2 mmol/L and serum glucose of 2.1 mmol/L. Despite IV fluids, his electrolytes have not showed much improvement. Which of the following investigations is most likely to give you the diagnosis?

   a. ADH
   b. Dehydroepiandrosterone (DHEA)
   c. Cortisol and ACTH levels
   d. IGF-1
   e. Abdominal CT scan

66. A 65-year-old woman is brought in by her family for progressive fatigue and confusion. Past medical history is notable for ovarian cancer. Physical examination reveals dry mucous membranes. Blood tests show an elevated adjusted serum calcium of 3.2 mmol/L, a low-normal albumin level, a low-normal phosphorus level and elevated alkaline phosphatase. What is the initial step in the management of hypercalcemia of malignancy?
   a. Fluid restriction
   b. Bisphosphonates intravenously
   c. Phosphate depletion
   d. Aggressive rehydration
   e. Diuresis with furosemide

67. A previously fit and well 30-year-old woman presents to her GP with a 3-month history of amenorrhoea. Clinical examination is unremarkable and urine beta human chorionic gonadotropin is negative. Subsequent blood tests show fasting morning prolactin levels of 350 mg/L. What is the most appropriate next step for this patient?
   a. Pituitary MRI
   b. Head CT
   c. Bromocriptine
   d. Surgical intervention
   e. Radiation therapy

68. A 35-year-old woman who is 8 months postpartum presents to her GP with palpitations, sweats, agitation and weight loss. On examination she has evidence of lid lag and tachycardia. There is a diffusely enlarged painless goitre with an audible bruit. Subsequent blood tests show normal erythrocyte sedimentation rate level but 'abnormal' thyroid function tests. What is the most likely diagnosis?
   a. Graves disease
   b. Postpartum thyroiditis
   c. Hashimoto thyroiditis
   d. de Quervain thyroiditis
   e. Thyroid tumour

69. A 45-year-old woman sees her GP after noticing a lump in her neck. Following a series of investigations, a diagnosis of thyroid malignancy is suspected. Which of the following is a characteristic of thyroid malignancy?
   a. Solid cold nodules
   b. Cystic cold nodules

c. Increased thyroxin level
d. Increased TSH level
e. None of the above

70. A 65-year-old man presents to the emergency department with acute confusional state preceded by a 4-day history of fevers, cough and breathlessness. Antibiotics were commenced for treatment of community-acquired pneumonia. Results from confusion screen showed low TSH, T4 and T3 levels. He is not known to have any preexisting thyroid diseases. Which of the following statements is incorrect?
   a. The abnormal findings on thyroid function tests are not related to thyroidal illness.
   b. The most prominent alterations are low serum T3.
   c. The highest incidence of low TSH values occurs in the most severely ill group.
   d. Most patients who are critically ill have reduced T4 levels.
   e. Thyroid hormone replacement is used to correct the low serum levels.

EXTENDED-MATCHING QUESTIONS (EMQs)

Pituitary disease

Each answer can be used once, more than once or not at all.

   a. Pituitary apoplexy
   b. Sheehan syndrome
   c. Empty sella syndrome
   d. Kallmann syndrome
   e. Pituitary tumour
   f. Syphilis
   g. Haemochromatosis
   h. Sarcoidosis
   i. Lymphocytic hypophysitis
   j. Anorexia

For each scenario below, choose the most likely corresponding option from the list given above.

   1. Associated with loss of smell and colour blindness.
   2. Associated with severe blood loss following childbirth.
   3. A middle-aged woman presenting with sudden-onset headaches, nausea and visual disturbances.
   4. A 37-year-old obese woman with known hypertension presenting with sudden-onset headaches. A head MRI scan reveals an unusually small pituitary gland.

5. A middle-aged man presenting with enlarged hands and feet. On further questioning he complains of visual disturbances and headaches.

Thyroid disease

Each answer can be used once, more than once or not at all.

   a. Hashimoto thyroiditis
   b. Lymphocytic thyroiditis
   c. Dyshormonogenesis
   d. Myxoedema coma
   e. Graves disease
   f. Plummer disease
   g. de Quervain thyroiditis
   h. Thyroid cancer
   i. Thyroid crisis
   j. Toxic multinodular goitre

For each scenario below, choose the most likely corresponding option from the list given above.

   1. Overactivity of the thyroid gland associated with fever and neck pain.
   2. A common cause of hyperthyroidism associated with immunoglobulin G (IgG) antibodies.
   3. A common cause of hypothyroidism associated with autoantibody formation and goitre formation.
   4. A middle-aged woman presenting with enlargement of the thyroid gland and a markedly raised serum calcium.
   5. A woman with known hyperthyroidism presenting with fever, tachycardia and restlessness following radioactive iodine therapy.

Diabetic complications

Each answer can be used once, more than once or not at all.

   a. Background retinopathy
   b. Maculopathy
   c. Preproliferative retinopathy
   d. Proliferative retinopathy
   e. Symmetrical sensory neuropathy
   f. Autonomic neuropathy
   g. Acute painful neuropathy
   h. Diabetic mononeuropathy
   i. Diabetic amyotrophy
   j. Mononeuritis multiplex

For each scenario below, choose the most likely corresponding option from the list given above.

   1. A common form of neuropathy affecting the toes and soles of the feet.
   2. Associated with cotton wool spots and venous beading.

3. Associated with blot haemorrhages and yellow-coloured exudates.
4. A diabetic patient complaining of wasting of his quadriceps muscles.
5. A diabetic patient presenting with a burning sensation in his anterior lower limbs that is generally worse at night.

Drugs

Each answer can be used once, more than once or not at all.

a. Glibenclamide
b. Tolbutamide
c. Metformin
d. Acarbose
e. Rosiglitazone
f. Repaglinide
g. Protamine insulin
h. Insulin lispro
i. Insulin aspart
j. Pioglitazone

For each scenario below, choose the most likely corresponding option from the list given above.

1. Associated with diarrhoea and abdominal bloating. This agent may also result in elevated serum transaminase levels.
2. Associated with diarrhoea and lactic acidosis.
3. First-line agent in the treatment of type II diabetes in obese individuals.
4. A drug that works via closure of K$^+$ adenosine triphosphate (ATP) channels but is best avoided in elderly people.
5. An insulin-releasing agent developed from glibenclamide.

Investigations

Each answer can be used once, more than once or not at all.

a. Thyroid function tests
b. Oral glucose tolerance test
c. Plasma aldosterone levels
d. Serum urea and electrolytes
e. Short synacthen test
f. Long synacthen test
g. Dexamethasone suppression test
h. Urine and plasma osmolality
i. Fasting blood glucose
j. 24-Hour urinary collection of metanephrines

For each scenario below, choose the most likely corresponding option from the list given above.

1. A middle-aged man presenting with enlargement of his hands and feet.

2. A 34-year-old obese gentleman presenting with a plethoric complexion and purple-coloured striae on his abdomen.
3. Associated with sudden-onset headaches, palpitations and sweating.
4. A middle-aged woman presenting with weight loss and lethargy. Examination reveals hyperpigmentation of oral mucosa and skin creases.
5. A 45-year-old man presenting with increased urinary frequency and thirst. Blood glucose levels are normal.

Diabetes

Each answer can be used once, more than once or not at all.

a. Acanthosis nigricans
b. Diabetes insipidus
c. Diabetic ketoacidosis (DKA)
d. Fasting serum glucose of >7.1 mmol/L
e. Glycosylated haemoglobin
f. Hyperosmolar nonketotic coma
g. Pyoderma gangrenosum
h. Random serum glucose >7.1 mmol/L but below 12 mmol/L
i. Type 1 diabetes mellitus
j. Type 2 diabetes mellitus

For each scenario below, choose the most likely corresponding option from the list given above.

1. A patient presents with polydipsia and polyuria, often drinking 15–20 L of fluid per day. Fasting serum glucose is 5.2 mmol/L; serum osmolarity is reduced.
2. A 56-year-old man presents with a 1-week history of polyuria and polydipsia; he has been drinking copious amounts of cola to rehydrate himself and feels very thirsty. Serum glucose is 37 mmol/L.
3. A 14-year-old boy presents with a 2-day history of lethargy, shortness of breath and polydipsia. His GP started amoxicillin for a chest infection 3 days ago. On examination he is very dehydrated, smells of nail varnish remover and is making deep sighing breaths.
4. A patient is diagnosed with impaired glucose tolerance.
5. This diagnosis is associated with a total lack of insulin production and presents in the young.

The pancreas and diabetes

Each answer can be used once, more than once or not at all.

a. Type 2 diabetes
b. Gestational diabetes mellitus
c. Hyperosmolar hyperglycaemic state (HHS)
d. DKA

e. The metabolic syndrome
f. Maturity-onset diabetes of the young (MODY)
g. Hypoglycaemia

For each scenario below, choose the most likely corresponding option from the list given above.

1. A 60-year-old woman whose recent-onset diabetes is entirely controlled by diet, metformin and sulphonylureas.
2. A 15-year-old girl with diabetes who is known to suffer from a mutation in the glucokinase gene.
3. A 50-year-old man suffering from mild fasting hyperglycaemia, hypertriglyceridaemia and central adiposity who has deranged function tests.
4. A 10-year-old boy who is found in his room drowsy, vomiting, severely dehydrated, suffering from acidotic breathing (Kussmaul breathing).
5. A 42-year-old pregnant woman with hyperglycaemia who has a family history of noninsulin-dependent diabetes and has previously given birth to a large baby.

The adrenal glands
Each answer can be used once, more than once or not at all.

a. Phaeochromocytoma
b. Conn syndrome
c. Renal artery stenosis
d. Cushing syndrome
e. Congenital adrenal hyperplasia
f. Addison disease
g. Bartter syndrome

For each scenario below, choose the most likely corresponding option from the list given above.

1. A 45-year-old woman with buccal hyperpigmentation, weakness, abdominal pain, hyperkalaemia and hypernatraemia.
2. A 36-year-old man with a hypochloremic metabolic alkalosis, low serum renin and a mass in the adrenal glands on MRI.
3. A 30-year-old female who presents with tachycardia, excessive sweating, pallor and weight loss. She was diagnosed with hypertension but it has been difficult to control despite medications.
4. A rheumatology patient on long-term steroids who presents with weight increase, moon face, menstrual irregularity and purple striae.
5. A young girl presenting with virilism and hirsutism.

Haematology 8

SINGLE BEST ANSWER (SBA) QUESTIONS

1. A 70-year-old man attends his routine anticoagulation clinic appointment for international normalized ratio (INR) check and warfarin dosing. He has been on long-term warfarin for permanent atrial fibrillation for 10 years. His INR is 7.2 but he is well in himself with normal vital signs and no recent bleeding. What is the most appropriate management for this patient?
   a. Discontinue use of warfarin for 3 days and recheck INR
   b. Oral administration of 1 mg of vitamin K
   c. Intravenous administration of 10 mg of vitamin K
   d. Intravenous administration of 1 mg of vitamin K
   e. Reduce dose of warfarin

2. A 75-year-old man was referred to the haematology department by his general practitioner (GP) following a recent blood test which showed a platelet count of 90×10^9/L. Which of the following conditions is NOT a known cause for the development of thrombocytopaenia?
   a. Myelodysplastic syndromes
   b. Chemotherapy
   c. *H*aemolysis, elevated *l*iver enzymes and *l*ow *p*latelet count (HELLP) syndrome
   d. Proinflammatory cytokines
   e. Liver cirrhosis

3. A middle-aged obese man presents with a headache, dizziness, tinnitus and visual disturbance. On examination you note a plethoric complexion and evidence of hepatosplenomegaly. Routine blood tests reveal a haemoglobin (Hb) of 202 g/L, a white cell count of 22×10^9/L and a platelet count of 405×10^9/L. Further investigations reveal a raised red cell volume and uric acid level. What is the next most appropriate step in management?
   a. Chemotherapy
   b. Radioactive phosphorus
   c. Allopurinol
   d. Venesection
   e. Lipid-lowering agents

4. A 56-year-old man presents with weight loss and lethargy. Routine blood tests reveal a Hb of 101 g/L, a white cell count of 14×10^9/L and a platelet count of 410×10^9/L. Blood film examination reveals 'tear drop'-shaped red cells. What is the most likely diagnosis?
   a. Myelodysplasia
   b. Chronic myeloid leukaemia

   c. Myelofibrosis
   d. Polycythaemia
   e. Chronic lymphocytic leukaemia (CLL)

5. A 5-year-old girl is brought by her mother to the emergency department after noticing multiple bruises on her arms and legs, and two episodes of nosebleeds. She has recently recovered from an upper respiratory tract infection. She has no other symptoms and there is no relevant family history. What is the most important investigation to establish the diagnosis?
   a. Prothrombin time (PT)
   b. Partial thromboplastin time (PTT)
   c. Bleeding time
   d. Peripheral blood film
   e. INR

6. A 65-year-old woman receives a blood transfusion following a recent episode of haematemesis. Within minutes, her blood pressure falls to 105/65 mmHg. She begins to itch and complain of difficulty in breathing. On examination you note swelling of her lips and face. After stopping the blood transfusion, what is the next most appropriate step in management?
   a. Adrenaline
   b. Hydrocortisone
   c. Antihistamines
   d. Colloids
   e. Crystalloids

7. A 66-year-old woman has problems at work due to lateness and reduced performance. You suspect that her problems might arise from excessive alcohol. Which haematological test is likely to be most helpful in supporting the diagnosis?
   a. Blood film
   b. Erythrocyte sedimentation rate
   c. Mean corpuscular volume (MCV)
   d. Platelet count
   e. White cell count

8. A 31-year-old woman presents to accident and emergency having cut her hand while preparing dinner. At the time she mentioned that it was bleeding and so she bandaged her hand herself before coming to hospital. You remove the bandage and notice the bleeding has stopped. What factor is most likely to have initiated the clotting process?
   a. Factor X
   b. Factor XIII

c. Factor V
d. Factor VII
e. Factor VIII

9. A 15-year-old girl presents with bruising, epistaxis and heavy periods. She has recently recovered from a viral infection. Physical examination is unremarkable. What is the most appropriate initial investigation?
   a. Platelet count
   b. Antiplatelet antibodies
   c. Megakaryocyte count
   d. Hb level
   e. Bleeding time

10. A 75-year-old man presents to his GP with a history of easy bruising and lower back pain. Examination reveals no obvious abnormality. Chest radiograph reveals multiple lytic lesions. Serum protein electrophoresis reveals a paraprotein band at the gamma zone. Bone marrow biopsy shows the presence of plasma cell infiltrate >10%. Peripheral blood film reveals numerous rouleaux formations and plasma cells. Which of the following is likely to be diagnosed?
    a. CLL
    b. Monoclonal gammopathy of uncertain significance (MGUS)
    c. Multiple myeloma
    d. Solitary plasmacytoma
    e. Waldenstrom macroglobulinaemia

11. A middle-aged man has been diagnosed with a bleeding disorder. He is unsure of the name of the condition. However, he remembers the consultant informing him that there are two main bleeding disorders which affect males and that he suffers from the most common one. What is the next most appropriate step in management?
    a. Factor X injection
    b. Factor IX injection
    c. von Willebrand factor injection
    d. Factor VIII injection
    e. Factor VII injection

12. A 35-year-old man presents with multiple bruises on his arms. He is deeply jaundiced and has recently been found to have gallstones and a dilated biliary tree on ultrasound examination. Abnormalities of the following clotting factors are likely to be responsible for his bruising EXCEPT?
    a. Factor II
    b. Factor VII
    c. Factor IX
    d. Factor X
    e. Factor V

13. An overweight 56-year-old woman returns from a trip to Hong Kong. She complains of a swollen left leg. On examination you note calf tenderness and iliofemoral venous distension. What is the most appropriate initial investigation?
    a. Doppler ultrasound
    b. Venography
    c. Ventilation perfusion scan
    d. Platelet count
    e. Coagulation screen

14. A 13-year-old African boy who recently arrived in the UK to join his parents presents to the GP with a facial distortion for the past 10 months from a lesion involving his jaw. On examination he has an enlarged right mandibular mass. Biopsy of one of the lymph nodes reveals many lymphocytes of similar size and morphology, with some macrophages. Infection with which of the following organisms is most likely to be associated with development of the boy's facial lesion?
    a. Adenovirus
    b. Cytomegalovirus
    c. Epstein–Barr virus
    d. Human immunodeficiency virus (HIV)
    e. Human T-lymphotropic virus type 1 (HTLV-1)

15. A middle-aged man is started on unfractionated heparin for a suspected deep vein thrombosis. What is the most appropriate method for monitoring this drug?
    a. PT
    b. INR
    c. Activated partial thromboplastin time (APTT)
    d. Platelet count
    e. Thrombin time

16. A middle-aged man comes into hospital for routine surgery. A preoperative full blood count shows mild anaemia and a raised white blood count of 30×10^9/L, 90% of which are mature lymphocytes. On examination he has small clusters of mobile, firm lymph nodes the size of peas in the posterior cervical triangle and an easily felt spleen. What is the most likely diagnosis?
    a. CLL
    b. Hodgkin disease
    c. Infectious mononucleosis
    d. Myelofibrosis
    e. Viral throat infection

17. A 35-year-old woman presents with slight bruising on her arms. She is currently taking digoxin and warfarin having been diagnosed with atrial fibrillation. Her INR is 7.6. What is the next most appropriate step in management?
    a. Stop warfarin and give vitamin K
    b. Stop warfarin and give protamine sulphate

c. Stop warfarin and give fresh frozen plasma
d. Stop warfarin completely
e. Reduce the current dose of warfarin

18. A middle-aged man presents with a sore throat and bruising of his lower limbs. On examination you note evidence of lymphadenopathy and hepatosplenomegaly. A bone marrow aspirate confirms the presence of abnormal myeloid cells. What additional finding is most likely to confirm a diagnosis of acute myeloid leukaemia?
    a. Blast cells
    b. Philadelphia chromosome
    c. Auer rods
    d. Smear cells
    e. T(15;17) translocation

19. A 45-year-old gentleman is diagnosed with acute leukaemia. The consultant explains to him that he will need to commence chemotherapy. He informs the patient of the possibility of acute tumour lysis syndrome as a consequence of tumour death following treatment. The consultant then turns to you and asks you to explain the most common biochemical disturbances of the syndrome to the patient. The following are all common disturbances EXCEPT?
    a. Hyperkalaemia
    b. Hyperuricaemia
    c. Hyperphosphataemia
    d. Hypocalcaemia
    e. Hyponatraemia

20. The defence system of the small intestine consists of T and B lymphocytes. B lymphocytes are responsible for producing antibodies which act in the gut lumen. Which is the main antibody that is produced?
    a. Immunoglobulin G (IgG)
    b. IgA
    c. IgM
    d. IgE
    e. IgD

21. A middle-aged gentleman is diagnosed with acute promyelocytic leukaemia. What is the next most appropriate step in management?
    a. Cytosine arabinoside
    b. Daunorubicin
    c. Methotrexate
    d. All-*trans* retinoic acid
    e. Bone marrow transplant

22. A 45-year-old man presents with fever, weight loss and night sweats. On examination you note evidence of splenomegaly. Routine blood investigations reveal an Hb of 102 g/L, a white cell count of 105×10^9/L

and a platelet count of 154×10^9/L. He undergoes bone marrow testing which reveals the presence of the Philadelphia chromosome. What is the most likely diagnosis?
    a. Chronic myeloid leukaemia
    b. Acute promyelocytic leukaemia
    c. Acute lymphoblastic leukaemia
    d. Acute myeloid leukaemia
    e. CLL

23. A 25-year-old male from Thailand was found to have mild microcytic anaemia with normal serum iron levels. Further genetic analysis reveals that he has α-thalassaemia trait due to the presence of *cis*-deletion of the α-globin genes on chromosome 16. Which of the following is most likely to be seen on the peripheral blood film?
    a. Bite cells
    b. Heinz bodies
    c. Pappenheimer bodies
    d. Schistocytes
    e. Target cells

24. A 40-year-old man is diagnosed with leukaemia. The consultant explains that his condition is associated with involvement of the central nervous system. What is the most likely diagnosis?
    a. Chronic myeloid leukaemia
    b. Acute promyelocytic leukaemia
    c. Acute lymphoblastic leukaemia
    d. Acute myeloid leukaemia
    e. CLL

25. A 49-year-old man presents with fever, weight loss and night sweats. Bone marrow testing confirms the diagnosis of chronic myeloid leukaemia. What is the next most appropriate step in management?
    a. Hydroxyurea
    b. Bone marrow transplantation
    c. Tyrosine kinase inhibitors
    d. Radiotherapy
    e. Alpha interferon

26. A 65-year-old woman presents with lethargy and a sore throat. On examination you note evidence of bruising. Routine blood investigations reveal a white cell count of 17×10^9/L, an Hb of 90 g/L and a platelet count of 75×10^9/L. A blood film reveals the presence of excess lymphocytes. You suspect a diagnosis of CLL. What additional finding would help to confirm such a diagnosis?
    a. Blast cells
    b. Philadelphia chromosome
    c. Auer rods
    d. Smear cells
    e. T(15;17) translocation

27. A 24-year-old woman presents with fever, night sweats and weight loss. On examination you note enlargement of her cervical lymph nodes. Which investigation is most likely to lead to a diagnosis?
    a. Blood count
    b. Liver function tests
    c. Computed tomography chest and abdominal scan
    d. Chest X-ray
    e. Lymph node biopsy and histology

28. A 17-year-old girl from Nigeria is brought into the emergency department with 2-day history of worsening abdominal pain and bilateral hip pain in the absence of any trauma. This is her third presentation with similar symptoms in 1 year. She required opioids for pain control during her previous admissions. Her Hb has always been low and is 70 g/L on this admission, with a high reticulocyte count. What is the most likely diagnosis?
    a. Spherocytosis
    b. Megaloblastic anaemia
    c. Sickle cell disease (SCD)
    d. Sideroblastic anaemia
    e. Thalassaemia

29. A 23-year-old man complains of fever and night sweats. On examination you note enlargement of his cervical lymph nodes. He comments that when he drinks alcohol he experiences pain at the site of these nodes. What is the most likely diagnosis?
    a. Non-Hodgkin lymphomas
    b. Burkitt lymphoma
    c. Mucosa-associated lymphoid tissue (MALT) lymphoma
    d. Hodgkin disease
    e. Sézary syndrome

30. A 17-year-old female presents to the GP complaining of feeling tired all the time. On further questioning, she admits to having heavy periods. Routine blood tests are done which show a Hb of 79 g/L and an MCV of 72.6 fL. What would the likely management plan be?
    a. Vitamin B_{12} injections
    b. Thiamine tablets
    c. Iron tablets
    d. Vitamin C supplements
    e. Folate supplements

31. A 28-year-old man is suspected of suffering from a form of lymphoma. A lymph node biopsy is performed and histology confirms the presence of Reed–Sternberg cells. What is the most likely diagnosis?
    a. Non-Hodgkin lymphomas
    b. Hodgkin disease

    c. Burkitt lymphoma
    d. MALT lymphoma
    e. Sézary syndrome

32. A man with newly diagnosed Hodgkin disease comes to see his GP. He has been reading about the condition on the Internet and came across a section on 'B symptoms'. He asks the GP what they are. What is the most likely example of a 'B symptom'?
    a. Chest pain
    b. Cough
    c. Headache
    d. Haematuria
    e. Night sweats

33. A woman with newly diagnosed Hodgkin disease is being commenced on chemotherapy. The following are all important factors when determining treatment choice EXCEPT?
    a. Stage
    b. Involved sites
    c. Age
    d. Bulk of lymph nodes involved
    e. Presence or absence of 'B symptoms'

34. A 47-year-old man presents with lethargy and a sore throat. On examination you note evidence of bruising and enlargement of cervical lymph nodes. A lymph node biopsy is performed and histology confirms the diagnosis as low-grade non-Hodgkin lymphoma. The following are all features of low-grade disease EXCEPT?
    a. Involvement of the bone marrow
    b. The disease is incurable with conventional chemotherapy
    c. Middle-aged people are affected
    d. Older-aged people are affected
    e. Involvement of the gastrointestinal tract in all cases

35. A 68-year-old woman presents to the GP feeling lethargic and more breathless than usual. Routine bloods are taken which show a Hb of 81 g/L and an MCV of 107.3 fL. What is the most likely cause of her anaemia?
    a. Iron-deficiency anaemia
    b. Anaemia of chronic disease
    c. Pernicious anaemia
    d. Haemolytic anaemia
    e. Thalassaemia

36. A middle-aged woman complains of epigastric pain in association with nausea and heartburn. Her GP refers her for an endoscopy which reveals evidence of gastric ulceration. Biopsies are taken and the histological diagnosis is of a lymphoma. A diagnosis

of lymphoma is made. What is the most likely type of lymphoma?

a. Non-Hodgkin lymphomas
b. Hodgkin disease
c. Burkitt lymphoma
d. MALT lymphoma
e. Sézary syndrome

37. A 12-year-old boy of African origin has recently moved with his family to the UK. The family go to see the GP as they are worried that their child is not eating well. He comments that he has slight pain in his jaw and that it feels numb. After appropriate investigation, he is found to have a lymphoma. What is the most likely type?

a. Non-Hodgkin lymphoma
b. Hodgkin disease
c. Burkitt lymphoma
d. MALT lymphoma
e. Sézary syndrome

38. A 62-year-old man presents with nonspecific bone pain. He comments that his vision is not as good as it used to be and that he often gets up in the night to pass urine. Routine blood investigations reveal a Hb of 102 g/L, a calcium of 4.2 mmol/L, a urea of 17.7 mmol/L and a creatinine of 175 μmol/L. What is the most likely diagnosis?

a. Waldenstrom macroglobulinaemia
b. Multiple myeloma
c. Acute-on-chronic renal failure
d. Anaemia of chronic disease
e. Benign prostatic hypertrophy

39. You suspect multiple myeloma in a 67-year-old man. Which initial investigation is most likely to lead to a diagnosis?

a. Urea and electrolytes
b. Bone profile
c. Platelet count
d. Protein electrophoresis
e. Liver function tests

40. A 19-year-old girl complains of heavy periods. On examination you note that her hair and nails are brittle. Routine blood investigations reveal a Hb of 98 g/L. What is the most likely diagnosis?

a. Vitamin B_{12}-deficiency anaemia
b. Folate-deficiency anaemia
c. Iron-deficiency anaemia
d. Anaemia of chronic disease
e. Aplastic anaemia

41. A 25-year-old woman presents with fatigue and lethargy. Routine blood investigations reveal a Hb of 96 g/L, an MCV of 72 fL and a ferritin of 4 μg/L. You

request a blood film. The following are all likely to be noted on the blood film EXCEPT?

a. Microcytosis
b. Macrocytosis
c. Hypochromia
d. Anisocytosis
e. Poikilocytosis

42. A 35-year-old man with known Crohn disease complains of feeling tired. Routine blood investigations reveal a Hb of 102 g/L, a serum iron of 7 μmol/L and a ferritin of 123 μg/L. What is the most likely diagnosis?

a. Anaemia of chronic disease
b. Folate-deficiency anaemia
c. Iron-deficiency anaemia
d. Haemolytic anaemia
e. Aplastic anaemia

43. A 60-year-old vegan woman presents with generalized fatigue and malaise. Routine blood investigations reveal a Hb of 82 g/L. What is the most likely diagnosis?

a. Anaemia of chronic disease
b. Folate-deficiency anaemia
c. Vitamin B_{12}-deficiency anaemia
d. Haemolytic anaemia
e. Aplastic anaemia

44. A 65-year-old woman is diagnosed with macrocytic anaemia. On examination you note a sore tongue. Her medical history includes autoimmune thyroid disease. Which investigation is most likely to lead to a diagnosis?

a. Blood count
b. Vitamin B_{12} level
c. Serum folate level
d. Parietal cell autoantibodies
e. Intrinsic factor autoantibodies

45. A 25-year-old woman presents with symptoms of anaemia. There is a family history of coeliac disease. Investigations reveal a reduced serum B_{12} of 102 ng/L. What is the most likely cause of her anaemia?

a. Ileal Crohn disease
b. Pernicious anaemia
c. Coeliac disease
d. Small intestinal bacterial overgrowth
e. Dietary deficiency

46. A 45-year-old man is diagnosed with anaemia. A blood film reveals the presence of megaloblasts. What is the next most appropriate step in management?

a. Vitamin B_{12} replacement
b. Folate replacement

c. Vitamin B_{12} and folate replacement
d. Iron replacement
e. Blood transfusion

47. A middle-aged gentleman comes to see his GP complaining of lethargy and shortness of breath. He has recently undergone mitral valve replacement following a diagnosis of mitral valve stenosis. Routine blood investigations reveal he is anaemic. The GP suspects a diagnosis of haemolytic anaemia. The following are features of haemolytic anaemia EXCEPT?
a. Increased serum bilirubin
b. Increased serum lactate dehydrogenase
c. Decreased reticulocyte count
d. Low haptoglobins
e. Presence of methaemalbumin

48. A 2-year-old boy of Middle Eastern origin is referred to the paediatric outpatient department by his GP following an abnormal blood count. The GP mentions that there is a strong family history of thalassaemia. On examination you note evidence of an enlarged maxilla and prominent frontal bones. What is the most likely diagnosis?
a. Alpha thalassaemia
b. Beta thalassaemia minor
c. Beta thalassaemia intermedia
d. Beta thalassaemia major
e. SCD

49. A 19-year-old girl with known SCD presents to the accident and emergency department with severe bone and chest pain following a viral infection. On examination you note she is mildly dehydrated. Her blood pressure and pulse are stable and oxygen saturation is 99% on room air. What is the next most appropriate step in management?
a. Fluid replacement
b. Analgesia
c. Oxygen
d. Antibiotics
e. Aspirin

50. A 34-year-old woman with systemic lupus erythematosus is found to be anaemic. Which investigation is most likely to lead to a diagnosis?
a. Coombs test
b. Serum ferritin level
c. Blood film
d. Vitamin B_{12} level
e. Serum folate level

51. A patient with newly diagnosed autoimmune haemolytic anaemia is started on treatment. The haematologist notes that the patient's autoantibodies attach to RBCs at a temperature of 29°C. Which management plan would you instigate first?
a. Steroids
b. Splenectomy
c. Azathioprine
d. Avoidance of cold exposure
e. Cyclophosphamide

52. A 55-year-old woman with inguinal lymphadenopathy presented to the GP, and a subsequent diagnosis of Hodgkin disease was made. Which of the following associated findings in Hodgkin disease would give the worst prognosis?
a. Cervical and inguinal lymphadenopathy
b. Just inguinal lymphadenopathy
c. Mediastinal and inguinal lymphadenopathy
d. Mediastinal, inguinal lymphadenopathy and night sweats
e. Mediastinal, inguinal lymphadenopathy and pruritis

53. A 42-year-old man is diagnosed with warm antibody autoimmune haemolytic anaemia. Which of the following antibodies are components of this form of anaemia?
a. IgG
b. IgA
c. IgM
d. IgD
e. IgE

54. A 35-year-old man presents with new-onset severe pains in his fingers when he goes outside in the cold, as well as going numb and cold. He had a recent bout of pneumonia. Laboratory investigation reveals the presence of IgM autoantibodies and a diagnosis of Raynaud phenomenon was made. Peripheral blood film showed no abnormalities. What is the most likely diagnosis?
a. Cold autoimmune haemolytic anaemia
b. Malaria
c. Paroxysmal cold haematuria
d. Paroxysmal nocturnal haematuria
e. Warm autoimmune haemolytic anaemia

55. A 44-year-old woman was diagnosed with type A atrophic gastritis after presenting with tiredness for over 6 months.
a. Decreased serum ferritin
b. Decreased serum folate
c. Increased neutrophil segmentation
d. Increased haematocrit
e. Microcytic RBCs

56. A 30-year-old mother who is a carrier for haemophilia A sees her GP with concerns that her 3-year-old child may have the condition. She reports that her child bruises easily and his knees get very swollen when he falls over. Which one of the following tests of haemostasis is more sensitive for this disease?
   a. Bleeding time
   b. PT
   c. INR
   d. APTT
   e. Platelet count

EXTENDED-MATCHING QUESTIONS (EMQs)

Anaemia
Each answer can be used once, more than once or not at all.

   a. Iron deficiency
   b. Vitamin B_{12} deficiency
   c. Aplastic anaemia
   d. Paroxysmal nocturnal haemoglobinuria
   e. Autoimmune haemolytic anaemia
   f. Glucose-6-phosphate dehydrogenase deficiency
   g. SCD
   h. Thalassaemia
   i. Hereditary spherocytosis
   j. Hereditary elliptocytosis

For each scenario below, choose the most likely corresponding option from the list given above.

   1. Associated with a pancytopenia and a hypocellular bone marrow.
   2. An autosomal dominant condition associated with increased red cell osmotic fragility.
   3. Associated with jaundice and splenomegaly. The blood film may demonstrate the presence of cigar-shaped blood cells.
   4. An X-linked disorder associated with neonatal jaundice and haemolysis due to ingestion of fava beans.
   5. A type of anaemia which occurs due to deficiency of CD59 and delay accelerating factor proteins.

Lymphadenopathy
Each answer can be used once, more than once or not at all.

   a. Epstein–Barr virus
   b. Cytomegalovirus
   c. Lymphoma
   d. Leukaemia
   e. Tuberculosis
   f. HIV
   g. Toxoplasmosis
   h. Sarcoidosis
   i. Carcinoma
   j. Rheumatoid arthritis

For each scenario below, choose the most likely corresponding option from the list given above.

   1. A disease of young adults associated with a sore throat, headache and a macular rash.
   2. A viral infection associated with depletion of CD4 helper lymphocytes.
   3. Characterized by malignant B and T lymphocytes with symptoms of anaemia, infection and bleeding.
   4. Associated with neoplastic cell formation in the bone marrow as result of a variety of genetic and environmental factors.
   5. A form of herpes virus that may result in fever, lethargy, diarrhoea and vomiting.

Splenomegaly
Each answer can be used once, more than once or not at all.

   a. Schistosomiasis
   b. Leukaemia
   c. Myelofibrosis
   d. Malaria
   e. Tuberculosis
   f. Rheumatoid arthritis
   g. Gaucher disease
   h. Kala-azar
   i. Endocarditis
   j. Typhoid

For each scenario below, choose the most likely corresponding option from the list given above.

   1. A disease associated with snail vectors which release cercariae that penetrate the skin to cause a papular rash.
   2. A condition prevalent in Asia and associated with dry wart-like hyperpigmented skin lesions.
   3. A disease widespread in the tropics associated with RBC rupture by sporozoites.
   4. A lipid storage disease known to cause thrombocytopenia, bone pain and neurodegenerative effects.
   5. A middle-aged woman presenting with abdominal pain, diarrhoea and confusion. On examination you note the presence of rose spots on the trunk.

SURGERY QUESTIONS

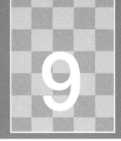
SINGLE BEST ANSWER (SBA) QUESTIONS

1. A 23-year-old woman presents to accident and emergency after being stabbed in the back with a knife. On examination you note weakness in her right limb and loss of proprioception below the level of the injury site. You also note loss of temperature and pain on the opposite side below the site of injury. What is the most likely diagnosis?
   a. Central cord syndrome
   b. Posterior cord syndrome
   c. Anterior cord syndrome
   d. Brown-Séquard syndrome
   e. Spinal shock

2. A 5-year-old boy is admitted to accident and emergency following contact with a hot pan. On examination you note erythema and mottling of his right hand. His blood pressure is 100/60 mmHg and pulse rate 65 beats/min. You decide to initiate fluid resuscitation but find it difficult to obtain good access in both his arms. You fast bleep the registrar and while waiting you note that his blood pressure is quickly dropping. What is the next most appropriate step in management bearing in mind the child's age?
   a. Central line
   b. Venous cut down
   c. Femoral line
   d. Arterial line
   e. Intraosseous needle in the proximal tibia

3. A 29-year-old man was involved in a road traffic accident during which he received a blow to the front of his chest from the steering column. On examination he had a tender sternum, the pulse was 120 beats/min, blood pressure 80/60 mmHg, jugular venous pressure + 20 cm water and the heart sounds were faint. What is most likely to confirm the diagnosis?
   a. Arterial blood gases
   b. Electrocardiogram (ECG)
   c. Echocardiogram
   d. Serum creatinine
   e. Ventilation–perfusion scan

4. A 32-year-old man presents with a 2-day history of sudden-onset pain in the right iliac fossa. On examination you note guarding and rebound tenderness localized to an area approximately one-third of the distance from the anterior superior iliac spine and umbilicus on the right side of his abdomen. What is being described here?
   a. Grey Turner sign
   b. Cullen sign
   c. McBurney point
   d. Rovsing sign
   e. Murphy sign

5. A 55-year-old man presents to accident and emergency following a stabbing to his chest. On examination you note an open wound on the right side of his chest. The patient is severely breathless. His oxygen saturation is 85% on room air. You apply an occlusive dressing to his wound, taping three of the four sides to the skin. His oxygen saturation begins to improve. What is the most likely diagnosis?
   a. Tension pneumothorax
   b. Open pneumothorax
   c. Massive haemothorax
   d. Flail chest
   e. Cardiac tamponade

6. A 26-year-old woman presents with sudden-onset right iliac fossa pain. On examination you note that when pressure is applied to her left iliac fossa, the patient complains of increased pain in her lower right side. What is being described here?
   a. Grey Turner sign
   b. Cullen sign
   c. McBurney point
   d. Rovsing sign
   e. Murphy sign

7. A 32-year-old woman presents with lower right-sided abdominal pain. She describes the pain as initially being centralized and associated with nausea. Routine blood investigations reveal a white cell count of 23×10^9/L. A urine dipstick reveals 3+ leucocytes. Which investigation is least useful in establishing the diagnosis?
   a. Abdominal X-ray
   b. Abdominal ultrasound
   c. Pregnancy test
   d. Abdominal computed tomography (CT) scan
   e. Pelvic ultrasound

8. A 45-year-old boxer is brought to accident and emergency following a blow to his head which left him unconscious. In the department, he regains consciousness but later deteriorates dramatically.

An urgent CT head scan is ordered which confirms the diagnosis. What is the most likely diagnosis?
a. Extradural haematoma
b. Subdural haematoma
c. Contusion
d. Intracerebral haemorrhage
e. Axonal injury

9. A 42-year-old man presents with generalized abdominal pain and vomiting. He comments that he has not opened his bowels for the past 2 days. On examination you note severe abdominal distension and tinkling bowel sounds. An abdominal X-ray is ordered which reveals distended loops of small bowel. What is the next most appropriate step in management?
a. Nasogastric decompression and normal saline intravenously (IV)
b. Surgery
c. Nasogastric decompression
d. Nasogastric decompression and dextrose IV
e. Normal saline IV

10. A 67-year-old woman presents to the accident and emergency department after collapsing in a shopping centre. She is pale, sweaty and complains of severe back pain. On examination she has a heart rate of 150 beats/min, blood pressure of 80/40 mmHg and a tender, expansile, pulsatile mass in her epigastrium. What is the most appropriate management for this woman?
a. Abdominal CT scan
b. Abdominal ultrasound scan
c. Erect chest X-ray and plain abdominal films
d. Serum amylase
e. Take patient to theatre

11. A 35-year-old chronic alcohol abuser complains of upper abdominal pain radiating to his back. On examination you note tenderness and guarding in the epigastrium. Which investigation is most likely to lead to a definitive diagnosis?
a. Abdominal CT scan
b. Abdominal X-ray
c. Chest X-ray
d. Abdominal ultrasound
e. Liver function tests

12. A 32-year-old woman is admitted to accident and emergency following a stabbing to her left chest. On examination she is notably breathless. Her left chest is dull to percussion and breath sounds are absent. What is the most likely diagnosis?
a. Tension pneumothorax
b. Open pneumothorax
c. Massive haemothorax

d. Flail chest
e. Cardiac tamponade

13. A 32-year-old man presents with severe abdominal pain radiating to his back. On examination you note notable tenderness and guarding in the epigastric region. In addition, you note evidence of bruising around the umbilicus. What is the term most likely used to describe this finding?
a. Grey Turner sign
b. Cullen sign
c. McBurney point
d. Rovsing sign
e. Murphy sign

14. A 75-year-old chronic alcoholic presents to accident and emergency following a fall. On examination she appears drowsy and her Glasgow Coma Scale (GCS) drops from 12 to 8. You order an urgent CT head scan. What is the most likely diagnosis?
a. Extradural haematoma
b. Subdural haematoma
c. Contusion
d. Intracerebral haemorrhage
e. Axonal injury

15. A 42-year-old man presents with severe colicky pain in his right loin radiating to his groin. On examination you note tenderness in the right loin. A urine dipstick is performed which is positive for blood. What is the next most appropriate initial investigation?
a. Abdominal ultrasound
b. Abdominal X-ray
c. Abdominal CT scan
d. 24-Hour urine collection
e. IV urogram

16. A middle-aged obese gentleman presents with severe right upper quadrant abdominal pain after a Chinese take away. On examination you note tenderness in his epigastrium and right upper quadrant. Which investigation is most likely to establish the actual diagnosis?
a. White cell count
b. Abdominal ultrasound
c. Liver function tests
d. Abdominal X-ray
e. Serum amylase

17. A 52-year-old building contractor is brought to accident and emergency having fallen from a height onto his chest. He is notably breathless and in severe pain. On examination you note crepitus on chest palpation and paradoxical movement of the lower segment of his right chest. What is the most likely diagnosis?

a. Tension pneumothorax
b. Open pneumothorax
c. Massive haemothorax
d. Flail chest
e. Cardiac tamponade

a. Pancreatitis
b. Large bowel obstruction
c. Large bowel perforation
d. Cholecystitis
e. Hepatitis

18. A 65-year-old hypertensive patient presents to accident and emergency with sudden-onset central abdominal pain radiating to his back. On examination you note evidence of generalized severe abdominal tenderness and a pulsatile mass. Routine observations reveal a pulse rate of 129 beats/min and a blood pressure of 75/40 mmHg. What is the next most appropriate step in management?
a. IV access and fluid resuscitation with Gelofusine
b. IV access and blood resuscitation
c. Abdominal CT scan
d. Abdominal ultrasound
e. Immediate transfer for surgery while simultaneously performing resuscitation

19. A 55-year-old woman presents with pain and numbness in her right leg. Her past medical history includes atrial fibrillation. On examination of her right leg you note absent pulses, pallor and a reduction in temperature as compared with her left limb. Routine observations reveal an irregular pulse of 125 beats/min, a blood pressure of 105/65 mmHg and an oxygen saturation of 96% on room air. Following initial resuscitation, what is the next most appropriate step in management?
a. ECG
b. Digoxin
c. Embolectomy
d. IV fluids
e. Oxygen

20. An elderly patient presents with left iliac fossa pain and vomiting. On examination you note evidence of tenderness in the left iliac fossa and peritonism. Routine blood investigations demonstrate a white cell count of 22×10^9/L. What is the most likely diagnosis?
a. Diverticulitis
b. Ulcerative colitis
c. Sigmoid volvulus
d. Small bowel obstruction
e. Large bowel obstruction

21. A middle-aged obese gentleman presents with right upper quadrant pain. Abdominal examination reveals evidence of severe tenderness in the right upper quadrant. Routine observations reveal a temperature of 38.5°C. Blood tests confirm a white cell count of 16×10^9/L and a C-reactive protein level of 135 mg/L. What is the most likely diagnosis?

22. A 35-year-old woman presents with lower left-sided abdominal discomfort that is severe in nature. She denies any gastrointestinal symptoms. Abdominal examination confirms evidence of lower abdominal tenderness. Routine blood investigations reveal a normal white cell count and C-reactive protein. Serum beta human chorionic gonadotropin is negative. What is the most likely diagnosis?
a. Diverticulitis
b. Ovarian cyst
c. Uterine cyst
d. Sigmoid volvulus
e. Ectopic pregnancy

23. A 15-year-old boy presents with sudden-onset severe pain in his left scrotum and vomiting. On examination you note marked tenderness on palpation. Elevation of the scrotum did not improve the pain. A urine dipstick proves normal. What is the most likely diagnosis?
a. Epididymitis
b. Hydrocele
c. Orchitis
d. Appendicitis
e. Testicular torsion

24. A 25-year-old sexually active male presents with scrotal swelling and pain. On examination you note evidence of scrotal erythema. A urine dipstick proves positive for leucocytes. What is the most likely diagnosis?
a. Epididymitis
b. Hydrocele
c. Orchitis
d. Appendicitis
e. Testicular torsion

25. A 32-year-old man presents to accident and emergency following a stabbing to his left chest. On examination he is severely breathless with a respiratory rate of 30 breaths/min. There is right-sided deviation of his trachea with hyperresonance on percussion and absent breath sounds on the left side. You insert a large-bore IV cannula through the second intercostal space midclavicular line. What is the most likely diagnosis?
a. Tension pneumothorax
b. Open pneumothorax
c. Massive haemothorax
d. Flail chest
e. Cardiac tamponade

EXTENDED-MATCHING QUESTIONS (EMQs)

Trauma

Each answer can be used once, more than once or not at all.

a. Airway obstruction
b. Cardiac tamponade
c. Flail chest
d. Haemothorax
e. Myocardial infarction
f. Open pneumothorax
g. Pulmonary contusion
h. Ruptured diaphragm
i. Ruptured oesophagus
j. Ruptured spleen
k. Tension pneumothorax
l. Traumatic aortic rupture

For each scenario below, choose the most likely corresponding option from the list given above.

1. An unconscious 30-year-old male with weak pulse who previously complained of left-sided pleuritic chest pain. Examination reveals the left chest to be hyperresonant to percussion, with decreased breath sounds.
2. A 20-year-old girl is brought in with a stab wound to the right side of her chest. She is in respiratory distress and air can be heard moving through the defect in the chest wall.
3. A 60-year-old man is hit by a lorry while out walking his dog. He has injured his chest and is in obvious respiratory distress. Initial observations show that he has a pulse of 120 beats/min, a blood pressure of 120/60 mmHg and a respiratory rate of 45 breaths/min. Examination reveals paradoxical chest wall movement.
4. A 3-year-old girl who has been eating peanuts and who now has a cough and stridor.
5. A 38-year-old man is brought into accident and emergency after a high-speed road traffic accident. He has chest pain and a blood pressure of 70/50 mmHg and a widened mediastinum on his chest X-ray.

Acute abdomen 1

Each answer can be used once, more than once or not at all.

a. Appendicitis
b. Pancreatitis
c. Renal colic
d. Abdominal aortic aneurysm (AAA)
e. Thoracic aortic aneurysm
f. Dissecting aortic aneurysm
g. Peptic ulcer disease
h. Bowel obstruction
i. Biliary colic
j. Perforated viscus

For each scenario below, choose the most likely corresponding option from the list given above.

1. Associated with colicky abdominal pain, vomiting and absent bowel movement.
2. A patient presenting with generalized abdominal tenderness with evidence of free gas on an erect chest X-ray.
3. Associated with colicky abdominal pain in the left flank with radiation to the groin. Abdominal signs are usually minimal. The pain may be so severe as to interrupt one's breath.
4. A medical student presents with severe upper abdominal tenderness and a serum amylase greater than four times the normal limit.
5. Associated with sudden-onset severe tearing chest pain radiating to the back. A chest X-ray demonstrates evidence of a widened mediastinum.

Glasgow Coma Scale

Each answer can be used once, more than once or not at all.

a. 6
b. 7
c. 8
d. 9
e. 10
f. 11
g. 12
h. 13
i. 14
j. 15

For each scenario below, choose the most likely corresponding option from the list given above.

1. Obeys commands, with normal speech and spontaneous eye movement.
2. Flexes to pain, with incomprehensible sounds and no eye movement.
3. Withdraws to pain with confused speech and eyes that open to pain.
4. No motor response with normal speech and spontaneous eye movement.
5. Inappropriate speech associated with obeying commands and eyes opening on command.

Acute abdomen 2

Each answer can be used once, more than once or not at all.

a. Acute pancreatitis
b. Acute pyelonephritis
c. Biliary peritonitis
d. Mesenteric adenitis
e. Perforated appendix
f. Perforated peptic ulcer
g. Perforated sigmoid diverticulus
h. Ruptured AAA
i. Small bowel obstruction
j. Superior mesenteric artery occlusion

For each scenario below, choose the most likely corresponding option from the list given above.

1. A 25-year-old man is admitted with severe upper abdominal pain radiating to the back. He has nausea and vomiting and is clearly dehydrated. He returned from holiday in Ayia Napa earlier today.
2. A 33-year-old woman is admitted with a 24-hour history of nausea, vomiting and absolute constipation. Her abdomen is tympanic with increased high-pitched bowel sounds.
3. A 57-year-old man is admitted with onset of abdominal pain initially in the left upper quadrant. He has been self-medicating with ibuprofen after spraining his left ankle playing squash. On examination the abdomen is rigid with no bowel sounds.
4. A 24-year-old woman is admitted with fever, rigors and severe back pain radiating to her left groin.
5. A 10-year-old boy is admitted with right iliac fossa pain of several hours' duration. Initially, he has guarding and rebound tenderness. Pressing in the right iliac fossa also elicits the same pain. He rapidly progresses to having a tense abdomen.

Perioperative care 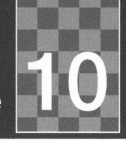 10

SINGLE BEST ANSWER (SBA) QUESTIONS

1. A 54-year-old woman is 2 days post an open appendicectomy for perforated appendicitis. She is reviewed on the ward round and comments that she is still experiencing abdominal soreness. On examination she is notably tender over the lower abdomen. The nurses inform you that she has a temperature of 38.9°C, a blood pressure of 100/54 mmHg and a pulse rate of 95 beats/min. Her blood results reveal a white cell count of 21 × 10⁹/L and C-reactive protein (CRP) of 154 mg/L. What is the most likely diagnosis?
   a. Cardiogenic shock
   b. Hypovolaemic shock
   c. Septic shock
   d. Obstructive shock
   e. Anaphylactic shock

2. A 55-year-old woman with severe intermittent claudication is admitted for an elective arteriogram and possible angioplasty of her right leg. She has a past medical history of rheumatoid arthritis and mildly impaired renal function. Current medication includes penicillamine. Admission blood investigations reveal a urea of 12.8 mmol/L and creatinine of 163 μmol/L with previous results being in a similar range. However, following the arteriogram, her urea and creatinine levels have increased to 32.8 mmol/L and 363 μmol/L, respectively. What is the most likely cause of her acute renal failure?
   a. Age
   b. Minimal fluid intake
   c. Radiological contrast nephropathy
   d. Penicillamine
   e. Past medical history of renal failure

3. You are a house officer in breast surgery and are clerking in a 45-year-old woman who is being admitted for excision of a benign breast lump. She has no known past medical or surgical history. Which investigation is most highly recommended prior to her surgery?
   a. Full blood count
   b. Electrocardiogram (ECG)
   c. Chest X-ray
   d. Urea and electrolytes
   e. None of the above

4. You are a house officer in general surgery and are clerking in a 65-year-old man who is being admitted electively for an inguinal hernia repair. His past medical history includes chronic obstructive pulmonary disease. He states that he had a chest X-ray around 6 weeks ago. Which investigation is most highly recommended prior to his surgery?
   a. Full blood count
   b. ECG
   c. Chest X-ray
   d. Urea and electrolytes
   e. Clotting screen

5. A 32-year-old man is complaining of increasing pain 2 days post inguinal hernia repair. He is currently prescribed paracetamol 1 g four times a day. What is the next most appropriate step in management?
   a. Codeine
   b. Tramadol
   c. Morphine
   d. Co-codamol
   e. Diclofenac

EXTENDED-MATCHING QUESTIONS (EMQs)

Postoperative complications
Each answer can be used once, more than once or not at all.

   a. Atelectasis
   b. Anastomotic dehiscence
   c. Constipation
   d. Deep vein thrombosis
   e. Gravitational oedema
   f. Haematoma
   g. Pneumonia
   h. Pseudo-obstruction
   i. Urinary retention
   j. Wound infection

For each scenario below, choose the most likely corresponding option from the list given above.

   1. A 45-year-old man complains of increasing pain in the groin following a right inguinal hernia repair 5 days previously. On examination, the wound is red, swollen and tender.

2. A 70-year-old man who had a hip replacement 5 days previously complains of generalized abdominal discomfort. He has vomited four times, his bowels have not functioned for 5 days and he feels thirsty and has not passed urine for 8 hours. On examination, his abdomen is grossly distended and tympanitic, but there is no tenderness and he has decreased bowel sounds. The rectum is empty.

3. An 83-year-old woman had an emergency laparotomy for a bleeding duodenal ulcer 18 hours previously. She has become borderline pyrexial, and pulse oximetry shows saturation of 90% on 2 L of oxygen. Her blood pressure is normal, but her pulse rate is 110 beats/min. Her respiratory rate is 20 breaths/min and she has decreased breath sounds at the right base.

4. A 72-year-old woman who has had an anterior resection of the rectum suddenly develops severe abdominal pain 4 days postoperatively. On examination, she is unwell, with a pyrexia of 38°C, blood pressure of 100/60 mmHg, abdominal distension, a discharging wound and peritonism.

5. A 62-year-old woman develops discomfort of the right lower leg 7 days after a hysterectomy for carcinoma of the uterus. On examination, she has a pyrexia of 37.5°C and bilateral ankle oedema (right > left).

Preoperative investigations

Each answer can be used once, more than once or not at all.

a. Arterial blood gases
b. Blood glucose
c. Carotid Doppler scan
d. Chest X-ray
e. Clotting screen
f. Coronary angiogram
g. Echocardiogram
h. ECG
i. Liver function tests
j. Spirometry
k. Troponin

For each scenario below, choose the most likely corresponding option from the list given above.

1. A 72-year-old woman has been admitted for a mastectomy. She gives a history of well-controlled hypertension for which she is on medication. On examination she looks well, and the examination of the cardiovascular system reveals an ejection systolic murmur in the aortic area.

2. A 50-year-old woman is admitted for a routine repair of a femoral hernia. She has chronic asthma for which she has been taking medication on a regular basis, but it is not always well controlled.

3. A 76-year-old patient is admitted as an emergency with symptoms of obstructive jaundice. An ultrasound shows the presence of a gallstone in the common bile duct. She is about to undergo an endoscopic retrograde cholangiopancreatography.

4. A 66-year-old man is admitted for a coronary artery bypass operation. During routine clerking, he describes an episode when he temporarily lost the vision in his right eye and some weakness of his arm, which has now recovered completely.

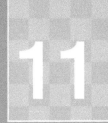
SINGLE BEST ANSWER (SBA) QUESTIONS

1. A term baby is born with a vitelline duct still present. His baby check was normal and he was discharged 2 days after birth. He remains well until he attends university at 19 years of age, when he develops colicky abdominal pain. What is the likely cause?
   a. Appendicitis
   b. Meckel diverticulum
   c. Exomphalos
   d. Gastroschisis
   e. Atresia

2. A 78-year-old female is admitted to the surgical assessment unit with severe, sudden-onset, abdominal pain for the past 3 days, along with bloody diarrhoea for the past 24 hours. She has a medical history of atrial fibrillation. Blood samples are unremarkable apart from an elevated lactate. What is the most likely diagnosis?
   a. Ulcerative colitis
   b. Colorectal carcinoma
   c. Angiodysplasia
   d. Crohn disease
   e. Ischaemic bowel

3. A 10-month-old baby was admitted to the children's ward with vomiting. The parents said he seemed generally unwell, crying more than usual and drawing his knees up to his chest. When the nurses changed his nappy, they noticed that his stools were loose, and looked redder than normal. What is the diagnosis?
   a. Pyloric stenosis
   b. Gastroenteritis
   c. Intussusception
   d. Gastro-oesophageal reflux disease (GORD)
   e. Duodenal atresia

4. A 21-year-old female presents to the hospital with sudden-onset acute abdominal pain. On examination she is tender in the right iliac fossa with guarding. She has tachycardia and is hypotensive. What would be your initial management?
   a. Abdominal X-ray
   b. Pregnancy test
   c. Intravenous (IV) fluids
   d. Urine dipstick
   e. Abdominal ultrasound

5. A 46-year-old female presents to accident and emergency (A&E) with severe upper abdominal pain. On examination she is tender in the right upper quadrant and her sclera looks jaundiced. Her temperature is 38.2°C. Her blood samples showed a raised alkaline phosphatase and bilirubin. What is the most likely diagnosis?
   a. Liver abscess
   b. Gallstone ileus
   c. Appendicitis
   d. Viral hepatitis
   e. Cholangitis

6. A 68-year-old male was referred for an urgent clinic appointment after a change in bowel habit. Colonoscopy and biopsy confirmed colorectal adenocarcinoma, which was resected. Histology showed spread to the muscle layer and bowel wall without any involvement of lymph nodes. What Dukes staging is this?
   a. Dukes A
   b. Dukes B
   c. Dukes C1
   d. Dukes C2
   e. Dukes D

7. A 70-year-old male presented with central intermittent abdominal pain for the past 3 weeks. On examination he had mild epigastric tenderness without any signs of peritonitis. He is a known heavy smoker and mentioned that he had recently had an ultrasound scan done on his neck as an investigation for dizzy spells. What is the most likely cause?
   a. Mesenteric ischaemia
   b. Chronic pancreatitis
   c. Duodenal ulcer
   d. Gastric carcinoma
   e. Appendicitis

8. A 5-week-old baby was brought into A&E vomiting. The mother reported a 3-day history of vomiting large amounts following every feed. The baby was born at 39 weeks without any complications and had been putting weight on well postbirth. On examination the doctor could palpate a sausage-shaped mass in the right upper quadrant. What is the most likely diagnosis?
   a. Pyloric stenosis
   b. Neonatal jaundice
   c. Duodenal atresia
   d. Diaphragmatic hernia
   e. Acute gastritis

9. A 67-year-old male noticed a swelling in the right groin region that appears to 'come and go'. On examination there is a reducible 2 × 2 cm mass that appears to lie inferior to the inferior gastric vessels. The hernia reappears on coughing, even when pressing. What hernia is this most likely to be?
   a. Incisional hernia
   b. Direct inguinal hernia
   c. Indirect inguinal hernia
   d. Femoral hernia
   e. Umbilical hernia

10. A 46-year-old female presented to the general practitioner (GP) with a change in bowel habit for the past 2 months. She is having looser stools than normal with blood mixed in with the stools. There is no history of any abdominal pain. What would be your first-choice investigation?
    a. Abdominal X-ray
    b. Faecal occult blood
    c. Abdominal computed tomography (CT)
    d. Ultrasound abdomen
    e. Colonoscopy

11. A 58-year-old male, who has a long medical history of achalasia, presents with symptoms of weight loss and worsening dysphagia. He is referred for an urgent oesophagogastroduodenoscopy, which shows a lesion in the upper third of the oesophagus suspicious for oesophageal cancer. What is the likely histological type to be shown on biopsy?
    a. Adenocarcinoma
    b. Lymphoma
    c. Small cell carcinoma
    d. Squamous cell carcinoma
    e. Melanoma

12. A 65-year-old woman presents with sudden-onset left iliac fossa pain, fever and vomiting. Which investigation is most likely to lead to a diagnosis?
    a. Colonoscopy
    b. Abdominal ultrasound
    c. Abdominal and pelvic CT scan
    d. Abdominal X-ray
    e. White cell count (WCC) and C-reactive protein (CRP)

13. A 55-year-old man presents with rectal bleeding and abdominal discomfort. A colonoscopy is performed which reveals the presence of a tumour in the sigmoid colon. Further assessment and staging confirm a colonic adenocarcinoma with probable local lymph node involvement. What is the next most likely step in management?
    a. Surgery
    b. Chemotherapy

c. Surgery and adjuvant chemotherapy
d. Radiotherapy
e. Palliative treatment

14. A 24-year-old obese woman presents to A&E with sudden-onset severe right upper quadrant pain. On examination you note notable tenderness in the right upper quadrant with guarding. Which investigation is most likely to lead to a diagnosis?
    a. WCC
    b. CRP
    c. Liver function tests
    d. Abdominal X-ray
    e. Abdominal ultrasound

15. A 25-year-old weightlifter presents with a lump near the right side of his groin. On examination you note the lump reduces upwards and laterally and moves downwards and medially on release. In addition, you note the lump is controlled by pressure over the deep ring. What is the most likely diagnosis?
    a. Indirect inguinal hernia
    b. Direct inguinal hernia
    c. Femoral hernia
    d. Richter hernia
    e. Sliding hernia

16. A 53-year-old man presents with a lump near his groin. On examination you note it reduces immediately on lying down and reaches full size immediately on standing. You ask the patient to cough and notice it protrudes straight. It is not controlled by pressure over the deep ring. What is the most likely diagnosis?
    a. Indirect inguinal hernia
    b. Direct inguinal hernia
    c. Femoral hernia
    d. Richter hernia
    e. Sliding hernia

17. A 35-year-old woman presents with a lump in her groin. On examination you note the lump is below and lateral to the pubic tubercle. What is the most likely diagnosis?
    a. Indirect inguinal hernia
    b. Direct inguinal hernia
    c. Femoral hernia
    d. Richter hernia
    e. Sliding hernia

18. A 25-year-old woman complains of pain at the navel. On examination you note an obvious swelling at the site of the umbilicus, which she says has been present since birth. What is the most likely diagnosis?
    a. Umbilical hernia
    b. Femoral hernia

c. Richter hernia

d. Sliding hernia

e. Paraumbilical hernia

19. A 43-year-old man presents with epigastric pain and associated nausea. On examination you note a palpable swelling in the midline which is tender and irreducible. What is the most likely diagnosis?
    a. Epigastric hernia
    b. Umbilical hernia
    c. Paraumbilical hernia
    d. Richter hernia
    e. Sliding hernia

20. A 42-year-old woman presents with a lump at the lateral edge of the rectus sheath. What is the most likely diagnosis?
    a. Epigastric hernia
    b. Umbilical hernia
    c. Spigelian hernia
    d. Paraumbilical hernia
    e. Richter hernia

21. A 65-year-old woman presents with a 2-day history of abdominal discomfort and vomiting. In addition, she complains of right-sided hip pain. An abdominal X-ray is ordered which confirms evidence of small bowel obstruction. She undergoes an emergency laparotomy. What is the most likely diagnosis?
    a. Epigastric hernia
    b. Obturator hernia
    c. Umbilical hernia
    d. Paraumbilical hernia
    e. Richter hernia

22. An elderly man presents with left-sided abdominal pain and dark red rectal bleeding. His medical history includes ischaemic heart disease. He is known to smoke 40 cigarettes per day over a 30-year period. On examination you note obvious distension of his abdomen. Routine observations demonstrate a blood pressure of 105/65 mmHg and a pulse rate of 130 beats/min. He is apyrexial. What is the most likely diagnosis?
    a. Lymphocytic colitis
    b. Ulcerative colitis
    c. Ischaemic colitis
    d. Diverticulitis
    e. Microscopic colitis

23. A 65-year-old man presents with sudden-onset abdominal pain. On further questioning, he comments that he has not opened his bowels for 3 days and has been vomiting intermittently. On examination his abdomen is grossly distended and he is notably tender throughout. A plain radiograph

of his abdomen demonstrates evidence of sigmoid volvulus. What is the next most appropriate step in management to achieve definitive resolution?
    a. Emergency laparotomy
    b. Flexible sigmoidoscopic decompression with a flatus tube
    c. IV fluids
    d. Nasogastric tube insertion
    e. IV fluids and insertion of a nasogastric tube

24. A middle-aged woman presents with bleeding when opening her bowels. She comments that the blood is bright red in nature and can be seen on the toilet paper and in the pan following defecation. A proctoscopy is performed which helps confirm the diagnosis. Which management plan would you suggest first?
    a. Review in 2 months
    b. Barron banding
    c. Surgery
    d. Cryotherapy
    e. Injection sclerotherapy

25. A 55-year-old man presents to his GP complaining of perianal discomfort. On examination you note a discrete swelling in the perianal margin. It is painful on palpation and has the appearance of a small blackcurrant. What is the most likely diagnosis?
    a. Perianal haematoma
    b. Haemorrhoid
    c. Thrombosed haemorrhoid
    d. Tumour
    e. Hidradenitis suppurativa

26. A middle-aged man presents with pain on defecation. He comments that the pain occurs during defecation and can continue for some time afterwards. On examination you note the presence of a midline fissure. He has had this symptom for the last 12 weeks. What is the next most appropriate step in management?
    a. Lateral internal sphincterotomy
    b. Botulinum A toxin injection
    c. Oral diltiazem
    d. Topical glyceryl trinitrate ointment
    e. Surgical sphincter dilatation

27. A 40-year-old woman is suspected of suffering from faecal incontinence. Which investigation is most likely to lead to a diagnosis?
    a. Abdominal ultrasound scan
    b. Barium enema
    c. Anorectal physiology studies
    d. Abdominal magnetic resonance imaging (MRI) scan
    e. Colonoscopy

28. A middle-aged man presents with episodes of recurrent perianal pain and swelling. He reports ongoing purulent discharge between such episodes. Inspection of the perineum reveals the presence of circular granulation tissue which exudes pus on digital compression from within the rectum. What is the most likely diagnosis?
    a. Abscess
    b. Hidradenitis suppurativa
    c. Pilonidal cyst
    d. Fistula in ano
    e. Pilonidal sinus

29. A 35-year-old man presents to A&E at 3 AM following an episode of severe vomiting. He complains of sudden-onset chest and neck pain. On examination you note the presence of crepitus in his suprasternal notch. What is the first initial investigation in the emergency department?
    a. Endoscopy
    b. Anteroposterior and lateral chest X-ray
    c. Chest CT scan
    d. Gastrograffin swallow
    e. Barium swallow

30. A 10-year-old boy presents to A&E following ingestion of household bleach. He complains of severe pain in his mouth and stomach. Routine observations reveal a temperature of 38.5°C, a blood pressure of 105/65 mmHg and a pulse rate of 135 beats/min. What is the next most appropriate initial investigation?
    a. Endoscopy
    b. Chest CT scan
    c. Chest X-ray
    d. Barium swallow
    e. Oesophageal manometry

31. A 45-year-old man presents complaining of difficulty in swallowing liquid and solid food. A barium swallow is performed which demonstrates a narrowed portion within the lower end of his oesophagus. An upper gastrointestinal (GI) endoscopy excludes the presence of organic pathology. Which therapeutic option is most likely to relieve his symptoms in the long term?
    a. Antispasmodics
    b. Balloon dilatation
    c. Heller myotomy
    d. Botulinum toxin
    e. Proton pump inhibitors

32. A 48-year-old woman presents with right upper quadrant pain. On examination you note a slight yellow discolouration of her skin and sclerae. Abdominal examination reveals tenderness across the upper abdomen. What is the next most appropriate initial investigation?

a. Abdominal CT scan
b. Abdominal X-ray
c. Abdominal ultrasound scan
d. Abdominal MRI scan
e. Endoscopic retrograde cholangiopancreatography (ERCP)

33. A 70-year-old woman presents with a 1-week history of abdominal discomfort and weight loss. She has a known history of hepatitis C. On examination you note evidence of moderate hepatomegaly. An ultrasound scan demonstrates an isolated lesion in her liver. Which additional investigation is most likely to confirm a diagnosis?
    a. Serum bilirubin
    b. Serum alkaline phosphatase
    c. International normalized ratio
    d. Prothrombin time
    e. Serum alpha-fetoprotein

34. A 43-year-old man presents with right upper quadrant pain. On examination you note tenderness and guarding in the right upper quadrant. Routine observations reveal a temperature of 38.5°C. Routine blood investigations demonstrate a WCC of 17×10^9/L and CRP of 98 mg/L. What additional sign is this patient most likely to demonstrate?
    a. Cullen sign
    b. Grey Turner sign
    c. Rovsing sign
    d. Boas sign
    e. Trousseau sign

35. An 80-year-old woman presents with abdominal pain and weight loss. An abdominal CT scan is performed which confirms the diagnosis of pancreatic cancer with distant metastases. What is the next most likely step in management?
    a. Surgery
    b. Palliative therapy
    c. Radiotherapy
    d. Chemotherapy
    e. Surgery and chemotherapy

36. A 50-year-old man presents with epigastric pain, vomiting and weight loss. He is a heavy drinker and admits to consuming half a bottle of vodka each day over a 10-year period. On examination you note a purple-coloured periorbital skin rash and a palpable lymph node in the left supraclavicular fossa. What is the next most appropriate investigation?
    a. Abdominal CT scan
    b. Abdominal ultrasound scan
    c. Endoscopy and biopsy
    d. Laparoscopy
    e. Abdominal X-ray

37. An elderly man presents with rectal bleeding and weight loss. A colonoscopy is performed which demonstrates a mass in his sigmoid colon. Biopsies are taken and histology confirms the presence of a cancer that extends into the muscularis mucosa, with no involvement of regional lymph nodes or distant metastases. What is the most likely histological diagnosis?
   a. Dukes stage A
   b. Dukes stage B
   c. Dukes stage C
   d. Dukes stage D
   e. Dukes stage E

EXTENDED-MATCHING QUESTIONS (EMQs)

Gastrointestinal bleeding
Each answer can be used once, more than once or not at all.

   a. Anal fissure
   b. Colonic carcinoma
   c. Crohn disease
   d. Diverticular disease
   e. Duodenal ulcer
   f. Gastric carcinoma
   g. Haemorrhoids
   h. Laryngeal carcinoma
   i. Mallory–Weiss tear
   j. Oesophageal varices

For each scenario described below, choose the SINGLE most likely diagnosis from the above list of options. Each option may be used once, more than once or not at all.

   1. A 60-year-old man presents with altered bowel habit, crampy abdominal pain and blood mixed in with his stools.
   2. A 40-year-old woman presents with a long history of indigestion, worse recently, black tarry stools and feeling light-headed.
   3. A 32-year-old woman presents to her GP following childbirth, worried about the fresh, painless red blood on the toilet paper.
   4. A 22-year-old medical student presents to A&E with haematemesis and chest pain following celebrations on passing his finals.
   5. A 17-year-old woman with cystic fibrosis presents to A&E vomiting profuse volumes of fresh blood.

Hernia
Each answer can be used once, more than once or not at all.

   a. Inguinal
   b. Pantaloon
   c. Paraumbilical
   d. Sciatic
   e. Cooper
   f. Incisional
   g. Richter
   h. Littre
   i. Spigelian
   j. Diaphragmatic

For each scenario below, choose the most likely corresponding option from the list given above.

   1. Associated with abdominal pain, notable distension and vomiting. It may result in perforation of the bowel.
   2. Seen commonly in newborn babies where, typically, the left side of the chest is occupied by the bowel.
   3. A hernia occurring through a part of the abdominal wall between the lateral border of the rectus abdominis and linea semilunaris, typically diagnosed by ultrasound.
   4. A combined indirect and direct hernia whereby the hernial sac protrudes on either side of the inferior epigastric vessels.
   5. A lump located near the groin which protrudes straight on coughing and is not controlled by pressure over the deep ring.

Upper gastrointestinal disorders
Each answer can be used once, more than once or not at all.

   a. Achalasia
   b. Diffuse oesophageal spasm
   c. Pharyngeal pouch
   d. Zollinger–Ellison syndrome
   e. Oesophagitis
   f. Duodenal ulcer
   g. Adenocarcinoma
   h. Squamous cell carcinoma
   i. Plummer–Vinson syndrome
   j. Atrophic gastritis

For each scenario below, choose the most likely corresponding option from the list given above.

   1. A condition known to cause severe gastroduodenal ulceration due to excessive gastrin secretion.
   2. A tumour of the lower third of the oesophagus thought to be the result of longstanding reflux disease.
   3. A motility disorder of the oesophagus characterized by a 'rat tail' segment at the lower oesophageal sphincter.
   4. Associated with severe epigastric discomfort particularly at night and relieved by food.
   5. A condition associated with iron-deficiency anaemia and swallowing difficulties.

Lower gastrointestinal disorders

Each answer can be used once, more than once or not at all.

a. Perianal abscess
b. Intussusception
c. Perianal haematoma
d. Haemorrhoids
e. Crohn disease
f. Angiodysplasia
g. Collagenous colitis
h. Ulcerative colitis
i. Anal fistula
j. Ischaemic colitis

For each scenario below, choose the most likely corresponding option from the list given above.

1. Associated with vomiting and the passage of redcurrant-like stool in children.
2. A bluish tender perianal swelling often resulting from constipation and straining.
3. Typically affects the right colon and associated with severe rectal bleeding. Colonoscopy may reveal the presence of dilated tortuous vessels and 'cherry red' areas.
4. A pan-intestinal inflammatory disorder associated with deep ulcers in the mucosa to give a cobblestone-like appearance.
5. Associated with left-sided abdominal pain and dark red rectal bleeding. Examination findings may demonstrate evidence of hypotension and abdominal distension. A barium enema may demonstrate thickening and blunting of the mucosal folds of the bowel.

Hepatobiliary disorders

Each answer can be used once, more than once or not at all.

a. Cholangitis
b. Hepatic haemangioma
c. Focal nodular hyperplasia of the liver
d. Cholangiocarcinoma
e. Hepatoma
f. Cholecystitis
g. Biliary colic
h. Acalculous cholecystitis
i. Pancreatitis
j. Hepatic abscess

For each scenario below, choose the most likely corresponding option from the list given above.

1. A patient presenting with recurrent pain in the right upper quadrant radiating to the tip of the scapula. There is no associated pyrexia.

2. A tumour presenting typically with painless jaundice, known to result commonly from primary sclerosing cholangitis.
3. A patient presenting with tenderness and guarding in the right upper quadrant with evidence of hyperaesthesia below the right scapula and pyrexia.
4. A patient presenting with abdominal pain, fever and jaundice as a result of *Escherichia coli* infection.
5. A female patient presenting with anorexia, ascites and abdominal discomfort with a background history of cirrhosis and long-term use of the oral contraceptive pill.

Abdominal pain

Each answer can be used once, more than once or not at all.

a. Acute appendicitis
b. Acute diverticulitis
c. Colorectal cancer
d. Crohn disease
e. Familial adenomatous polyposis
f. Perforated duodenal ulcer
g. Renal colic
h. Strangulated inguinal hernia
i. Ulcerative colitis
j. Testicular torsion

For each scenario below, choose the most likely corresponding option from the list given above.

1. A 19-year-old male who was previously fit and well presents with generalized abdominal pain for 3 days which is worsening, weight loss, diarrhoea and dysuria. He is most tender in the right iliac fossa. He has no appetite and has been feverish.
2. A 35-year-old man presents with 5 months of colicky abdominal pain, weight loss and bloody diarrhoea with mucus. He has also been suffering from lower back pain for the last few months.
3. A 37-year-old man presents with acute sudden right testicular pain which radiates to the right groin, and has blood +++ in his urine.
4. A 35-year-old man presents with red blood mixed in his stool and weight loss over the last 6 months. He had a colonoscopy 5 years ago, but is an infrequent attender to his GP. His father died of colorectal cancer aged 46.
5. A 60-year-old woman presents with a 2-day history of left iliac fossa pain and a significant (PR) bleed of bright red blood which fills the pan. She has had alternating diarrhoea and constipation over the last year.

Hernias

Each answer can be used once, more than once or not at all.

a. Congenital diaphragmatic hernia
b. Epigastric hernia
c. Femoral hernia
d. Incarcerated hernia
e. Incisional hernia
f. Inguinal hernia
g. Obturator hernia
h. Rolling hiatus hernia
i. Sliding hiatus hernia
j. Spigelian hernia
k. Umbilical hernia

For each scenario below, choose the most likely corresponding option from the list given above.

1. A 64-year-old labourer presents to his GP with increasing pain in his groin. He has had a lump for several years which usually disappears on lying. It no longer does so. On examination you can feel a mass in the right groin arising above the inguinal ligament. It is irreducible but bowel sounds are present.

2. A 57-year-old woman is referred to the surgeon who performed her laparoscopic cholecystectomy 2 years previously. She has developed a bulge, which on examination is in the midclavicular line in the right upper quadrant of the abdomen. It disappears on lying down and 'gurgles'.

3. A 92-year-old frail lady is admitted to hospital with severe abdominal pain, colicky in nature, with nausea and vomiting. A nasogastric tube is passed, but on abdominal X-ray, no bowel distension is seen. Close inspection of the film reveals the diagnosis.

4. A 31-year-old man presents to his GP with a mass in his left groin. It disappears on lying, is above the inguinal ligament and reappears on coughing. His brother had the same problem.

5. A 29-year-old woman presents to her GP with an abdominal mass following the birth of her first child. During her pregnancy, she had had an everted umbilicus and this has worsened after giving birth.

Acute abdominal pain

Each answer can be used once, more than once or not at all.

a. Acute appendicitis
b. Acute cholecystitis
c. Acute diverticulitis
d. Acute pancreatitis
e. Biliary colic
f. Large bowel obstruction
g. Perforated peptic ulcer
h. Perforated sigmoid diverticular disease
i. Small bowel obstruction
j. Urinary tract infection

For each scenario below, choose the most likely corresponding option from the list given above.

1. A 69-year-old woman presents with a 3-day history of constipation and constant pain in the left iliac fossa. The pain has suddenly become much worse and she has collapsed and been admitted to casualty. On examination she has a tachycardia and is hypotensive. There is severe lower abdominal pain with guarding throughout the mid- and lower abdomen.

2. A 50-year-old obese woman presents with epigastric pain. On examination, her temperature is 38.5°C. She is tender in the upper abdomen and Murphy sign is positive.

3. A 22-year-old woman presents with pain in the right iliac fossa. The patient is anorexic, has not vomited, but had some dysuria and frequency. Her temperature is 37.5°C. The patient is flushed and has localized guarding in the right iliac fossa and suprapubic region.

4. A 72-year-old man presents with increasing constipation. He has colicky lower abdominal pain and has not passed flatus for 24 hours. Examination reveals a distended abdomen which is tympanitic on percussion.

5. A 60-year-old man presents with a 48-hour history of sudden-onset epigastric pain radiating through to the back after an alcoholic binge. Examination reveals the patient to be apyrexial, tachycardic and normotensive. The patient is diffusely tender, with guarding in the epigastrium. An erect chest X-ray is normal, but the blood gas analysis reveals hypoxia.

Intestinal obstruction

Each answer can be used once, more than once or not at all.

a. Adhesions
b. Carcinoma caecum
c. Carcinoma rectum
d. Carcinoma sigmoid
e. Gallstone ileus
f. Intussusception
g. Pseudo-obstruction
h. Sigmoid volvulus
i. Strangulated femoral hernia
j. Strangulated inguinal hernia

For each scenario below, choose the most likely corresponding option from the list given above.

1. An 80-year-old man presents with a 4-day history of abdominal distension and pain. He is vomiting faeculent fluid. He has not been feeling well for 3 months and has lost 2 stone in weight. Clinical examination reveals visible peristalsis in the midabdomen, distension and a mass in the right iliac fossa.
2. A 68-year-old woman presents with colicky abdominal pain and vomiting. Examination shows that she is dehydrated, with abdominal distension and a lower midline scar from a perforated appendix. Plain abdominal film shows multiple distended small bowel loops and the presence of air in the biliary tree.
3. A 60-year-old man undergoes emergency lumbar disc decompression. Postoperatively, he is immobile. He becomes increasingly constipated and develops a distended abdomen. Plain abdominal films show a grossly distended colon down to the pelvic brim.
4. A 78-year-old man presents with a 3-day history of vomiting faeculent fluid. He has a grossly distended abdomen and a palpable mass in the right groin. The mass is firm, slightly tender and lies below and lateral to the pubic tubercle.
5. An 88-year-old woman with dementia is referred by her GP because she seems to be in pain and unwell. She has a long history of constipation. On examination, she has a grossly distended tympanitic abdomen which is nontender. The plain abdominal X-ray shows a large distended loop of colon.

Gastrointestinal bleeding

Each answer can be used once, more than once or not at all.

a. Angiodysplasia
b. Anterior duodenal ulcer
c. Caecal carcinoma
d. Crohn disease
e. Mallory–Weiss tear
f. Oesophageal varices
g. Posterior duodenal ulcer
h. Rectal carcinoma
i. Sigmoid carcinoma
j. Sigmoid diverticular disease

For each scenario below, choose the most likely corresponding option from the list given above.

1. An 82-year-old woman suffering with osteoarthritis of the hip is admitted with haematemesis and melaena. She has been taking ibuprofen in increasing amounts to control her hip pain.
2. A 77-year-old man presents with his fourth episode of acute rectal bleeding. The blood is a mixture of fresh blood and clots. On this occasion, the bleeding has been severe enough to require a 4-unit blood transfusion. A barium enema is undertaken and is normal.
3. A 56-year-old man presents with anaemia and weight loss. Examination reveals a mass in the right iliac fossa and hepatomegaly.
4. A 50-year-old alcoholic presents with melaena. On examination the patient is drowsy and hypotensive. Examination of the abdomen shows splenomegaly.
5. A 58-year-old man is admitted with acute onset of left iliac fossa pain. Recently, he has noticed he has had some vague abdominal pain and felt more constipated. On examination he is pyrexial, pale and has localized peritonism in the left iliac fossa. His abdomen is distended. Investigations show a haemoglobin (Hb) of 7 g/dL (hypochromic, microcytic) and a WCC of 18×10^9/L.

Oesophagogastric disorders

Each answer can be used once, more than once or not at all.

a. Achalasia
b. Duodenal ulcer disease
c. Gastric cancer
d. Gastric ulcer disease
e. GORD
f. *Helicobacter* atrophic gastritis
g. Mallory–Weiss tear
h. Oesophageal adenocarcinoma
i. Oesophageal squamous carcinoma
j. Pyloric stenosis

For each scenario below, choose the most likely corresponding option from the list given above.

1. A 45-year-old man presents with severe epigastric pain. The pain is most severe when he is hungry and often wakes him from sleep at night. The pain is relieved by eating and by taking milk and snacks. The patient has gained half a stone in weight since his symptoms started.
2. A 19-year-old student experiences worsening dysphagia for 3 months. She has lost a stone in weight and has had two courses of antibiotics for a persistent chest infection.
3. A 55-year-old vagrant man has had a long history of recurrent episodes of epigastric pain. He presents with weight loss and severe vomiting. On admission, he is noted to be dehydrated and abdominal examination demonstrates a succussion splash.
4. A 65-year-old man presents with a long history of indigestion self-treated with antacids, but progressive dysphagia and weight loss for

3 weeks. On examination, the patient is anaemic and is markedly cachectic.

5. A 27-year-old man is admitted to the casualty with frank haematemesis. He has been on his stag weekend and after consuming large amounts of alcohol, has been vomiting repeatedly, and has some epigastric pain.

Foregut investigations

Each answer can be used once, more than once or not at all.

a. Abdominal ultrasound
b. Barium meal
c. Barium swallow
d. Chest X-ray
e. CT scan
f. ERCP
g. Endoscopic ultrasonography
h. Gastroscopy
i. Laparoscopy
j. Magnetic resonance scanning

For each scenario below, choose the most likely corresponding option from the list given above.

1. A 55-year-old man presents with flatulent dyspepsia, fatty food intolerance and right upper quadrant pain.
2. A 65-year-old man is diagnosed with oesophageal adenocarcinoma. The surgeon wishes to stage the local extent of the tumour and to assess whether there is local lymph node spread or invasion of the thoracic aorta.
3. A 70-year-old man presents with painless obstructive jaundice. He has undergone assessment by ultrasonography, showing a mass in the head of the pancreas. The surgeon wishes to stage the tumour.
4. An 80-year-old man presents with intermittent cervical dysphagia and has a soft swelling on the left side of his neck. He coughs and splutters after eating and often aspirates liquids.
5. A 59-year-old man has carcinoma of the stomach. He is suitable for surgical resection but the surgeon wants to exclude peritoneal seedlings before undertaking a laparotomy.

Abdominal mass

Each answer can be used once, more than once or not at all.

a. Appendix mass
b. Caecal carcinoma
c. Crohn disease
d. Diverticular abscess
e. Empyema of the gallbladder
f. Hepatomegaly
g. Mucocoele of the gallbladder
h. Ovarian carcinoma
i. Ovarian cyst
j. Sigmoid carcinoma
k. Sigmoid volvulus
l. Uterine fibroids

For each scenario below, choose the most likely corresponding option from the list given above.

1. A 69-year-old woman presents to her GP with a history of fatigue for 3 months, and 4 days of colicky abdominal pain and vomiting. Examination shows that she is pale and dehydrated, with a mass in the right iliac fossa.
2. A 72-year-old woman presents with a 3-week history of increasing discomfort in her lower abdomen. She has not opened her bowels for 5 days but has passed flatus. On examination, she looks pale and dehydrated and the abdomen is distended and tympanitic. There is an irregular nontender mass in the left iliac fossa region.
3. A 25-year-old woman presents with acute onset of generalized abdominal pain. She has been unwell for about 2 months and has lost half a stone in weight. On examination, she looks unwell, has a pyrexia and a tender mass felt in the right iliac fossa with diffuse tenderness in the lower abdomen.
4. A 67-year-old man is seen in the outpatient clinic following an episode of severe colicky upper abdominal pain which has settled to leave some discomfort. He has a history of 'indigestion' after fatty food and alcohol intake of at least 4 units a day. On examination, he is slightly jaundiced, apyrexial and, on abdominal examination, has a smooth, nontender mass in the right hypochondrium.
5. A 45-year-old woman complains to her GP of tiredness and a dragging sensation in the lower abdomen. She has noticed that her clothes do not fit as well. On examination, she is anaemic and her abdomen is distended with a mass consistent with the size of an 18-week pregnancy in the suprapubic region.

Groin lump

Each answer can be used once, more than once or not at all.

a. False aneurysm
b. Femoral artery aneurysm
c. Femoral hernia
d. Inguinal hernia

e. Lymphocoele
f. Lymphoma
g. Malignant lymphadenopathy
h. Psoas abscess
i. Obturator hernia
j. Reactive lymphadenopathy
k. Saphena varix
l. Soft tissue sarcoma

For each scenario below, choose the most likely corresponding option from the list given above.

1. An 80-year-old woman presents with a 2-day history of a lump in the left groin. It has been associated with colicky abdominal pain, vomiting and abdominal distension. Examination reveals a red, tender, irreducible lump below and lateral to the pubic tubercle. The abdomen is distended, with high-pitched 'tinkling' bowel sounds.
2. A 75-year-old lady presents with a 3-month history of a right groin lump. It becomes painful when she walks, but disappears when she rests. Examination reveals a right groin lump with cough impulse. It reduces to a point above and medial to the pubic tubercle. She also has long-standing varicose veins.
3. A 70-year-old woman presents with a pretibial laceration but also mentions that she has a 4-week history of a lump in the right groin. It is completely painless but has gradually increased in size during this period. She had a melanoma excised from her right calf 2 years previously. Examination reveals a firm, nontender, irregular lump below and lateral to the pubic tubercle.
4. An 80-year-old woman with recent onset of a leg ulcer presents with a painless lump in her right groin. She has recently had a femoral angiogram. On examination, there is a 3 × 2 cm pulsatile lump.

Rectal bleeding

Each answer can be used once, more than once or not at all.

a. Anal carcinoma
b. Anal fissure
c. Anal skin tags
d. Angiodysplasia
e. Crohn disease
f. Haemorrhoids
g. Meckel diverticulum
h. Peptic ulceration
i. Rectal adenocarcinoma
j. Rectal villous adenoma
k. Sigmoid carcinoma
l. Sigmoid diverticular disease
m. Ulcerative colitis

For each scenario below, choose the most likely corresponding option from the list given above.

1. A 60-year-old woman presents with fresh rectal bleeding, diarrhoea, profuse mucous discharge, tenesmus and lethargy. Investigations show that she is anaemic (Hb 10 g/dL) and has a potassium of 2.2 mmol/L.
2. A 50-year-old woman presents with a short history of painful, fresh rectal bleeding. She has a history of cervical intraepithelial neoplasia (CIN). On examination, she has a single indurated painful ulcer in the perianal region.
3. A 5-year-old girl's mother brings her to the GP because of increasing problems with constipation and she has noticed some fresh blood on her clothes.
4. An 80-year-old man is admitted as an emergency with acute onset of profuse, painless, dark red rectal bleeding. He is normally fit and well and has no history of bowel problems. On examination, he is pale, cold, clammy, hypotensive and his abdomen is nontender.

Cardiothoracics and vascular surgery 12

SINGLE BEST ANSWER (SBA) QUESTIONS

1. A 75-year-old man, recently found to have an abdominal aortic aneurysm (AAA) on a routine abdominal ultrasound scan, sees his general practitioner (GP) to find out more about the risks of the condition. Which of the following factors is not considered a high risk of rupture of AAA?
   a. Chronic obstructive pulmonary disease
   b. Heavy smoking
   c. Fusiform shape of aneurysm
   d. Poorly controlled hypertension
   e. Size increase by 0.6 cm/year

2. A 65-year-old woman has a history of increasing angina pectoris which led to coronary artery bypass surgery 3 years ago. She has generally done well since the surgery; she has reduced her cigarette smoking, but still smokes and leads a sedentary lifestyle. In addition to emphasizing smoking cessation and recommending an exercise program, which one of the following would be most effective for managing this patient's intermittent claudication?
   a. Aspirin
   b. Cilostazol
   c. Clopidogrel
   d. Ginkgo biloba
   e. Pentoxifylline

3. A 62-year-old man presents to his GP with a 1-month history of bilateral leg pain after walking 1 mi (1.6 km). The pain disappears following a period of rest. He has mildly raised blood glucose and cholesterol levels which are treated by lifestyle modification. He is a smoker with a 40-pack year history and drinks 16 units of alcohol per week. His blood pressure is 135/85 mmHg. What is the most likely cause of this condition in this patient?
   a. Alcohol
   b. Diabetes mellitus
   c. Hypercholesterolaemia
   d. Hypertension
   e. Smoking

4. A middle-aged man presents with sudden-onset back pain and difficulty in swallowing. On examination his blood pressure is stable at 126/76 mmHg and pulse rate regular at 82 beats/min. What is the most likely diagnosis?
   a. Thoracic aortic aneurysm
   b. False aneurysm
   c. AAA
   d. Mycotic aneurysm
   e. Popliteal aneurysm

5. A 42-year-old woman presents with sudden-onset abdominal and back pain. An abdominal computed tomography (CT) scan is arranged which confirms the presence of an AAA. The patient is referred for surgery. Postoperatively the patient complains of weakness in her lower limbs. What is the most likely aetiological cause for this weakness?
   a. Vertebral artery damage
   b. Cervical radicular artery damage
   c. Thoracic radicular artery damage
   d. Iliac artery damage
   e. Artery of Adamkiewicz damage

6. A 63-year-old woman with a history of ischaemic heart disease presents to the GP with pain in her legs. She states that she gets cramping pains in her buttocks and thighs when she tries to exercise. On examination her femoral pulses are absent and there is wasting of her thighs and buttocks. Which of the following conditions has caused this patient's symptoms?
   a. AAA
   b. Aortoiliac occlusive disease
   c. Cauda equina syndrome
   d. Inferior vena cava thrombosis
   e. Peripheral artery disease (PAD) affecting both femoral arteries

7. A 35-year-old woman presents to accident and emergency (A&E) with a 3-hour history of acute left leg pains. Her past medical history is notable for previous ischaemic heart disease and diabetes. Which one of the following is a potential source of embolism causing acute ischaemia of the lower limb?
   a. Amniotic fluid
   b. Cerebral thrombus
   c. Fat embolism
   d. Gun shot
   e. Mural thrombus

8. A 36-year-old man presents to his GP. On abdominal examination the GP notes a pulsatile mass. The GP suspects an AAA. What is the next most appropriate initial investigation?
   a. Abdominal X-ray
   b. Abdominal ultrasound
   c. Abdominal magnetic resonance imaging scan
   d. Abdominal CT scan
   e. Echocardiography

9. You are on a post-take ward round when you assess a patient recently diagnosed with an aneurysm. Your consultant informs you that the patient presented with a painful, tender pulsatile mass associated with a temperature of 38.2°C. What is the most likely diagnosis?
   a. Thoracic aortic aneurysm
   b. False aneurysm
   c. AAA
   d. Mycotic aneurysm
   e. Popliteal aneurysm

10. A 65-year-old male is diagnosed with an AAA following an asymptomatic screen. It is 4.2 cm in diameter. Which of the following is the best form of management for this patient?
    a. Annual abdominal ultrasound scans
    b. Annual abdominal CT scans
    c. Endovascular aneurysm repair
    d. No further treatment required
    e. Open surgical repair

11. You are on a ward round when your consultant shows you a patient recently diagnosed with an aneurysm. He tells you that the patient developed the aneurysm in his femoral artery following a recent angiogram.
    a. Thoracic aortic aneurysm
    b. Popliteal aneurysm
    c. AAA
    d. Mycotic aneurysm
    e. False aneurysm

12. A 45-year-old smoker presents with a tight cramp-like pain in his left calf. He comments that the pain is worse on walking and eases at rest. What is the next most appropriate initial investigation?
    a. Duplex ultrasound
    b. Ankle brachial pressure index
    c. Angiography
    d. Magnetic resonance (MR) angiography
    e. Intravascular ultrasound

13. A 54-year-old hypertensive patient presents with a tight cramp-like pain in his left calf. He comments that the pain is worse on walking and eases at rest. What is the next most appropriate step in management?
    a. Cilostazol
    b. Angioplasty
    c. Surgery to restore arterial inflow
    d. Hypertension control
    e. Watchful waiting

14. A 55-year-old man is brought to A&E with his wife as a result of sudden-onset right-sided weakness. His past medical history includes diabetes, hypertension, hypercholesterolaemia and one previous stroke. On examination you note the presence of a bruit in his carotids. You arrange an urgent carotid doppler which confirms carotid artery stenosis. You refer the man to the on-call vascular surgeon who agrees to perform a carotid endarterectomy. You explain to the patient's wife that there is a risk of potentially damaging his cranial nerves. What is the most likely cranial nerve complication of a carotid endarterectomy?
    a. Cranial nerve V
    b. Cranial nerve VII
    c. Cranial nerve III
    d. Cranial nerve XI
    e. Cranial nerve XII

15. A 75-year-old male presents to his GP with a dull backache that has been worsening over the last 3 months. On examination a pulsatile and expansile mass can be felt at the level of the umbilicus. Which of the following investigations would be most sensitive in confirming the underlying diagnosis?
    a. Abdominal X-ray
    b. Abdominal ultrasound
    c. Ankle brachial pressure index
    d. CT scan of the abdomen
    e. CT venogram

16. A 65-year-old woman presents with an aching sensation in both her lower legs. She comments that this is mainly relieved by elevating her legs. On examination you note the presence of tortuous dilated veins on the back of her legs. You suspect a diagnosis of varicose veins. What is the next most appropriate initial investigation?
    a. Handheld Doppler assessment of sapheno-femoral competence
    b. Venous duplex imaging
    c. Venography
    d. Plethysmography
    e. Leg X-ray

17. A 55-year-old obese woman presents with an aching sensation in both her lower legs. On examination you note the presence of varicose veins. Which management plan would you instigate first?
    a. Surgery
    b. Endovenous laser therapy
    c. Radiofrequency ablation
    d. Compression stockings
    e. Regular exercise

18. A middle-aged, overweight man presents with bilateral leg swelling. On examination you note evidence of ulceration and fissuring. There is no notable evidence of infection. He comments that there is a family history of Milroy disease. What is the next most appropriate step in management?
    a. Antibiotics
    b. Compression stockings
    c. Homans procedure
    d. Charles procedure
    e. Liposuction

19. An 87-year-old woman with known atrial fibrillation (AF) presents to A&E with severe diffuse abdominal pain and tenderness. The patient has a blood pressure of 87/56 mmHg and a heart rate of 145 beats/min. Initial blood tests show an increasing serum lactate and a raised serum amylase. Which of the following investigations is most useful in confirming the underlying diagnosis?
    a. Abdominal X-ray and erect chest X-ray
    b. Colonoscopy with biopsy
    c. CT scan abdomen without contrast
    d. Flexible sigmoidoscopy
    e. MR angiography

EXTENDED-MATCHING QUESTIONS (EMQs)

Vascular disorders

Each answer can be used once, more than once or not at all.

a. AAA
b. Thoracic aortic aneurysm
c. Dissecting aortic aneurysm
d. Compartment syndrome
e. Thromboangiitis obliterans
f. Raynaud disease
g. Raynaud phenomenon
h. Varicose veins
i. Thrombophlebitis migrans
j. Deep venous thrombosis

For each scenario below, choose the most likely corresponding option from the list given above.

1. Typically affects young men who smoke. The condition is progressive unless one stops smoking.
2. A disease of young women whereby arteries of the fingers and toes are reactive and enter spasm in response to the cold. There is often no underlying vascular disease.
3. Inflammation of a vein associated with pain, tenderness and redness. There is often an association with connective tissue disease.
4. Associated with a pulsatile mass on abdominal examination with possible evidence of calcification on abdominal X-ray.
5. A condition associated with severe tearing central chest pain radiating to the back. Blood pressure is often unequal in both arms.

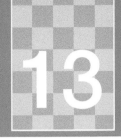

Orthopaedics   13

SINGLE BEST ANSWER (SBA) QUESTIONS

1. A 13-year-old male who is active in sports most of the year presents with bilateral anterior knee pain that is worse in the right knee. An examination reveals tenderness and some swelling at the tibial tubercles. Which one of the following is true regarding this patient's condition?
   a. Bilateral symptoms are unusual
   b. Corticosteroid injection of the tibial tubercle is a safe and effective treatment
   c. It is almost never seen in adults
   d. Radiographs should always be ordered to rule out other conditions
   e. Treatment with a straight leg cylinder cast for 6 weeks is often needed

2. A 14-year-old boy presents to accident and emergency (A&E) complaining of sudden-onset pain in his right limb. On examination you note his right limb is red, tender and notably swollen. In addition, you observe he is unwilling to move his limb. Routine blood investigations reveal a white cell count of 23×10^9/L and C-reactive protein (CRP) of 98 mg/L. What is the most common aetiological cause for this presentation?
   a. *Streptococcus pyogenes*
   b. *Haemophilus influenzae*
   c. *Salmonella*
   d. *Staphylococcus aureus*
   e. *Brucella*

3. An 8-year-old boy presents with a painful left limb. On examination you note he is pyrexic with a temperature of 38.2°C. You suspect a diagnosis of acute osteomyelitis. Which investigation is most likely to lead to a diagnosis?
   a. Magnetic resonance imaging (MRI) of the affected limb
   b. Plain limb X-ray
   c. Erythrocyte sedimentation rate (ESR)
   d. White cell count
   e. CRP

4. A 69-year-old man with Paget disease presents with a painful right leg. He comments that it is particularly painful when walking. A plain limb X-ray reveals evidence of bone destruction and a 'sunray'-like appearance of his right femur. What is the most likely diagnosis?
   a. Osteoid osteoma
   b. Chondroma

c. Ewing sarcoma
d. Osteoclastoma
e. Osteosarcoma

5. A 48-year-old woman known to have systemic lupus erythematosus (SLE) presents to her general practitioner (GP) with a 3-month history of progressive right hip pain, which is most severe during physical activity. She denies a history of trauma. She has been taking paracetamol for 2 months with partial relief only. She has also been on 20 mg of prednisolone for a lupus flare 6 months ago. Clinical examination shows pain with movement, but otherwise unremarkable. A plain X-ray of the pelvis and hip is unremarkable. Which of the following is the most appropriate next step in the management of this patient?
   a. Reassurance that pain will resolve
   b. Advise patient to continue taking regular paracetamol and follow-up in 1 month
   c. Discontinue the steroids and start methotrexate
   d. Switch to intravenous steroids
   e. Order an MRI of the hip

6. A 45-year-old manual worker presents to his GP with a painful right shoulder made worse by movement. On examination you note palpable crepitus; his pain is reproduced on cross body stressing of the right shoulder. What is the most likely diagnosis?
   a. Subacromial impingement
   b. Acromioclavicular osteoarthritis
   c. Rotator cuff tear
   d. Calcific tendinitis
   e. Frozen shoulder

7. A woman presents to her GP with a painful right shoulder. On examination you note that her pain can be reproduced with shoulder abduction and external rotation. What is the most likely diagnosis?
   a. Subacromial impingement
   b. Acromioclavicular osteoarthritis
   c. Rotator cuff tear
   d. Calcific tendinitis
   e. Frozen shoulder

8. A 70-year-old woman complains of bilateral gradual knee pain on most days of the past few months. She complains of stiffness in the morning that lasts for a few minutes and a creaking sensation at times in the right knee. On examination there is a small effusion, diffuse crepitus and limited flexion of both knees.

Joint tenderness is more prominent over the medial joint line bilaterally. Which one of the following is characteristic of osteoarthritis of the knee?

a. Greater frequency in men than in women
b. Increased pain with rest
c. A direct correlation between radiographic changes and pain severity
d. Reduction of pain with repair of associated meniscal tears
e. Reduction of pain with muscle strengthening

9. A rugby player presents to his GP complaining of a painful left shoulder following a local match. On examination you note reduced active but full passive movement. In addition, you note evidence of muscle wasting and tenderness on palpation. What is the most likely diagnosis?

a. Subacromial impingement
b. Acromioclavicular osteoarthritis
c. Rotator cuff tear
d. Calcific tendinitis
e. Frozen shoulder

10. A middle-aged woman presents with a painful right elbow. She comments that the pain starts over the outer side of her elbow and radiates down her forearm. In addition, she states that she finds it difficult to open door handles. What is the next most appropriate step in management?

a. Steroid injections
b. Paracetamol
c. Nonsteroidal antiinflammatory drugs (NSAIDs)
d. Surgery
e. Tramadol

11. An 80-year-old woman falls in the geriatrics ward whilst mobilizing with the physiotherapist. A lower limb fracture is suspected. On examination her leg and foot are externally rotated compared with the opposite limb and there is some shortening. What is the most likely affected structure?

a. Ankle
b. Neck of the femur
c. Rami of the pelvis
d. Shaft of the femur
e. Tibia

12. A man presents to his GP complaining of numbness in his ring and little finger of his right hand. What is the most likely nerve involved in this presentation?

a. Radial
b. Ulnar
c. Median
d. Brachial
e. Musculocutaneous

13. An 11-year-old overweight boy presents with a limp in his right leg and groin pain. Physical examination reveals that his right leg is shorter than his left. X-ray reveals widening of the growth plate. What is the most likely diagnosis?

a. A slipped femoral epiphysis
b. Perthes disease
c. Osteoarthritis
d. Osteogenic sarcoma
e. Osteomyelitis

14. A man presents to his GP complaining of being unable to extend his right wrist. What is the most likely nerve involved in this presentation?

a. Radial
b. Ulnar
c. Median
d. Brachial
e. Musculocutaneous

15. A middle-aged chronic alcohol abuser complains of being unable to extend his ring and little finger of his right hand. What is the most likely diagnosis?

a. Ulnar nerve palsy
b. Dupuytren contracture
c. Brachial nerve palsy
d. Carpal tunnel syndrome
e. Trigger finger

16. A middle-aged woman presents to her GP complaining that her right middle finger 'catches' as she bends it. What is the most likely diagnosis?

a. Ulnar nerve palsy
b. Dupuytren contracture
c. Brachial nerve palsy
d. Carpal tunnel syndrome
e. Trigger finger

17. A 69-year-old retired construction worker presents with a 2-week history of lower back pain. He comments that it is severe in nature and radiates down both legs. Today, he is unable to pass urine and has reduced perianal sensation on neurological testing. Which investigation is most likely to lead to a diagnosis?

a. Plain spine X-ray
b. Computed tomography (CT) spine
c. MRI spine
d. Myeloma screen
e. Prostate-specific antigen

18. An 18-year-old man presents with knee pain. This came on suddenly as a sharp pain while he was turning quickly during a football match 1 week ago. Since then, his knee has been swollen, he has been unable to completely straighten his leg and has

experienced painful locking of his knee. Which of the following is the most likely diagnosis?

a. Anterior cruciate ligament tear
b. Meniscal tear
c. Osteoarthritis
d. Patella tendon rupture
e. Suprapatellar effusion

19. A 65-year-old woman presents with pain in her right hip. She comments that the pain is particularly worse on walking and at the end of the day. On examination you note crepitus on movement and reduced active and passive range of movement. You suspect the possibility of osteoarthritis. Which investigation is most likely to lead to a diagnosis?

a. Plain hip X-ray
b. ESR
c. CRP
d. Rheumatoid factor
e. Full blood count

20. A 35-year-old man is diagnosed with right knee haemarthrosis following a football injury. What is the most common aetiological cause for this condition?

a. Peripheral meniscal tear
b. Capsular tear
c. Anterior cruciate ligament rupture
d. Osteochondral fracture
e. Posterior cruciate ligament rupture

21. A 16-year-old male presents with ongoing pain around his knee. On examination there is clear localized swelling and tenderness. An X-ray of the knee shows periosteal elevation (known as Codman triangle) and underlying bone destruction with new bone formation, described as 'sunray spicules'. Which of the following is the most likely underlying condition?

a. Ewing sarcoma
b. Giant-cell tumour
c. Osgood–Schlatter disease
d. Osteosarcoma
e. Secondary metastases to the bone cortex

22. A teenager presents to A&E with severe pain in his right knee following a football injury. He comments that he heard a loud crack and then found it too difficult to run. On examination you note the right knee is red and swollen in appearance. What is the most likely diagnosis?

a. Peripheral meniscal tear
b. Capsular tear
c. Anterior cruciate ligament rupture
d. Osteochondral fracture
e. Posterior cruciate ligament rupture

23. A middle-aged woman presents to A&E with pain in her left knee following a head-on car crash. On examination you note displacement of the tibia on application of a posterior force. What is the most likely diagnosis?

a. Peripheral meniscal tear
b. Capsular tear
c. Anterior cruciate ligament rupture
d. Osteochondral fracture
e. Posterior cruciate ligament rupture

24. A 65-year-old retired physical education teacher presents to her GP with lower back pain, radiating into her thighs and buttocks. The pain is worse on walking downhill and alleviated by cycling. Lower limb neurological examination reveals diminished ankle and knee reflexes. Which of the following investigations is most likely to confirm the diagnosis?

a. X-ray of the lumbar region
b. CT scan of the lumbar region
c. MRI of the lumbar region
d. Rheumatoid factor
e. Electromyography

25. An 8-month-old boy is brought to the GP for a postnatal check. On examination the GP notes asymmetry of groin skin creases. Further assessment reveals an unstable dislocatable right hip. An ultrasound scan confirms the diagnosis. What is the next most appropriate step in management?

a. Pavlik harness
b. von Rosen splint
c. Femoral osteotomy
d. Open/closed reduction and immobilization
e. Plaster immobilization

26. A 9-year-old boy presents with a limp and generalized ache of his right hip. A hip X-ray reveals a smaller femoral head epiphysis and widening of the joint space on the right side. What is the most likely diagnosis?

a. Developmental dysplasia of the hip
b. Perthes disease
c. Slipped upper femoral epiphysis (SUFE)
d. Irritable hip
e. Osteoarthritis

27. A 12-year-old boy of African descent presents with acute-onset left-sided hip pain and a limp. A hip X-ray reveals displacement of the femoral head. What is the most likely diagnosis?

a. Developmental dysplasia of the hip
b. Perthes disease
c. SUFE
d. Irritable hip
e. Osteoarthritis

28. Which of the following nerves is most at risk of being damaged following a shoulder dislocation?
    a. Accessory nerve
    b. Axillary nerve
    c. Median nerve
    d. Radial nerve
    e. Ulnar nerve

EXTENDED-MATCHING QUESTIONS (EMQs)

Fractures

Each answer can be used once, more than once or not at all.

    a. Clavicle
    b. Humeral neck
    c. Humeral shaft
    d. Scaphoid
    e. Distal radius
    f. Pelvis
    g. Femoral shaft
    h. Intracapsular neck of femur
    i. Tibial
    j. Scapula

For each scenario below, choose the most likely corresponding option from the list given above.

1. Commonly seen in osteoporotic postmenopausal ladies who fall on an outstretched hand.
2. Occurs as a result of falling on an outstretched arm. May be associated with radial nerve injury.
3. Associated with external rotation and shortening of the leg.
4. Swelling and pain on wrist movement. Notably difficult to diagnose on an X-ray.
5. Associated with damage to the medial femoral circumflex artery.

Fracture complications

Each answer can be used once, more than once or not at all.

    a. Crush syndrome
    b. Compartment syndrome
    c. Algodystrophy
    d. Nonunion
    e. Malunion
    f. Contracture
    g. Compensation neurosis
    h. Fat embolus
    i. Pneumonia
    j. Renal stone

For each scenario below, choose the most likely corresponding option from the list given above.

1. An elderly woman complaining of a productive cough and shortness of breath following a hip fracture.
2. Occurs typically on day 3 after the fracture is sustained. Associated features include confusion, dyspnoea and hypoxia.
3. Failure of fracture healing within the expected period. Typically seen with scaphoid fractures.
4. A serious condition associated with increased tissue pressure, vascular occlusion and soft tissue necrosis.
5. A condition whereby a fracture unites in a nonanatomical position and is associated with poor fracture healing.

Orthopaedic clinical examination

Each answer can be used once, more than once or not at all.

    a. Detects osteoarthritis of the thumb
    b. Discriminates between a muscular and a bony flat foot deformity
    c. Identifies an Achilles tendon rupture
    d. Tests for a fixed flexion deformity of the hip
    e. Tests for a fixed flexion deformity of the lumbar spine
    f. Tests for laxity of the anterior cruciate ligament
    g. Tests for torn medial menisci
    h. Tests for a torn posterior cruciate ligament
    i. Tests for an unstable shoulder girdle
    j. Tests for weak ipsilateral hip abductor muscles

For each scenario below, choose the most likely corresponding option from the list given above.

1. Anterior draw test
2. Thomas test
3. Trendelenburg test
4. Schober test
5. Apprehension test
6. Lachman test
7. McMurray test

Knee injuries

Each answer can be used once, more than once or not at all.

    a. Anterior cruciate ligament rupture
    b. Bucket handle tear of meniscus
    c. Dislocation of the knee
    d. Lateral collateral ligament rupture
    e. Medial collateral ligament rupture
    f. Meniscal tear
    g. Patella fracture
    h. Patella ligament rupture
    i. Posterior cruciate ligament rupture
    j. Tibial plateau fracture

For each scenario below, choose the most likely corresponding option from the list given above.

1. A 13-year-old girl presents with locking of the knee, having sustained previous knee injuries while playing netball. Arthroscopy diagnoses and treats the condition successfully.
2. A 37-year-old man is hit side on by a van while riding his motorbike. You, the orthopaedic senior house officer, are called to see the man after several attempts at reducing his patella have failed. There is obvious deformity of the knee. X-ray shows medial displacement of the femur on the tibia.
3. A 52-year-old lady is involved in a car accident. She is hit by an uninsured driver as she crosses the road to work. Her knee is very painful and she is unable to bear weight. X-ray demonstrates the abnormality, which is reported as 'Schatzker grade 3'.
4. A 32-year-old man is brought into A&E having injured his right knee in a strong tackle playing football. The mechanism of injury is unclear. On examination pulses are present, there is no posterior sag but anterior draw is positive.
5. A 30-year-old professional woman is brought into A&E. She fell down some stairs at a conference, landing on her right knee. She is in pain and is unable to straight leg raise.

Skin, joint and bone infections

Each answer can be used once, more than once or not at all.

a. *Escherichia coli*
b. *Pseudomonas aeruginosa*
c. *Proteus mirabilis*
d. Group A streptococcus
e. *S. aureus*
f. Coliforms
g. *Pasteurella multocida*
h. *Mycobacterium tuberculosis*
i. *Streptococcus pneumoniae*
j. *Bacteroides fragilis*

For each scenario below, choose the most likely corresponding option from the list given above.

1. A builder with olecranon bursitis.
2. Necrotizing fasciitis of the leg following a trivial injury.
3. Prosthetic hip infection.
4. An infected cat bite on the hand.
5. A foot infection after stepping on a nail while wearing trainers.

Ear, nose and throat

SINGLE BEST ANSWER (SBA) QUESTIONS

1. A 54-year-old woman recently travelled to Cornwall for a scuba diving trip. Since her return, she has noted brief intermittent episodes of vertigo not associated with nausea or vomiting. She is concerned, however, because these episodes occurred after sneezing or coughing and then a couple of times after straining while lifting something. She has had no hearing loss, and no vertigo with positional changes such as bending over or turning over in bed. The most likely cause of this patient's vertigo is which of the following?
   a. Benign paroxysmal positional vertigo
   b. Ménière disease
   c. Multiple sclerosis triggered by a rapid change in climate
   d. Perilymphatic fistula
   e. Vestibular neuronitis

2. A 35-year-old man presents with a lump between his thyroid notch and hyoid bone which moves upwards on tongue protrusion. What is the most likely diagnosis?
   a. Lymphoma
   b. Thyroglossal cyst
   c. Branchial cyst
   d. Carotid body tumour
   e. Carcinoma

3. An 18-year-old woman presents with a cyst in the upper anterior border of her sternocleidomastoid muscle. What is the most likely diagnosis?
   a. Lymphoma
   b. Thyroglossal cyst
   c. Branchial cyst
   d. Carotid body tumour
   e. Carcinoma

4. A 45-year-old male presents with a 3-day history of increasing cough, sinus pressure and low-grade fever. His past medical history is positive only for hypertension. What is the most appropriate initial step in patient care?
   a. 7-Day course of amoxicillin
   b. 10-Day course of levofloxacin
   c. Explaining that most cases of sinusitis resolve without treatment

   d. High-dose pseudoephedrine and increase fluid intake
   e. Ordering sinus X-rays (XRs) to determine the most appropriate course of care

5. A 75-year-old man with a 20-year history of type 2 diabetes mellitus presents to his general practitioner (GP) with constant and severe right ear pain. Otoscopic examination shows offensive-smelling purulent otorrhoea. There is also a red lesion at the external auditory canal. A biopsy of this lesion is subsequently performed, and histology reveals presence of granulation tissue. Which of the following agent is the most likely cause?
   a. *Escherichia coli*
   b. *Pseudomonas aeruginosa*
   c. *Haemophilus influenzae*
   d. *Proteus vulgaris*
   e. *Staphylococcus aureus*

6. A middle-aged man presents with a lump in his neck. On examination you note it is oval, nontender and pulsatile in nature. What is the most likely diagnosis?
   a. Lymphoma
   b. Thyroglossal cyst
   c. Branchial cyst
   d. Carotid body tumour
   e. Carcinoma

7. A 76-year-old man complains of swollen neck glands. On examination you note swelling and tenderness of both his parotid glands and the presence of purulent saliva on gentle palpation of his parotids. What is the most likely diagnosis?
   a. Lymphoma
   b. Pleomorphic adenoma
   c. Parotitis
   d. Parotid calculi
   e. Adenolymphoma (Warthin tumour)

8. A 65-year-old man presents with a painless mass in his right parotid gland. He comments that he has noticed the mass grow slowly over time. What is the most likely diagnosis?
   a. Lymphoma
   b. Pleomorphic adenoma
   c. Parotitis
   d. Parotid calculi
   e. Adenolymphoma (Warthin tumour)

9. A patient presents complaining of facial flushing following parotid surgery to remove a pleomorphic adenoma. She states that whenever she is eating, she develops an erythematous rash on her cheek and starts sweating. She also experiences a burning pain in the distribution of the rash. What is the most likely underlying diagnosis?
   a. Facial nerve palsy
   b. Frey syndrome
   c. Heerfordt syndrome
   d. Salivary fistula
   e. Staphylococcal infection

10. A 67-year-old woman presents with a painless mass in her left parotid gland. She comments that she has noticed the mass grow slowly over time but did not feel it was anything to worry about as it was not painful in nature. What is the most likely diagnosis?
    a. Lymphoma
    b. Pleomorphic adenoma
    c. Parotitis
    d. Parotid calculi
    e. Adenolymphoma (Warthin tumour)

11. A 25-year-old man presents with mild discomfort and occasional pain in his right ear. On examination you note some discharge from his ear. He comments that there has been no change in his hearing. What is the most likely diagnosis?
    a. Otitis externa
    b. Otitis media
    c. Mastoiditis
    d. Glue ear
    e. Otosclerosis

12. A 4-year-old boy is brought to his GP by his mother. She comments that he has been tearful and complains of pain in his right ear. She also mentions that it seems as if he is unaware of his surroundings. On examination the GP notes a red-coloured, tense-looking ear drum. What is the most likely diagnosis?
    a. Otitis externa
    b. Otitis media
    c. Mastoiditis
    d. Glue ear
    e. Otosclerosis

13. A 5-year-old boy is brought to his GP by his mother after complaining of pain in his right ear. She comments that he is continually crying and tugging on his right ear. On examination the GP notes a red-coloured ear drum. Routine observations demonstrate a temperature of 38.5°C. What is the next most appropriate step in management?
    a. Clarithromycin
    b. Erythromycin

   c. Ibuprofen
   d. Paracetamol
   e. Amoxicillin

14. A 6-year-old girl is brought to her GP by her mother. Her mother comments that her right ear is giving her trouble and that she appears inattentive at times. On examination the GP notes the eardrum is yellow in colouration and that it has been drawn inwards. What is the most likely diagnosis?
    a. Otitis externa
    b. Otitis media
    c. Mastoiditis
    d. Glue ear
    e. Otosclerosis

15. A middle-aged man complains of hearing loss and ringing in his right ear. You first perform the Rinne test and note that air conduction is better than bone conduction, but both are notably reduced as compared with normal. On performing the Weber test, you note that the sound is localized to his left ear. What is the most likely diagnosis?
    a. Ménière disease
    b. Otitis externa
    c. Acoustic neuroma
    d. Otitis media
    e. Otosclerosis

16. A 45-year-old man presents to his GP with tinnitus, hearing loss and a sensation that the room is spinning around him. The GP prescribes an antihistamine which helps to relieve his symptoms. What is the most likely diagnosis?
    a. Ménière disease
    b. Otitis externa
    c. Acoustic neuroma
    d. Otitis media
    e. Otosclerosis

17. A 36-year-old man presents to accident and emergency with a nose bleed. As you begin to assess the patient you notice the bleeding has increased in severity. He comments that he is feeling slightly dizzy and light-headed. He is hypotensive and tachycardic. Which management plan would you instigate first?
    a. Topical cocaine
    b. Cauterization of the bleeding vessel
    c. Ribbon gauze
    d. Large-bore cannula insertion and blood samples for urgent cross match
    e. Introduction of an epistaxis balloon

18. A 15-year-old woman presents with sneezing and nasal discharge having been playing in the nearby fields. Her GP informs her that she is suffering from allergic rhinitis. Which management plan would you instigate first?
    a. Intranasal antrostomy
    b. Radical antrostomy
    c. Antibiotics
    d. Oral antihistamines
    e. Steroid nasal spray

19. An elderly gentleman presents with difficulty in swallowing. He states that his initial mouthful of either solid or liquid food is fine, but then progressively gets more difficult. In addition, he states experiencing bouts of coughing episodes at night. What is the most likely diagnosis?
    a. Achalasia
    b. Diffuse oesophageal spasm
    c. Oesophageal carcinoma
    d. Pharyngeal pouch
    e. Systemic sclerosis

20. An elderly gentleman is diagnosed with squamous cell carcinoma of the neck. What is the most common risk factor for development of such a condition?
    a. Epstein–Barr virus (EBV)
    b. Smoking
    c. Human papillomavirus
    d. Gastro-oesophageal reflux disease
    e. Asbestos

21. An 18-year-old patient has a smooth lump on the left side of his neck. It is situated in the anterior triangle, under the anterior border of the sternocleidomastoid muscle and roughly one-third of the way down the sternocleidomastoid muscle. Which of the following is the most likely diagnosis?
    a. Brachial cyst
    b. Carotid artery aneurysm
    c. Chondroma
    d. Dermoid cyst
    e. Thyroglossal cyst

EXTENDED-MATCHING QUESTIONS (EMQs)

Neck swellings

Each answer can be used once, more than once or not at all.

a. Branchial cyst
b. Branchial sinus
c. Carotid body tumour
d. Parotitis
e. Sjögren syndrome
f. Pleomorphic adenoma
g. Adenolymphoma
h. Carcinoma
i. Thyroglossal cyst
j. Cystic hygroma

For each scenario below, choose the most likely corresponding option from the list given above.

1. An autoimmune condition associated with dry eyes and parotid swelling.
2. A hard, irregular, craggy lump noted within the parotid gland. There is often associated facial nerve involvement.
3. A slow-growing mass which pulsates and has a potential for malignant transformation.
4. A discharging cavity which presents anteriorly to the lower third of the sternocleidomastoid muscle.
5. A soft painless mass which transilluminates brightly and typically presents in the anterior triangle of the neck.

Neck lumps

Each answer can be used once, more than once or not at all.

a. Branchial cyst
b. Carotid artery aneurysm
c. Carotid body tumour
d. Cervical rib
e. Cystic hygroma
f. Lymph nodes
g. Pharyngeal pouch
h. Thyroglossal cyst
i. Thyroid goitre
j. Torticollis

For each scenario below, choose the most likely corresponding option from the list given above.

1. A midline lump that moves on swallowing and upon tongue protrusion. It has been present since birth.
2. Multiple lumps in the anterior triangle which do not move upon swallowing. There are similar lumps in the axilla.
3. A painless, transilluminable lump in a 25-year-old man which arises from beneath the anterior border of sternocleidomastoid in its upper third.
4. An anterior triangle lump in a 70-year-old man which does not move up on swallowing. The patient presented with a recent history of dysphagia and had not noticed the lump before.
5. A swelling which crosses the midline and has an irregular surface. It moves on swallowing but not on tongue protrusion. The patient is thin, anxious and tachycardic.

Neck swellings

Each answer can be used once, more than once or not at all.

a. Anaplastic carcinoma of the thyroid
b. Benign tumour of parotid (pleomorphic adenoma)
c. Branchial cyst
d. Papillary carcinoma of the thyroid
e. Pharyngeal pouch
f. Riedel thyroiditis
g. Solitary thyroid nodule
h. Submandibular calculus
i. Thyroglossal cyst
j. Virchow node

For each scenario below, choose the most likely corresponding option from the list given above.

1. A 56-year-old woman complains of an intermittent swelling under her jaw on the left side. The swelling increases in size and becomes painful when she eats.

2. A 70-year-old woman presents with a 2-month history of a swelling in the front of the neck. There has been a rapid increase in the size of the lump. She has become hoarse. On examination, she is noted to have an audible wheeze and there is a large hard mass in the lower anterior part of the neck.

3. A 60-year-old man presents with a $4 \times 2\,\text{cm}^2$ mass to the left of the midline in the lower neck. The mass is oval with a smooth surface. It moves upwards on swallowing.

4. A 14-year-old girl presents with a swelling on the left side of the neck. It is painless but has been slowly increasing in size. On examination, there is a smooth $5 \times 5\,\text{cm}^2$ swelling arising from beneath the anterior aspect of the upper third of the sternomastoid muscle.

5. A 65-year-old man presents with difficulty with swallowing, weight loss and vomiting. On examination he is cachexic, with a firm swelling in the left supraclavicular fossa.

SINGLE BEST ANSWER (SBA) QUESTIONS

1. A 47-year-old married male comes to your clinic complaining of right testicular pain that developed quickly over the last 24 hours. He has a recent history of having a catheter put in post-appendectomy. He reports no fever, dysuria, or urethral discharge. His abdominal examination is normal but he has an enlarged, exquisitely tender right hemi-scrotum. A urinalysis is normal and his white blood cell count is 13 × 10^9/L. Testicular ultrasonography shows increased blood flow in the affected testicle and epididymis. What is the most appropriate initial treatment in this patient?
   a. Ceftriaxone
   b. Clindamycin
   c. Famciclovir
   d. Ofloxacin
   e. Urgent urology review

2. A 75-year-old male with a past medical history of gout and a recent chemotherapy regimen presents with right flank pain. He tells you the pain was rapid in onset and radiates to his groin. Laboratory analysis shows microscopic haematuria. A renal ultrasound (USS KUB) is negative but a noncontrast computed tomography (CT) scan is diagnostic. Which of the following should be used to prevent this condition from occurring again?
   a. Citrate
   b. Sodium restriction
   c. Penicillamine
   d. Thiazide diuretics
   e. Surgery

3. A 62-year-old man presents with sudden onset loin pain, urinary frequency and dysuria. On examination he is pyrexic, with a temperature of 38.2°C. He appears notably confused. What is the next most appropriate initial investigation?
   a. Urinalysis and culture
   b. Abdominal ultrasound
   c. Intravenous urogram
   d. Abdominal X-ray
   e. Prostate specific antigen (PSA)

4. An 82-year-old man presents with a 3-month history of weak stream, straining and hesitancy. Examination reveals a severely enlarged prostate. A urinalysis is normal and the PSA level is 4.2 μg/L (3.0 nanograms/mL). Which amongst the following options is the correct treatment for benign prostatic hyperplasia (BPH)?
   a. α-Adrenergic antagonists that reduce the smooth muscle tone
   b. β-Reductase agonist that increase smooth muscle tone
   c. β-Reductase agonist that reduce smooth muscle tone
   d. 5α-Reductase inhibitors that reduce smooth muscle tone
   e. 5α-Reductase inhibitors that increase smooth muscle tone

5. A 23-year-old woman presents with urinary frequency and dysuria. Routine observations confirm a temperature of 38.7°C. Blood cultures are taken which demonstrate the growth of gram-negative organisms. Which management plan would you instigate first?
   a. Oral antibiotics
   b. Intravenous antibiotics
   c. Oral fluids
   d. Urinary catheterization
   e. Analgesia

6. A previously fit and well 22-year-old student presents to his general practitioner (GP) with an incidental finding of a painless testicular lump. He has a past medical history of an undescended testis at birth. Clinical examination shows a hard, nontender mass on his left testis which does not transilluminate. Which of the following tests will have to be performed to investigate this mass?
   a. Testicular ultrasound
   b. CT scan of lungs, abdomen and pelvis
   c. Alpha-fetoprotein (AFP)
   d. β-Human chorionic gonadotropin (β-HCG)
   e. All of the above

7. A 45-year-old man presents with urinary frequency, dysuria and haematuria. On examination you note suprapubic tenderness. What is the most likely diagnosis?
   a. Pyelonephritis
   b. Interstitial cystitis
   c. Prostatitis
   d. Acute cystitis
   e. Epididymo-orchitis

8. A previous fit and well 45-year-old man presents to the emergency department with a 1-day history of severe left sided loin pain radiating to his groin. Plain abdominal radiograph reveals a left ureteral calculus. Urinalysis shows a trace of blood but nil else. What is the most likely composition of his calculus?
   a. Cystine
   b. Uric acid
   c. Calcium oxalate
   d. Magnesium-ammonium phosphate
   e. Iron deposits

9. A 41-year-old man presents with urinary frequency, dysuria and urgency. Urine cultures are taken which reveal no bacterial organisms. What is the most likely diagnosis?
   a. Pyelonephritis
   b. Interstitial cystitis
   c. Prostatitis
   d. Acute cystitis
   e. Epididymo-orchitis

10. A 62-year-old man presents with urinary frequency and dysuria. On examination you note tenderness in the lower abdomen. On rectal examination you note tenderness on palpation of his prostate. What is the most likely diagnosis?
    a. Pyelonephritis
    b. Interstitial cystitis
    c. Prostatitis
    d. Acute cystitis
    e. Epididymo-orchitis

11. A 31-year-old man presents with an acute onset severe, colicky right flank pain radiating down into the groin. Over the past 3 days he has increased frequency, dysuria and haematuria. Which of the following is the most common metabolic abnormality associated with this patient's condition?
    a. Hypercalciuria
    b. Increased urine citrate
    c. Hyperuricaemia
    d. Alkaline urinary pH
    e. Hypernatraemia

12. A fit and well 55-year-old man sees his GP for advice. Both his father and uncle suffer from prostate cancer, and he is concerned that he might also be at risk. He has read some information regarding PSA and is requesting the blood test to screen for prostate cancer. Which of the following statements is not true regarding PSA?
    a. PSA is a protein produced by cells of the prostate gland
    b. PSA is sensitive and specific for prostate cancer

c. PSA is elevated in prostatitis
d. PSA is elevated in BPH
e. PSA is used to monitor the recurrence of prostate cancer

13. A 25-year-old sexually active man presents with testicular pain and vomiting. On examination you note his testicles are swollen and tender. A urine dipstick reveals 3+ leucocytes, 2+ nitrites but no blood. What is the most likely diagnosis?
    a. Pyelonephritis
    b. Interstitial cystitis
    c. Prostatitis
    d. Acute cystitis
    e. Epididymo-orchitis

14. A 70-year-old man sees his GP with a 1-month history of painless haematuria, urinary frequency and mild pelvic and lower back discomfort. He recalls a transient episode of haematuria in his childhood when he lived in West Africa. Clinical examination is unremarkable. What is the most likely diagnosis?
    a. Transitional cell carcinoma of urinary bladder
    b. Adenocarcinoma of urinary bladder
    c. Acute infection of urinary bladder
    d. Squamous cell carcinoma of urinary bladder
    e. Stone in the urinary bladder

15. A 49-year-old woman presents with loin pain and haematuria. On examination you note a mass in her right loin. Which investigation is most likely to lead to a diagnosis?
    a. Urea and electrolytes
    b. Abdominal CT scan
    c. Chest X-ray
    d. Intravenous urogram
    e. Urinalysis

16. A 50-year-old man presents to his GP with a 1-month history of dull ache within the right side of his scrotum, which he describes as a 'dragging sensation'. Clinical examination reveals a nontender, twisted mass along the right spermatic cord that feels like a bag of worms, which does not change in size in the supine position. The rest of the scrotal examination is unremarkable. What is the most important investigation in this case?
    a. PSA blood test
    b. Plain chest radiograph
    c. Plain abdominal radiograph
    d. Urinalysis
    e. CT of the abdomen

17. A middle-aged man is recently diagnosed with renal cell carcinoma of his left kidney without evidence of distant metastasis. What is the next most appropriate step in management?
    a. Embolization of the renal artery
    b. Radiotherapy
    c. Chemotherapy
    d. Radical nephrectomy
    e. Hormonal treatments

18. A 26-year-old man presents with severe colicky pain in his right loin which radiates to his right groin. A urine dipstick is positive for blood. An intravenous urogram is requested which demonstrates a ureteric stone approximately 3 mm in size. Following appropriate analgesia, which management plan is most appropriate in the first instance?
    a. Extracorporeal shockwave lithotripsy
    b. Percutaneous nephrolithotomy
    c. Open surgical removal
    d. Ureteric stenting
    e. Allow for the stone to pass spontaneously

19. A 26-year-old man presents with severe colicky pain in his right loin which radiates to his right groin. A urine dipstick proves positive for blood and nitrites. An intravenous urogram is requested which demonstrates a ureteric stone approximately 4 mm in size. Which management plan would you instigate first?
    a. Analgesia
    b. Commence an α-blocker
    c. Open surgical removal
    d. Arrange referral for extracorporeal shockwave lithotripsy
    e. Antibiotics

20. A 68-year-old man presents to the urology outpatients clinic with urinary urgency and frequency which is worse when he exercises. This has gradually worsened over a period of weeks. What is the most likely diagnosis?
    a. A bladder cancer
    b. A bladder stone
    c. A renal stone
    d. Prostatitis
    e. Urinary infection

21. A 65-year-old smoker presents with painless haematuria. Routine examination proves unremarkable. Routine blood investigations reveal a urea of 15.4 mmol/L and creatinine of 154 μmol/L. You suspect a diagnosis of bladder cancer. What is the next most appropriate initial investigation?
    a. Cystoscopy and biopsy
    b. Chest X-ray
    c. Intravenous urogram

    d. Abdominal magnetic resonance imaging scan
    e. Abdominal CT scan

22. A 60-year-old man presents with painless haematuria. A cystoscopy confirms the presence of a tumour in his bladder, which is malignant on biopsy. He undergoes a staging CT scan which confirms involvement of the superficial muscle and no evidence of distant metastases. What is the next most appropriate step in management?
    a. Radical cystectomy
    b. Radiotherapy
    c. Systemic chemotherapy
    d. Transurethral resection
    e. Watchful waiting

23. A 72-year-old man presents with urinary frequency and nocturia. You suspect a diagnosis of BPH. According to the International Prostate Symptom Score, his symptoms are classified as mild. What is the next most appropriate step in management?
    a. Watchful waiting
    b. Radical prostatectomy
    c. Radiotherapy
    d. 5α-Reductase inhibitors
    e. α-Blockers

24. You are called to see a 65-year-old man following a transurethral resection of the prostate (TURP). He has lost consciousness and is having uncontrolled rhythmic tonic clonic movements of his arms and legs. Which of the following is most likely to be the cause of his symptoms?
    a. Hypernatraemia
    b. Hyperkalaemia
    c. Hyponatraemia
    d. Hypokalaemia
    e. Withdrawal of anaesthetic drugs

25. A 35-year-old man presents with a lump in his scrotum. On examination the lump is translucent and nontender. You find it difficult to identify the testes and epididymis separately. What is the most likely diagnosis?
    a. Hydrocele
    b. Epididymo-orchitis
    c. Epididymal cyst
    d. Testicular tumour
    e. Testicular torsion

26. A 24-year-old man presents with a lump in his scrotum. On examination the lump is non-translucent and extremely tender. You find it difficult to identify the testes and epididymis. What is the most likely diagnosis?
    a. Hydrocele
    b. Epididymo-orchitis
    c. Epididymal cyst

d. Testicular tumour
e. Testicular torsion

27. A 56-year-old male presents to his GP with a fever and backache. He also complains of a poor stream when urinating. A rectal (PR) examination reveals a tender and boggy prostate which is of a regular size. Which of the following drugs should this patient be prescribed?
   a. Amoxicillin
   b. Ciprofloxacin
   c. Doxazosin
   d. Finasteride
   e. Trimethoprim

28. A 60-year old male patient presents with painless haematuria after being referred by the GP. Urinary cytology was positive. What is the most likely diagnosis?
   a. A clear cell renal cancer
   b. A renal transitional cell cancer
   c. Adenocarcinoma of the bladder
   d. Prostatic adenocarcinoma
   e. Transitional cell cancer (TCC) of the bladder

29. A 32-year-old man presents with a lump in his scrotum. On examination the lump is translucent, separate from the testes and is nontender. What is the most likely diagnosis?
   a. Hydrocele
   b. Epididymo-orchitis
   c. Epididymal cyst
   d. Testicular tumour
   e. Testicular torsion

30. A 76-year-old man was seen in accident and emergency with abdominal discomfort. On examination he has a nontender, dome-shaped cystic mass dull to percussion reaching to the umbilicus. Investigation reveal Hb is 96g/L, serum urea is 15mmol/L, serum creatinine is 160mmol/L. What is the most appropriate next step in patient care?
   a. Abdominal CT scan
   b. Sigmoidoscopy
   c. Suprapubic aspiration
   d. X-ray of the abdomen
   e. Urinary catheterization

31. A 16-year-old boy presents with sudden onset severe pain in his left scrotum and vomiting. On examination you note evidence of scrotal erythema and tenderness on palpation; upon elevation of the scrotum, there is no relief of pain. A urine dipstick proves negative. What is the most likely diagnosis?
   a. Hydrocele
   b. Epididymitis
   c. Epididymal cyst

d. Testicular tumour
e. Testicular torsion

EXTENDED-MATCHING QUESTIONS (EMQs)

Scrotal swellings

Each answer can be used once, more than once or not at all.

   a. Direct inguinal hernia
   b. Epididymal cyst
   c. Hydrocele
   d. Hydrocele of the cord
   e. Indirect inguinal hernia
   f. Lipoma
   g. Lymph node
   h. Spermatocele
   i. Testicular tumour
   j. Varicocele

For each scenario below, choose the most likely corresponding option from the list given above.

1. A 40-year-old man presents with a tense lump in the scrotum which has appeared over the last 3 weeks and is mildly tender. It is transilluminable and the testis cannot be felt separately.
2. A 22-year-old man presents with a tender lump in his scrotum that his girlfriend noticed in the shower. He has lost a stone in weight over the last 2 months, and clinically, there is a lump attached to the testis.
3. A 30-year-old man presents with a large lump in the scrotum that came on a few days ago. It is large, tense and you cannot feel above it. It is nontender and non-transilluminable, and it has a cough impulse.
4. A 35-year-old man presents with a left-sided lump in the scrotum. He says that it disappears when he lies down. Upon palpation, the lump is inconsistent in nature and feels very mobile.

Lower urinary tract symptoms

Each answer can be used once, more than once or not at all.

   a. Acontractile bladder
   b. Benign prostatic hypertrophy
   c. Bladder neck stenosis
   d. Low-pressure, low-flow voiding
   e. Multiple sclerosis
   f. Prolapsed intervertebral disc
   g. Prostatic cancer
   h. Spinal canal stenosis
   i. Stress incontinence
   j. Urethral stricture

For each scenario below, choose the most likely corresponding option from the list given above.

1. A 70-year-old man presents with a 5-year history of a poor flow, hesitancy, frequency, nocturia and postmicturition dribbling. A flow rate showed a Q max of 7 mL/s with a voided volume of 270mL and a residual of 100mL.
2. A 40-year-old woman presents with urinary incontinence when coughing, sneezing and during her fitness class. She has had three children delivered vaginally. The first labour was prolonged and she had a repair of a second-degree tear.
3. A 16-year-old man presents with a long history of hesitancy and worsening urinary stream. He also complains of postmicturition dribbling, which may occur some minutes after he completes his normal void. He had a significant fall astride a bar injury as a child.
4. A 40-year-old woman presents with urinary frequency, urgency and episodes of urge incontinence. She had a transient episode of unilateral blindness 2 years prior to these new symptoms.
5. A 40-year-old man has a long history of intermittent low back pain but develops acute onset of difficulty passing urine. On examination he has a palpable bladder and an area of saddle anaesthesia.

Urological investigations

Each answer can be used once, more than once or not at all.

a. Urine dipstick
b. Cystoscopy
c. Serum PSA
d. Renal ultrasound scan
e. Abdominal CT scan
f. Serum urea and creatinine
g. Urodynamic studies (cystometrogram)
h. Abdominal X-ray of kidneys, ureters and bladder (KUB)
i. Intravenous urography
j. Renal aortography

For each scenario below, choose the most likely corresponding option from the list given above.

1. A patient presenting with dysuria and frequency. Routine observations reveal a temperature of 38.6°C.
2. A 25-year-old long-distance runner presenting with severe right-sided loin pain and vomiting.

3. A middle-aged man presenting with urinary hesitancy, a poor stream and terminal dribbling postmicturition with evidence of renal dysfunction.
4. A 75-year-old man presenting with urinary frequency, nocturia and weight loss. An irregular mass is evident on the prostate on digital examination.
5. A middle-aged female who has had five vaginal deliveries presenting with urinary leakage when coughing or laughing.

Urgent urological referrals

Each answer can be used once, more than once or not at all.

a. Benign prostatic hypertrophy
b. Cystitis
c. Epididymitis
d. Lymphoma
e. Priapism
f. Prostate cancer
g. Pyelonephritis
h. Seminoma of testis
i. Teratoma of testis
j. Testicular torsion
k. Ureteric colic
l. Urinary tract infection

For each scenario below, choose the most likely corresponding option from the list given above.

1. A 19-year-old man presents with a firm, nontender lump in his right testicle.
2. A 23-year-old woman presents with right-sided loin pain which radiates to the groin. The pain comes and goes in waves. She also complains of frequency of micturition. Dipstick urine test reveals 4+ blood. The only abnormality on examination is tenderness in the right loin.
3. An 88-year-old man presents via his GP with suprapubic pain and a history of frequency and passing only very small amounts of urine for 1 week. He has had long-standing problems with nocturia and poor stream. He has a tender palpable mass arising from the pelvis. His PSA is < 5ng/mL (NR 0–4ng/mL).
4. A 52-year-old man presents with a 3-day history of dysuria and frequency and a gradual onset of left testicular pain and swelling. Dipstick urine reveals 3+ blood, 2+ leukocytes and nitrites.

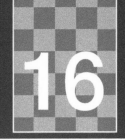

Breast surgery 16

SINGLE BEST ANSWER (SBA) QUESTIONS

1. A 45-year-old woman presents to her general practitioner (GP) with a unilateral erythematous, itchy rash around her nipple. On examination her nipple is inverted. Which of the following is the most likely diagnosis?
   a. Ductal carcinoma in-situ
   b. Infective mastitis
   c. Lobular carcinoma in-situ
   d. Medullary carcinoma
   e. Nipple eczema

2. A 35-year-old woman presents to her GP complaining of a lump in the upper outer quadrant of her right breast. She comments the lump becomes particularly tender before the start of her menstrual cycle. What is the most likely diagnosis?
   a. Localised fibroadenosis
   b. Fibroadenoma
   c. Cyst
   d. Fat necrosis
   e. Carcinoma

3. A 31-year-old woman presents complaining of a lump in her left breast. On examination you note the lump is nontender, rubbery and fairly mobile. What is the most likely diagnosis?
   a. Localised fibroadenosis
   b. Cyst
   c. Fat necrosis
   d. Fibroadenoma
   e. Carcinoma

4. A 67-year-old woman had her breast cancer removed with breast conserving surgery 2 weeks ago. Subsequently, she notices a painless lump beneath the incision. On examination she is apyrexial, the lump is nontender, firm and well circumscribed. What is the most likely diagnosis?
   a. Abscess
   b. Cystic disease
   c. Fat necrosis
   d. Fibroadenoma
   e. Recurrence of the cancer

5. A 35-year-old woman presents with a lump on her right breast. On examination you note the lump is tense and mobile. On fine-needle aspiration you note the production of a straw-coloured fluid. What is the most likely diagnosis?
   a. Localised fibroadenosis
   b. Fibroadenoma
   c. Fat necrosis
   d. Carcinoma
   e. Cyst

6. A 34-year-old woman smoker presents with a green-coloured discharge from both her nipples. On examination you note evidence of nipple retraction and breast lumpiness. What is the most likely diagnosis?
   a. Mammary duct ectasia
   b. Duct papilloma
   c. Galactorrhoea
   d. Duct carcinoma
   e. Paget disease

7. A middle-aged woman presents with a serous discharge from her right nipple. On examination the breast appears normal but on deep palpation the discharge is produced. What is the most likely diagnosis?
   a. Mammary duct ectasia
   b. Duct papilloma
   c. Galactorrhoea
   d. Duct carcinoma
   e. Paget disease

8. A 57-year-old woman has been recently diagnosed with breast cancer. Her GP comments she was at high risk due to her strong family history of breast cancer. The GP explains that particular chromosomes are linked to the condition. Which chromosome is most likely to be associated with breast cancer?
   a. Chromosome 14
   b. Chromosome 15
   c. Chromosome 16
   d. Chromosome 17
   e. Chromosome 18

9. A 45-year-old woman is concerned about developing breast cancer. She comes to see you asking when she will be called for a 'screening mammogram'. At what ages do women in the UK undergo screening as part of a National Programme?
   a. 50–70
   b. 45–59
   c. 55–69
   d. 46–60
   e. 56–70

10. A 54-year-old woman presents with a 5 cm lump in her right breast. On examination you note the presence of fixed, right-sided axillary nodes. There are no palpable supraclavicular or infraclavicular nodes. You refer her for tissue biopsies. The histology report confirms the presence of a moderately differentiated adenocarcinoma with no evidence of distant metastasis. According to the International Union against Cancer, what is the most likely staging classification of this presentation?
    a. Stage 1
    b. Stage 2
    c. Stage 3
    d. Stage 4
    e. Stage 5

11. A 52-year-old woman presents with a lump approximately 4 cm in size in her right breast. On examination you note no palpable nodes in her axilla, supraclavicular or infraclavicular region. Wide local excision and axillary node clearance confirm the presence of a well-differentiated cancer with no evidence of lymph node involvement. According to the International Union against Cancer, what is the most likely 5-year survival rate for this presentation?
    a. 84%
    b. 71%
    c. 59%
    d. 48%
    e. 18%

12. A 64-year-old woman presents with a lump in her left breast. On examination the lump is nontender and painless. In addition, you note dimpling of the skin and retraction of her left nipple. You refer her for urgent tissue biopsies, which confirm the presence of an adenocarcinoma with associated fibrosis. Having explained the diagnosis, you explain that this tumour is the most common type of tumour to affect women. What is the most likely diagnosis?
    a. Ductal
    b. Lobular
    c. Medullary
    d. Colloid
    e. Sarcoma

13. A 28-year-old woman presents with a lump on her right breast. On examination you note the lump is tense, discrete and mobile. You suspect the possibility of a breast cyst. Which investigation is the most appropriate in this scenario?
    a. Mammography
    b. Computed tomography chest scan
    c. Magnetic resonance imaging chest scan
    d. Ultrasound
    e. Chest X-ray

14. A 39-year-old woman is diagnosed with left-sided breast cancer. The tumour is confirmed as an oestrogen-receptor-negative, well-differentiated adenocarcinoma, approximately 6.5 cm in size. There is involvement of ipsilateral axillary nodes but no evidence of distant metastasis. She is referred to a breast surgeon who explains possible treatment options. What is the next most appropriate step in management?
    a. Neoadjuvant chemotherapy and surgical excision with axillary clearance
    b. Primary surgical excision of tumour without axillary dissection
    c. Radiotherapy
    d. Tamoxifen
    e. Herceptin

15. A middle-aged woman presents with a scaly red coloured rash affecting her right nipple and areola. She comments it is sore and has a tendency to bleed. What is the most likely diagnosis?
    a. Mammary duct ectasia
    b. Duct papilloma
    c. Galactorrhoea
    d. Duct carcinoma
    e. Paget disease

16. A 52-year-old woman presents with a fairly large painless lump in her left breast. On examination you note it appears fleshy and has a characteristic tear drop shaped appearance. What is the most likely diagnosis?
    a. Fibroadenoma
    b. Duct papilloma
    c. Phyllodes tumour
    d. Duct carcinoma
    e. Paget disease

EXTENDED-MATCHING QUESTIONS (EMQs)

Management of breast cancer
Each answer can be used once, more than once or not at all.

    a. Cyclophosphamide
    b. Trastuzumab (Herceptin)
    c. Tamoxifen
    d. Anastrozole
    e. Doxorubicin
    f. Raloxifene
    g. Vincristine
    h. Dexamethasone
    i. Paclitaxel
    j. Faslodex

For each scenario below, choose the most likely corresponding option from the list given above.

1. A therapeutic agent highly recommended in the treatment of lymph-node-positive HER2-positive breast cancer.
2. A selective oestrogen-receptor modulator drug useful in the treatment of breast cancer but associated with risks of endometrial cancer and pulmonary embolism.
3. An aromatase inhibitor useful in the treatment of early breast cancer in postmenopausal women.
4. A therapeutic agent useful in the treatment of breast cancer but known to cause left ventricular failure and pulmonary toxicity.
5. A therapeutic agent useful in the treatment of breast cancer but known to cause bladder cancer.

Breast lumps

Each answer can be used once, more than once or not at all.

a. Breast abscess
b. Cyst
c. Duct ectasia
d. Fat necrosis
e. Fibroadenoma
f. Fibrocystic change
g. Galactorrhoea
h. Lipoma
i. Mastitis
j. Papilloma

For each scenario below, choose the most likely corresponding option from the list given above.

1. A 19-year-old woman presents with a highly mobile lump in her breast. Fine-needle aspiration shows no malignancy.
2. A 28-year-old woman, four weeks postpartum, presents to her GP with a tender lump in the upper outer quadrant of her left breast. On examination it is ill-defined, erythematous and hot to touch.
3. A 38-year-old very anxious woman presents with a hard, irregular lump in her breast. On examination it is craggy and well-defined. Fine-needle aspiration shows no evidence of malignancy. On further questioning, she reveals that she was involved in a car crash 6 months previously.
4. A 42-year-old woman presents with a yellow-brown discharge from her nipples. On examination her discharge appears to be coming from multiple ducts. Examination is otherwise normal and mammography is unremarkable.
5. A 32-year-old woman presents with a lump in her breast which is painless. On examination it is well demarcated, fluctuant and transilluminable.

MEDICINE ANSWERS

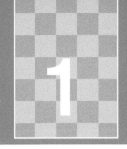

Cardiology 1

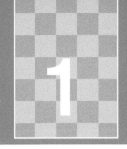

SBA ANSWERS

Question 1

D. Hypertrophic cardiomyopathy (HCM) is the most common cause of sudden cardiac death in young athletes in the UK. It is autosomal dominant with variable penetrance. Long QT syndrome is a cause of sudden death in the young athlete, but is less common. Wolff–Parkinson–White is caused by the presence of an abnormal accessory electrical conduction pathway between the atria and the ventricles. Electrical signals travelling down this abnormal pathway (known as the bundle of Kent) may stimulate the ventricles to contract prematurely, resulting in a unique type of supraventricular tachycardia (SVT) (referred to as an atrioventricular (AV) reciprocating tachycardia) but is less common than HCM.

Question 2

D. Treatment with spironolactone reduces mortality along with beta-blockers, ACE I, angiotensin receptor blockers (ARBs) and other aldosterone antagonists. Beta-blockers and ACE I reduce the degree of neurohormonal activation in heart failure. Beta-blockers are contraindicated in acute heart failure (HF), but are often used during stable period of HF to modulate the sympathetic system.

Question 3

A. Sick sinus syndrome is characterized by a time interval of greater than 2 seconds between consecutive P waves. The very slow P rate and relatively stable ventricular rate suggest a sinoatrial problem rather than an AV nodal problem. Thromboembolism is a feature and patients often require anticoagulation.

Question 4

C. Also known as Wenckebach phenomenon. This arrhythmia is characterized by an increasing PR interval until the P wave no longer conducts to the ventricles.

Question 5

D. Adenosine should be given to stop SVT or to slow down the conduction to reveal underlying rhythm. IV amiodarone can often be given for any supraventricular or ventricular tachycardias upon cardiology advice. However, it is not used to terminate SVT; adenosine is used instead. IV lignocaine can be given for VT with pulse if bisoprolol is contraindicated.

Question 6

C. Narrow complex regular tachycardia is invariably SVT. Slowing down the rhythm with IV adenosine may break the re-entrant circuit and back into normal rhythm. If there is response to adenosine, then the rhythm may slow down if it is atrial flutter (to reveal sawtooth pattern ECG). Lack of response to adenosine means underlying rhythm is likely sinus tachycardia or paroxysmal atrial tachycardia.

Question 7

B. First-degree heart block is the result of delayed atrioventricular conduction and is characterized by a PR interval greater than 0.22 seconds.

Question 8

E. Digoxin, with warfarin. Rate control is good for elderly patients, but this patient has a CHADSVASC risk score that needs anticoagulation too. The elderly patient is asymptomatic and has enlarged left atrium, which means that he has a smaller chance to cardiovert out of.

Question 9

D. Second-degree block is characterized by an intermittent failure or interruption of AV conduction but there is no increasing PR interval as is the case with Mobitz type 1 block.

Question 10

D. Treatment with statins as primary prevention should be offered to those at the highest risk of developing coronary heart disease. This patient is at risk now because of this mild elevation in lipid levels, borderline blood pressure and overweight. Alcohol consumption is associated with an increase in high-density lipoprotein cholesterol levels of as much as 9 to 13 mg/dL (0.23 to 0.34 mmol/L) when nondrinkers are compared with the highest consumers. The patient's hyperlipidaemia should be controlled by lifestyle modifications in the beginning for 4 to 6 months.

Question 11

E. Typical symptoms include blackouts and dizzy spells. Pacemaker insertion is the mainstay form of treatment.

Question 12

B. If someone is in ventricular fibrillation (on monitor or defib pads), then advanced life support (ALS) guidelines say that you need to shock in the first instance. Continue CPR until you establish the charge needed. Calcium chloride/gluconate and sodium bicarbonate IV administration are for hyperkalaemia. Carotid artery compression has no place in the ALSalgorithm.

Question 13

A. This is atrial flutter with 2:1 block and characterized by sawtooth flutter waves on the ECG.

Question 14

D. Selective coronary angiography is the definitive diagnostic test for evaluating the anatomic extent and severity of coronary artery disease. More importantly, you can treat it with balloon angioplasty to treat the lesion as well!

Question 15

E. The diagnosis is atrial flutter of recent onset and treated with electrical cardioversion in the first instance.

Question 16

E. Gastrointestinal distress such as bloating or indigestion, along with muscular imbalances and poor posture, can also irritate the vagus nerve causing palpitations, but this patient is not relating her symptoms to meals or to any intestinal problems.

Question 17

A. The diagnosis is AF. Current National Institute for Health and Clinical Excellence (NICE) guidelines state that beta-blockers are the initial choice of management for rate control.

Question 18

C. Thrombolytic therapy is indicated in patients with evidence of ST-segment elevation myocardial infarction (STEMI) or new left bundle-branch block presenting within 12 hours of the onset of symptoms, if there are no contraindications to fibrinolysis. Thrombolysis remains the treatment of choice in STEMI when primary percutaneous coronary intervention (PCI) cannot be performed within 90 minutes. The benefits of fibrinolytic therapy are well established during the initial 12 hours after symptom onset. The new guidelines mention that you should consider administration of a fibrinolytic agent in symptomatic patients presenting more than 12 to 24 hours after symptom onset with STEMI affecting a large area of myocardium or hemodynamic instability if PCI is not available.

Question 19

C. The diagnosis is an SVT. Carotid sinus massage is helpful in the acute situation. Other manoeuvres may include the Valsalva manoeuvre. Adenosine is used in the treatment of SVT but is contraindicated in this patient because of asthma.

Question 20

A. The diagnosis is pulseless electrical activity due to hypovolaemia. This is a nonshockable rhythm. Administration of colloid, saline or blood would be the next most appropriate step in management, followed by adrenaline 1 mg IV.

Question 21

B. The main features of cholesterol embolism include eosinophilia, purpura, livedo reticularis and renal injury. Usually occur in arteriopaths, or as a complication of coronary angiography, or following the commencement of anticoagulants/ thrombolytics. Treatment is supportive.

Question 22

B. Serial assessments of serum digoxin levels are not necessary in most patients. The radioimmunoassay was developed to assist in the evaluation of toxicity, rather than the efficacy of the drug. There appears to be little relationship between serum digoxin concentration and the drug's therapeutic effect. The dosage of digoxin should be 125–250mcg daily in the majority of patients. Higher doses (e.g., 375–500mcg) are rarely needed, especially as initial therapy for chronic heart failure.

Question 23

A. Typical features of mitral stenosis. Additional signs include a malar flush and tapping apex beat.

Question 24

C. This patient had a syncopal episode, which can be cardiogenic or neurogenic in origin. After the history review and physical examination, blood tests are usually sent to rule out anaemia, infections, hypocalcaemia or hypomagnesemia and an ECG must be performed. An ECG may show evidence of cardiac abnormalities such as Wolf–Parkinson–White syndrome, idiopathic hypertrophic subaortic stenosis or congenital prolonged QT syndrome.

Question 25

B. Typical features of mitral regurgitation. Additional signs include a displaced apex beat.

Question 26

D. Thiazide diuretics such as bendrofluazide can cause hypokalaemia. Afro-Caribbeans should have calcium channel blocker (CCB) as first-line antihypertensives. In cases of renal artery stenosis, ACE I is contraindicated as it may result in acute kidney injury. CCBs cause ankle swelling as a side effect.

Question 27

C. NICE no longer recommends aspirin as monotherapy to prevent stroke in people with AF (small benefit is offset by risk of bleeding). If the CHADSVASC score is 1 or greater, then NICE recommends offering anticoagulation. In this case, we have no documented AF on the ECG, and we just have one episode of self-reported palpitations. He should have a longer Holter monitor to see whether this is paroxysmal AF. His CHADSVASC score is 0 and does not warrant anticoagulation currently.

Question 28

C. Additional signs would include a slow rising carotid pulse.

Question 29

E. This is a hypertensive 'urgency' with minor end-organ damage (without papilloedema). The hypertension is longstanding, given by the ECG changes showing left ventricular hypertrophy. This will require a reduction in blood pressure (over hours) using oral agents with the goal of normal blood pressure within 24 to 48 hours. If there was haematuria (renal damage), papilloedema and mental changes, then IV therapy would need to be commenced instead.

Question 30

D. Additional signs would include a collapsing pulse, a displaced apex beat and a mid-diastolic murmur over the cardiac apex.

Question 31

C. Typical features of tricuspid regurgitation. Abdominal examination is likely to reveal an enlarged pulsatile liver.

Question 32

E. Enalapril is an ACE inhibitor. ACE inhibitors delay progression of diabetic kidney disease and are more effective than other medications in delaying the onset of kidney failure in patients who have hypertension and type 1 diabetes with macroalbuminuria.

Question 33

B. An echo is the first-line investigation in the diagnosis of cardiac murmurs.

Question 34

E. The diagnosis is mitral stenosis. A widened angle of carina (representing enlarged left atrium) on the chest X-ray can be seen.

Question 35

A. When patients present with severely elevated blood pressure (systolic blood pressure of 180 mmHg or greater, or diastolic blood pressure of 110 mmHg or greater), doctors need to differentiate hypertensive emergency from severely elevated blood pressure without signs or symptoms of end-organ damage (severe asymptomatic hypertension). Most patients who are asymptomatic but have poorly controlled hypertension do not have acute end-organ damage and, therefore, do not require immediate workup or treatment. Rapidly lowering blood pressure in A&E is unnecessary in asymptomatic patients and may be harmful (can cause watershed infarcts).

Question 36

B. The echocardiogram is the most useful investigation and may show regional wall abnormalities with ischaemia, valve abnormalities and pericardial thickening. A CXR will usually, but not always, show typical features of heart failure but will not usually demonstrate the cause.

Question 37

C. The patient is suffering from left-sided heart failure. CXR features include fluid in the right horizontal fissure, seen as a white line running over the anterior end of the fourth rib. There is no horizontal fissure in the left lung as there are only two lobes.

Question 38

A. Ischaemic heart disease is the most common cause of heart failure in the Western world.

Question 39

A. ACE I should be first-line therapy for someone with congestive heart failure. Propranolol is a rather dirty beta-blocker, and bisoprolol/metoprolol can be added once patient stabilized on ACE I. Verapamil (CCB) is not first-line to slow down the heart rate, beta-blockers are. Disopyramide is an antiarrhythmic medication used in the treatment of ventricular tachycardia. Phosphodiesterase inhibitors play no role in congestive heart failure. However, hydralazine/nitrates can be considered if patients cannot tolerate ACE I/ARB.

Question 40

E. The diagnosis is heart failure. Current guidelines state that ACE inhibitors are typically the first-line treatment in heart failure. However, as this patient is severely fluid overloaded, diuretics such as furosemide would be the first-line of treatment.

Question 41
B. This class of drug is known to cause hyperkalaemia.

Question 42
D. The diagnosis is pulmonary oedema. Furosemide is the most appropriate treatment. IV GTN (glyceryl trinitrate) may be added in if he does not respond to diuretics to reduce the cardiac preload.

Question 43
E. This patient exhibits atypical (noncardiac) chest pain and has no risk factors for coronary artery disease. Because the likelihood of coronary disease is very low, stress testing is not indicated.

Question 44
E. Low intake of folic acid is a risk factor for ischaemic heart disease.

Question 45
E. A patient with positional chest pain (occurs in conjunction with a viral infection) along with ECG changes (widespread ST changes), and a pericardial rub are consistent with a diagnosis of acute pericarditis.

Question 46
C. Such a syndrome is thought to be due in part to an abnormal coronary microcirculation. Angiograms are always normal.

Question 47
C. Hypertension may be primary, which may develop as a result of environmental or genetic causes, or secondary, which has multiple aetiologies, including renal, vascular and endocrine causes. Primary or essential hypertension (undetermined cause) accounts for 90% to 95% of adult cases and a small percentage of patients (2%–10%) have a secondary cause.

Question 48
E. Enoxaparin 1 mg/kg twice daily is the recommended dose in patients with evidence of acute coronary syndrome

Question 49
D. This patient presents with a stab wound to the chest and highly suspicious for penetrating cardiac trauma and cardiac tamponade. Always consider cardiac tamponade in a patient who presents with hypotension and silent heart sounds. Other features are neck vein distension – build-up of blood in the pericardium

elevates the pressure, which prevents blood outflow from neck veins into the mediastinum. Another feature is pulsus paradoxus, which is a blood pressure drop greater than 12 mmHg during inspiration. Normally, inspiration leads to a systolic blood pressure drop of up to 10 mmHg. Another commonly tested condition that can cause pulsus paradoxus is asthma or chronic obstructive pulmonary disease.

Question 50
B. The patient is experiencing angina, which is best treated by GTN in the first instance.

Question 51
B. Q waves indicate old infarcts and II, III and aVF indicate that it involves the right coronary artery, an inferior MI.

Question 52
E. Typical ECG changes of a posterior infarct.

Question 53
B. At present, the ICD is the most effective modality for preventing sudden death in high-risk patients with asymptomatic HCM. Because of its effects on decreasing dysrhythmias, amiodarone may decrease the risk of sudden death; however, the ICD is the most effective modality for the prevention of sudden death. Medications such as verapamil, beta-blockers and diltiazem are used for symptom management, but do not decrease the risk of sudden death.

Question 54
A. Troponin is the most appropriate investigation in individuals with chest pain as it is highly specific and sensitive for cardiac damage.

Question 55
B. ST elevation is an indication for PCI; however, if there are no PCI centres within 90 minutes of symptoms, then thrombolysis is second-line. Q waves suggest an old infarct. ST depression (V1–V3) might indicate acute true posterior MI; however, widespread STD is not an acute indication as it is likely to represent digitalis effect (it would be highly unlikely that an obstruction would affect so many coronary vessels globally).

Question 56
D. Aspirin 300 mg is the recommended immediate management in a suspected MI.

Question 57
A. According to the Duke criteria, the presence of a new murmur (or changing characteristic of an existing one) is a major criterion for infective endocarditis. Along with positive blood cultures, it would be diagnostic.

Question 58

D. Pericarditis is an early complication of an MI and typically occurs within the first 2–4 days.

Question 59

B. Congestive heart failure can cause mild jaundice due to hepatic congestion from excess fluid with hepatic venous system (deranged liver function tests will normalize once patient is off-loaded and back to dry body weight). Consider also eventual cardioversion for AF, which will increase ejection fraction and improve symptoms.

Question 60

D. This is the most likely organism to cause infective endocarditis in intravenous drug abusers and those with central venous lines.

Question 61

A. This is the most likely offending organism associated with dental diseases or procedures.

Question 62

E. Whilst all of the conditions give the patient a higher risk for infective endocarditis, NICE guidelines (2015) do not recommend prophylaxis antibiotics.

Question 63

A. A splenic abscess is more likely to be due to embolization of vegetations of fibrin and platelets.

Question 64

E. The most likely diagnosis is infective endocarditis typically confirmed by three sets of blood cultures in the first instance.

Question 65

A. Classic features of a dilated cardiomyopathy.

Question 66

C. Patients with Marfan syndrome often develop mitral valve prolapse or ascending aortic aneurysms (which can lead to fatal aortic dissections). As the ascending aorta dilates, the aortic valve annulus also stretches and may lead to regurgitation.

Question 67

B. Additional features include a jerky carotid pulse and an ejection systolic murmur.

Question 68

A. Classic presentation of pericarditis. Management is usually with nonsteroidal antiinflammatory drugs (NSAIDs) or corticosteroids.

Question 69

D. Symptoms of aortic stenosis are syncope, angina and dyspnoea. Usually presents in elderly patient. ECG shows left ventricular hypertrophy. Once you suspect aortic stenosis and patient has symptoms of angina, do echocardiography before ordering stress test as there is risk of sudden death. If stenosis is severe, take patient to cardiac cath to assess concomitant coronary artery disease and if planned for surgery, then both valvular surgery and coronary artery bypass grafting can be done at the same time.

Question 70

B. This patient has developed a pericardial effusion. Echo is diagnostic.

Question 71

C. According to current guidelines, ACE inhibitors are the first-line management of hypertension in diabetic patients.

Question 72

E. The Duke diagnostic classification for IE divides signs and symptoms into major and minor criteria. IE is diagnosed if patients have two major criteria, or one major and three minor criteria or five minor criteria. Microbiological evidence that is considered as minor criteria includes the following: positive blood culture that does not meet the requirements of a positive blood culture as mentioned in the major criteria, or serological evidence of active infection with an organism consistent with IE.

Question 73

C. Additional features include 'cotton wool' exudates.

Question 74

D. Infective endocarditis is most commonly due to *Streptococcus viridans*, which is a normal flora of the mouth and thus frequently enters the bloodstream after dental procedures. Preexisting valvular heart disease increases the risk of endocarditis and a new regurgitation murmur should raise suspicion as the pathogen can destroy valve leaflets.

Question 75

C. Many medications interfere with the absorption, metabolism and pharmacological action of ACE inhibitors. Of the choices given, the one most likely to do this is ibuprofen, a commonly used NSAID. NSAIDs may attenuate the haemodynamic actions of ACE inhibitors. NSAIDs reduce renal excretion of ACE inhibitors, with a corresponding increase in circulating drug concentrations.

Question 76

E. Enalapril is an ACE inhibitor. ACE inhibitors delay progression of diabetic kidney disease and are more effective than other medications in delaying the onset of kidney failure in patients who have hypertension and type 1 diabetes with macroalbuminuria. CCBs reduce cardiovascular events in patients with diabetes and hypertension; however, they may be inferior to other agents in some cardiovascular outcomes. Dihydropyridine and nondihydropyridine CCBs are less effective than ACE inhibitors and ARBs in slowing progression of diabetic kidney disease. Because CCBs may be inferior in some patient-oriented outcomes in those with diabetes, they should be reserved for patients who cannot tolerate preferred agents or those who need additional agents to achieve target blood pressure.

EMQ ANSWERS

Cardiac murmurs and added sounds

1. A   Aortic regurgitation. The early diastolic murmur is best heard at the left sternal edge, with the patient leaning forward and the breath held in expiration.
2. E   Mitral stenosis. Acquired mitral stenosis is usually due to rheumatic fever, now a very rare disease in the West, but still common in the developing world.
3. B   Aortic stenosis. Patients may also present with angina, even in the absence of severe coronary arterial disease, due to a combination of increased oxygen requirements and fixed flow obstruction.
4. D   Mitral regurgitation. This often occurs because of papillary muscle or chorda rupture.
5. I   Ventricular septal defect. A more common presentation is an asymptomatic ejection systolic murmur detected on routine examination.

Chest pain

1. A   Typical presentation of angina pectoris.
2. C   Classic features of a myocardial infarction. Additional features would include sweating, breathlessness, nausea and vomiting.
3. D   There may also be unequal blood pressure in both arms.
4. H   Classic description of costochondritis.
5. B   Pain may also radiate to the neck and shoulders.

Drugs

1. E   Captopril is an ACE inhibitor, which can lead to a cough due to inhibition of bradykinin metabolism. Other side effects include renal failure and angioedema.
2. E   ACE inhibitors such as captopril can affect renal function in patients with renovascular disease. This is due to elimination of efferent vasoconstriction which leads to a decrease in the glomerular filtration rate.
3. D   Typical side effects of CCBs.
4. C   Aspirin is regarded as the gold standard in the management of acute coronary syndrome.
5. A   This is due to bronchoconstrictive and vasoconstrictive effects.

Clinical features of cardiac disease

1. D   Classic features of mitral regurgitation.
2. E   Additional features would include Roth spots and Osler nodes.
3. F   The pink-coloured rings are characteristic of erythema marginatum seen typically in rheumatic fever. One would also expect to suffer from arthritis and cardiac murmurs.
4. A   Classic presentation of aortic stenosis.
5. I   Additional features include chest pain and dyspnoea.

Murmurs

1. H   Tricuspid regurgitation. He may have caught schistosomiasis in Egypt, affecting the tricuspid valve.
2. F   Mitral regurgitation. The apex is displaced.
3. J   Ventricular septal defect. Down syndrome with congenital heart defects.
4. A   Aortic regurgitation. Murmurs can be discriminated by the pattern of murmur, where it is loudest, and any features that make it louder (in this case sitting forward).
5. E   Graham Steell murmur. An uncommon murmur, typically associated with pulmonary regurgitation.

Symptoms of heart failure

1. G   Pulmonary fibrosis. This patient has been treated with diuretics and is hypovolaemic. He may have had pulmonary oedema; however, this has resolved. Pulmonary fibrosis may give very similar auscultatory findings to pulmonary oedema.
2. E   Paroxysmal nocturnal dyspnoea. These are episodes of acute breathlessness that usually occur at night and may result in the patient getting out of bed and pulling the window open. It happens in left heart failure due to fluid redistribution, but there are other causes.
3. D   Orthopnoea. Breathlessness occurring on lying flat; it is often described in terms of how many pillows a patient requires to get to sleep (e.g., 'four-pillow orthopnoea'). It is seen in left heart failure.
4. B   Cough. ACE inhibitors may cause a chronic cough that can persist for up to 1 month after cessation

of treatment; this is likely due to decreased bradykinin breakdown.

5. C Hepatomegaly. Hepatomegaly can be seen in right heart failure due to hepatic venous congestion. This can lead to a macroscopic 'nutmeg' appearance.

Electrocardiograph findings

1. G Posterior myocardial infarction. Because of lead placement, posterior myocardial infarction changes are the reverse of those elsewhere: dominant R waves equivalent to Q waves and ST depression instead of elevation.
2. F Pericarditis. These changes may be less marked as T-wave inversion. The widespread nature and saddle shape allow distinction from myocardial infarction.
3. E Inferior myocardial infarction.
4. D Digitalis effect. Complete (also known as third-degree) heart block: the ventricular escape rate of 45 beats/min, broad complex QRS and presence of P waves (which will be at a rate of 70 beats/min) confirm this diagnosis.
5. C Atrial flutter with 2:1 block. Any rhythm at 150 beats/min should prompt a search for 'sawtooth' P waves to exclude flutter.

Heart disease

1. H Infective endocarditis. Known valve disease plus a minor procedure leading to fever should be considered infective endocarditis until proven otherwise.

2. B Aortic stenosis. This gentleman has all three of the classical symptoms of aortic stenosis. He should be assessed for valve surgery, as the presence of these symptoms increases the risk of sudden cardiac death in these patients.
3. G Fibrinous pericarditis. This is suggested by the speed of postmyocardial infarction onset, relief by NSAIDs and classical ST changes.
4. F Dilated cardiomyopathy. This is associated with excess alcohol consumption. The clinical findings are classic with the mitral murmur caused by dilatation of the annulus.
5. E Cor pulmonale. This is suggested by the ankle swelling (sign of right heart failure) on top of chronic lung disease.

Chest pain

1. B Pulmonary embolus. Sinus tachycardia, right bundle-branch block and pleuritic chest pains should point you towards pulmonary embolus.
2. F Gastro-oesophageal reflux disease (GORD) (secondary to NSAID). Taking NSAIDs and having large body mass index are risk factors for GORD.
3. C Pericarditis.
4. E Rib fracture (with associated pneumothorax). CXR shows pneumothorax, which can give a pleuritic pain.
5. A Myocardial infarct (lateral). Elevated troponin and ST elevation point to lateral MI.

Gastroenterology 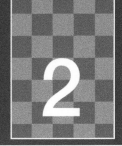 2

SBA ANSWERS

Question 1

D. Pancreatic cancer. The most likely diagnosis here is carcinoma of the head of the pancreas. The tumour obstructs the common bile duct causing jaundice and dark urine because of conjugated hyperbilirubinaemia. The faeces are pale due to a lack of stercobilinogen. Painless jaundice is typically the presenting feature of carcinoma of the head of the pancreas, along with weight loss. Hepatocellular carcinoma would not cause the change in stool colour.

Question 2

A. Columnar cells. Barrett oesophagus is when prolonged injury (due to acid reflux) results in the normal squamous epithelium of the lower oesophagus being replaced by columnar epithelium. This metaplastic change may be followed by dysplastic change, which predisposes to malignant transformation. The majority of patients present with a long history of reflux.

Question 3

A. Primary biliary cirrhosis. PBC is an autoimmune disorder and predominantly affects women, especially those aged 40–50. All patients with PBC have antimitochondrial autoantibodies and this, together with raised serum alkaline phosphatase, is diagnostic for the condition. Patients often present with pruritus and fatigue, and jaundice can be present at a later stage; some patients have xanthelasma.

Question 4

E. Haemochromatosis. Primary haemochromatosis is an autosomal recessive disorder characterized by the absorption of too much iron, which then accumulates (as haemosiderin) in the liver, pancreas, heart, pituitary and joints. The most common presentation is an incidental finding of abnormal liver enzymes or raised ferritin level. Symptoms are rare in women of child-bearing age as menstrual losses and pregnancy compensate for the excess iron absorption. Symptomatic presentation in males is usually in the fourth or fifth decade and can be obscure, such as loss of libido and hypogonadism, secondary to dysfunction of the pituitary gland or can include diabetes mellitus or arthritis.

Question 5

B. Vitamin B_1. Vitamin B_1 is also known as thiamine. Thiamine deficiency is very common in people who drink excess alcohol due to several factors. These patients generally have a poor oral diet, and thiamine is also a coenzyme in alcohol metabolism. It is essential that it is given quickly in patients who have decompensated liver failure as thiamine deficiency can lead to Wernicke encephalopathy. It is always given intravenously in the acute presentation as it is poorly absorbed orally in people who are alcohol dependent.

Question 6

D. Oesophageal candidiasis. Patients with diabetes are more prone to getting candidiasis as high sugar levels lead to better conditions for the yeast to grow. It is also only a short 10-day history, which also favours candidiasis over some of the more chronic conditions listed.

Question 7

A. Oesophageal varices. The examination findings here show evidence of liver disease. This helps point to the diagnosis of oesophageal varices as the cause of the upper GI bleed. In patients with cirrhosis of the liver and portal hypertension, the raised pressure in the portal system causes the site of a connection between the systemic and portal venous systems to open up and enlarge. The enlarged veins protrude into the lumen of the lower oesophagus and may burst, resulting in haematemesis. A man with this history could also be prone to a Mallory–Weiss tear without varices but there would usually be a history of retching or vomiting before blood appears and it would rarely cause large-volume haematemesis.

Question 8

B. Hepatic encephalopathy. Hepatic encephalopathy is a neurological disorder caused by metabolic failure of the hepatocytes and the shunting of blood around the liver (due to cirrhosis or after portocaval anastomosis). It may occur in both chronic and acute liver failure, and results in the exposure of the brain to abnormal metabolites, causing oedema and astrocyte changes. Symptoms include disturbances in consciousness (ranging from confusion to coma and death), asterixis (coarse flap of outstretched hand) and fluctuating neurological signs including seizures, muscular rigidity and hyperreflexia.

Question 9

C. Gilbert syndrome. The isolated rise in the bilirubin within the LFTs is suggestive of Gilbert syndrome. This is a congenital disorder caused by patients having a reduced amount of the enzyme UDP-glucuronyl transferase (UGT-1), which conjugates bilirubin with glucuronic acid. There is only a slight increase in serum bilirubin (unconjugated), often after prolonged starvation or intercurrent illness. The syndrome is asymptomatic, although some patients complain of fatigue.

Question 10

A. Giardiasis. Giardiasis, prevalent in the tropics, is an important cause of traveller's diarrhoea. It is caused by the flagellate protozoan *Giardia lamblia*, which lives in the duodenum and jejunum and is transmitted by the faecal–oral route. Patients may be asymptomatic, or alternatively, symptoms of diarrhoea, malabsorption and abdominal pain or bloating may develop within 1 or 2 weeks of ingesting cysts. Diagnosis is by stool microscopy, and treatment is with metronidazole. Hepatitis A can also be picked up when travelling abroad; however, this is usually asymptomatic, or presents as fever, jaundice and malaise.

Question 11

D. α_1-Antitrypsin deficiency. The history here of both chronic obstructive pulmonary disease and deranged LFT is suggestive of α_1-antitrypsin deficiency. α_1-Antitrypsin is a serum protein that is produced in the liver and has antiprotease effects. One in ten northern Europeans carries a deficiency gene, which is autosomal recessive in inheritance. Symptoms include basal emphysema in about 75% of homozygotes and liver cirrhosis in approximately 10%. Heterozygotes have an increased risk of developing emphysema if they smoke. None of the other diagnoses given have a link with respiratory disease.

Question 12

E. Gastric cancer. An enlarged supraclavicular lymph node of the left side of the body is also known as Virchow node. This is highly suggestive of carcinoma of the stomach. Patients with a palpable Virchow node should be referred for an upper GI endoscopy for further investigation.

Question 13

A. Hepatocellular carcinoma. A raised AFP is associated with hepatocellular carcinoma. In younger males, a raised AFP along with a raised β-human chorionic gonadotropin is also indicative of germ cell tumours. However, with hepatocellular carcinoma, the rest of the LFTs are often deranged as well.

Question 14

E. Mallory–Weiss tear. A Mallory–Weiss tear is a tear at the gastro-oesophageal junction. It is caused by prolonged retching or coughing and a sudden increase in intraabdominal pressure. It is most common in alcoholics and presents as haematemesis. All the other answers can cause an upper GI bleed, but the history given of prolonged vomiting preceding haematemesis is suggestive of a Mallory–Weiss tear.

Question 15

C. Viral illness. The raised WCC and raised lymphocyte count is suggestive of an acute viral illness, whilst the rise in the LFTs, in particular the transaminases, suggests a hepatitis type of picture. There are several causes of a viral hepatitis, which include Epstein–Barr virus and hepatitis A. Drugs such as antibiotics and alcohol can also cause a noninfective hepatitis. Further investigations to determine the exact cause would be required. In general, the treatment would be supportive.

Question 16

D. CT abdomen. When acute pancreatitis is diagnosed, the focus should be on the acute management. Once the patient has recovered from the initial attack, he/she requires further imaging to assess whether there has been any damage to the pancreas. In particular, the consultant is looking for any evidence of pancreatic necrosis. CT scan is the most appropriate investigation to view the pancreas properly and any soft tissue damage. CT is normally done prior to an MRI due to the lower cost and the lower levels of radiation to the patient.

Question 17

B. Chronic pancreatitis. Chronic pancreatitis is an ongoing inflammation of the pancreas accompanied by irreversible architectural changes. Alcohol consumption causes more than 85% of cases and is the most common cause of pancreatitis in developed countries. High-fat and high-protein diets amplify the damage done by alcohol. Other causes include idiopathic chronic pancreatitis; trauma and scar formation, leading to the obstruction of the main pancreatic duct; previous episodes of acute pancreatitis predispose to others although they may often be subclinical; cystic fibrosis resulting in protein plugs in the duct system; and hereditary forms of pancreatitis. Patients normally present with a history of prolonged ill-health with chronic epigastric pain, usually radiating through to the back.

Question 18

D. Crohn disease. In a young adult, the history of diarrhoea and weight loss should be investigated by a colonoscopy to look for inflammatory bowel disease (IBD). The presence of skip lesions in the colon indicates that Crohn is the most likely diagnosis. Crohn disease may affect any part of the GI tract from the mouth to the anus. Endoscopy usually shows skip lesions and deep ulcers and fissures in the mucosa. Ulcerative colitis usually starts in the rectum and it may extend proximally, although never beyond the colon. Unlike Crohn disease, which commonly shows skip lesions, ulcerative colitis is continuous. Areas of normal gut are not found between lesions.

Question 19

E. Cyclizine. Cyclizine is an antiemetic from the H_1 receptor antagonist class. These are effective against motion sickness, as these receptors are found in the vestibular nuclei, and against vomiting caused by substances acting in the stomach.

Question 20

C. Serum amylase. Diagnosis of acute pancreatitis is by measurement of serum amylase. It is normally greatly elevated (five times or more) in acute pancreatitis. The rest of the investigations are relevant once acute pancreatitis has been diagnosed. The U&Es and arterial blood gases should be done to ascertain the severity of the disease, using the Glasgow criteria. AXR may show an absent psoas shadow and an air-filled dilatation of the proximal jejunum. CT is typically done after the acute event to assess the degree of damage to the pancreas.

Question 21

A. Duodenal ulcer. The positive ^{14}C urea breath test is indicative of the presence of *Helicobacter pylori*, which is closely associated with peptic ulcer disease. The history given means the diagnosis is most likely to be a duodenal ulcer. With duodenal ulcers, classically the epigastric pain is said to be relieved by food or antacids and exacerbated by hunger. The epigastric pain with gastric ulcers is characteristically associated with food.

Question 22

A. Cefotaxime. Pseudomembranous colitis is caused by an overgrowth of *Clostridium difficile*, a bacillus which is carried by 2% of the population, asymptomatically. It usually occurs postantibiotic therapy, which suppresses the normal colonic flora allowing *C. difficile* to proliferate. Pseudomembranous colitis is associated mainly with broad-spectrum antibiotics;

however, cephalosporins are considered the highest-risk group. Cefotaxime is a third-generation cephalosporin antibiotic.

Question 23

A. Tropical sprue. Weight loss, diarrhoea and steatorrhea are classic symptoms for malabsorption. The colonoscopy findings of villous atrophy are suggestive initially of coeliac disease; however, you would expect the patient's symptoms to improve with a gluten-free diet. Tropical sprue is a chronic, progressive malabsorption in patients from the tropics (mainly the West Indies and Asia) associated with abnormalities of small intestinal structure and function. It is thought to have an infective cause. Like coeliac disease, there is villous atrophy, although obviously a gluten-free diet is of no help. Treatment is with broad-spectrum antibiotics.

Question 24

B. Sodium docusate. This patient's constipation has been caused by the strong opioids he is taking. His main problem is hard stools, so the first-line laxative should be a faecal softener. Sodium docusate is the only faecal softener in the answers given. If he is still having problems with constipation, then it would be appropriate to add in a different class of laxative.

Question 25

C. The diagnosis is GORD which is usually investigated by upper GI endoscopy as a first-line. However, in patients less than 55 years and without red flag symptoms or signs, it is reasonable to have a trial of treatment before proceeding with investigations.

Question 26

D. Proton-pump inhibitors, such as lansoprazole or omeprazole, are usually first choice for GORD. H_2 receptor antagonists can be added, but they suffer from tachyphylaxis, which means their utility diminishes with time and are often stopped after 2 weeks.

Question 27

A. A classic description of achalasia. This is a motility disorder associated with aperistalsis and failure of relaxation of the lower oesophageal sphincter. The tapered portion of the oesophagus is commonly referred to as a beak deformity.

Question 28

E. GORD is a risk factor for adenocarcinoma and not squamous cell carcinoma. The rest are risk factors for squamous cell carcinoma.

Question 29

C. A 'corkscrew' appearance is diagnostic of diffuse oesophageal spasm. Treatment often involves the use of calcium-channel blockers. Systemic sclerosis can cause peptic stricturing due to chronic GORD.

Question 30

C. Management of *Helicobacter pylori* infection involves a proton-pump inhibitor and two antibiotics. Common regimens include omeprazole, metronidazole and clarithromycin (penicillin allergic patients), or omeprazole, amoxicillin and clarithromycin.

Question 31

D. The diagnosis is most likely gastric cancer. The peri-orbital skin rash is classic of dermatomyositis which is associated with an underlying malignancy in some cases. An upper GI endoscopy for biopsy and diagnosis is the most appropriate investigation.

Question 32

E. Tar-coloured stool is commonly known as melaena, which is partially digested blood, and signifies an upper GI bleed. The most common cause of such a bleed is a peptic ulcer.

Question 33

A. Severe vomiting often leads to a tear in the oesophagus (Mallory–Weiss) and a subsequent bleed. Conservative approach is used initially, but if bleeding does not settle, then endoscopic management is indicated.

Question 34

C. Diclofenac is a nonsteroidal antiinflammatory drug and can cause peptic ulceration which may be complicated by bleeding or perforation.

Question 35

D. This patient is haemodynamically unstable and hence the first-line treatment would be IV access and urgent fluid resuscitation with saline or O-negative blood. Once haemodynamic stability has been achieved, upper GI endoscopy is needed.

Question 36

C. This patient has iron-deficiency anaemia and the initial investigation is an upper and lower GI endoscopy (top and tail) to look for a source of GI blood loss such as a malignancy.

Question 37

E. Coeliac disease is the most likely as it is common (1% of the population) and causes these symptoms. Other listed diagnoses are far less common, other than irritable bowel syndrome, which does not cause iron and folate deficiency.

Question 38

A. The first-line investigation to confirm coeliac disease is via endoscopy and biopsy. Positive IgA and tTG are not enough to confirm the diagnosis. In people who have IgA deficiency, a serologically positive result can be derived from any one of the IgG antibodies.

Question 39

C. These symptoms suggest small bowel bacterial overgrowth following recent surgery. The hydrogen breath test helps to demonstrate the presence of such organisms. Upon ingestion of glucose the bacteria will metabolize the sugar and produce hydrogen, which can then be subsequently measured in exhaled air.

Question 40

B. In cases of acute severe ulcerative colitis (by Truelove and Witt's severity index), IV hydrocortisone is the first-line treatment to induce remission, with ciclosporin as second-line if patients do not tolerate IV steroids. For patients not tolerating ciclosporin, infliximab is indicated instead.

Question 41

A. His symptoms suggest a flare-up of his Crohn disease and steroids are the most appropriate treatment to induce remission.

Question 42

D. Although dietary and lifestyle factors are thought to play an aetiological role, family history is the most important aetiological factor in this case.

Question 43

A. An ileoscopy would assess for recurrent Crohn disease, which is the most likely diagnosis.

Question 44

D. Sepsis is common with TPN. To confirm a source, both peripheral and central (Hickman) line blood cultures should be taken and TPN stopped until cultures are deemed negative.

Question 45

A. This patient has developed jaundice. Following liver biochemistry, a USS is the initial investigation to assess for biliary duct dilatation.

Question 46

B. Hepatitis A is commonly due to ingestion of contaminated water or food such as shellfish. Symptoms such as abdominal pain, diarrhoea and dark urine are characteristic of the condition, as is the timeline of 3 days.

Question 47

E. This patient has developed jaundice as a result of hepatitis C. Hepatitis C is known to cause cryoglobulinemia-mediated glomerulonephritis, which explains this patient's haematuria. Hepatitis B causes membranous and mesangiocapillary glomerulonephritis, which does not commonly result in haematuria.

Question 48

D. This patient most probably has a diagnosis of hepatitis A, which is commonly due to consumption of contaminated food such as shellfish or clams. Management is often conservative.

Question 49

C. Grade 3 encephalopathy comprises features of drowsiness, stupor and no evidence of communication.

Question 50

B. The suspected diagnosis is autoimmune hepatitis, which is more common in patients with other autoimmune conditions. This condition is associated with high titres of antinuclear antibodies. PBC causes elevated IgM levels.

Question 51

D. The best assessment of liver function in cirrhotic patients is prothrombin time. Therefore if there are no acute bleeding issues, gastroenterologists tend not to correct the international normalized ratio (INR) with vitamin K (within limits).

Question 52

A. With any GI bleed, an urgent endoscopy is the most appropriate initial management following adequate resuscitation of the patient.

Question 53

C. This patient has developed ascites. The initial management is with diuretics, such as spironolactone, and sodium restriction. Of course, alcohol cessation would be useful here.

Question 54

B. This patient has developed spontaneous bacterial peritonitis which is a complication of ascites in chronic liver disease. The most common organism in this condition is *Escherichia coli*. IV Tazocin is first-line therapy.

Question 55

E. The diagnosis is hepatic encephalopathy, confirmed by features of asterixis, fetor hepaticus and confusion.

The diagnosis is usually clinical, but an EEG will show characteristic changes if there is diagnostic uncertainty.

Question 56

D. The history suggests PBC, a condition known to affect middle-aged women. Serum AMAs are the first-line investigation as they are elevated in 90% to 95% of PBC with a specificity of 98%. Serum ANA can be elevated in 20%. IgM is elevated but is nonspecific.

Question 57

E. The diagnosis in this case is haemochromatosis based on the history and examination. From the listed options, serum ferritin is the most appropriate diagnostic tool.

Question 58

C. The diagnosis is alcoholic hepatitis in view of the presence of Mallory bodies. Stopping alcohol completely is the mainstay form of treatment to prevent the development of alcoholic cirrhosis.

Question 59

D. This patient is likely to be suffering from a primary hepatocellular carcinoma in view of his weight loss, presence of ascites and raised AFP level. USS or CT is the most appropriate diagnostic tool.

Question 60

D. The diagnosis is chronic pancreatitis. As a result of pancreatic lipase secretion reduction, this patient has developed steatorrhoea. Chronic pancreatitis is most appropriately investigated by abdominal CT scan.

Question 61

B. Pancreatic carcinoma has a poor prognosis. This lady is elderly and frail with metastatic disease and therefore is likely to have palliative treatment only.

EMQ ANSWERS

Liver problems

1. A Alcoholic liver disease. Classic signs of hepatic failure and hepatic encephalopathy.
2. G Metastatic liver disease. The patient needs an urgent ultrasound examination and possible liver biopsy; LFTs would not be particularly helpful at this stage.
3. B Biliary atresia. Prolonged jaundice (>2 weeks) should be investigated. Bilirubin accumulation will eventually cause hepatic failure if left untreated. Physiological jaundice should disappear by day 8 in normal births.

4. D Hepatitis A. The disease is endemic in many parts of the world, and transmission is via the orofaecal route, usually from consumption of contaminated water or food.

5. C Gallstones. In the classic presentation, the patient might also have dietary fat intolerance and flatulence.

Hepatobiliary disorders

1. G Haemochromatosis. This condition is associated with a triad of skin pigmentation, diabetes and hepatomegaly. Treatment is with venesection, initially weekly and then less frequently to maintain iron depletion.

2. B α1-Antitrypsin deficiency. This disorder can result in liver cirrhosis and emphysema. There is no specific treatment available.

3. J PBC. Such a disorder is most appropriately diagnosed by the presence of antimitochondrial antibodies. Treatment plans include the use of ursodeoxycholic acid and cholestyramine to help relieve pruritus.

4. A Wilson disease is associated with an error of copper metabolism. Treatment consists of copper chelating agents such as penicillamine or trientine.

5. F Primary sclerosing cholangitis is diagnosed following a liver biopsy which demonstrates evidence of polymorph infiltration of bile ducts and is associated with IBDs. An ERCP may also be useful in such cases and may demonstrate a bead-like appearance within the bile ducts as a result of stricture formation.

Gastrointestinal bleeding

1. C Haemorrhoids. Additional symptoms may include perianal irritation and itch. Treatment involves the use of sclerosant injections, elastic band ligation or surgical resection.

2. A This is a classic presentation of a Mallory–Weiss tear. Forceful vomiting has led to a tear in the oesophagus and a subsequent bleed.

3. B Angiodysplasia. There is a strong association with underlying cardiac disease, particularly aortic stenosis, possibly due to the shearing of the von Willebrand factor as they go across the stenosed valves. Replacement of the aortic valve can cure the problem.

4. G Reflux oesophagitis. Classic description of reflux disease.

5. E Duodenal ulcer. The gram-negative bacterium is most probably *Helicobacter pylori,* which is commonly associated with both gastric and duodenal ulcers.

Drugs

1. D Acamprosate is known to help reduce the craving experienced by alcohol-dependent patients. It is thought to interact with glutamate and gamma-aminobutyric acid (GABA) neurotransmitters to restore neuronal excitation and inhibition balance.

2. F Acute severe exacerbations involve the use of IV steroids in almost all cases. Ciclosporin can be given for patients who do not tolerate/refuse steroids.

3. B In view of his stroke, this patient is likely to have been prescribed aspirin. Aspirin is an antiplatelet drug and may be associated with an increased risk of GI bleeding.

4. A Omeprazole. This patient is likely to be suffering from GORD. Agents such as proton-pump inhibitors or alginate containing antacids are beneficial in such cases.

5. E The diagnosis is Crohn disease in view of histological findings. Mesalazine induces remission in this condition.

Dysphagia

1. I *Candida.* This patient is likely to be taking immunosuppressants to prevent rejection following her recent transplant. *Candida* infection is common in such patients and can lead to swallowing difficulties.

2. G Oesophageal web. These features are consistent with Plummer-Vinson syndrome. This condition is associated with ulceration and subsequent structuring or web-like formations in the upper oesophagus resulting in dysphagia.

3. E Pharyngeal pouch. Muscle dysmotility can lead to mucosal out pouching, which is commonly referred to as a pharyngeal pouch. Treatment is primarily surgical.

4. C Benign oesophageal stricture. Additional causes include reflux disease, ingestion of caustic substances and previous radiotherapy.

5. A Achalasia. Such radiological findings are classic of achalasia. A barium swallow often demonstrates a tapered lower end of the oesophagus.

Gastroenteritis

1. H *Staphylococcus aureus.* This organism is known to produce such symptoms as a result of the production of a heat-stable endotoxin. Treatment is usually supportive.

2. C *Bacillus cereus.* Vomiting in this case is commonly due to production of an emetic toxin. Diarrhoea typically occurs 8–16 hours following vomiting.

3. B *Campylobacter.* Symptoms last for approximately 1 to 2 weeks. Treatment involves the use of antibiotics such as erythromycin.

4. E   *Escherichia coli.* Additional features may include renal failure and anaemia. Avoidance of antibiotics is key as certain agents may lead to toxin production.
5. F   *Yersinia enterocolitica.* Diagnosis is often by serology and treatment is typically supportive.

Pancreatitis
1. E   Hyperlipidaemia. This is an uncommon cause of pancreatitis and is frequently seen in conjunction with alcohol excess. High triglycerides in the blood causes pseudohyponatraemia as only the sodium in the serum, rather than lipid, is measured.
2. D   Grey-Turner sign. Grey-Turner described his sign in acute haemorrhagic pancreatitis. This is an uncommon presentation now, but the sign may still be seen in trauma where there is retroperitoneal bleeding, in this case due to trauma of the pancreas as it comes into contact with the vertebral bodies.
3. F   Pancreatic divisum. Pancreatic divisum is relatively common and most patients are asymptomatic. Drainage of the ducts of Santorini and Wirsung by a minor papilla can lead to increased intraduct pressure leading to pancreatitis.
4. A   Alcohol. This is the most common cause of pancreatitis. Presentation may be delayed after a significant bout of drinking, as in this case.
5. C   Gallstones. This is the other common cause of pancreatitis (alcohol and gallstones making up around 95% of pancreatitis). The patient gives a history of biliary colic as her gallstone impacts in Hartmann's pouch.

Diarrhoea
1. G   Irritable bowel syndrome. This is the likely diagnosis in this patient; however, he should be monitored as he is the right age for a primary presentation of IBD.
2. H   Metformin. This is the likely culprit. Many drugs are associated with diarrhoea; however, it is common with metformin, especially at higher doses.
3. E   Diverticular disease. Colonoscopy is indicated to rule out a malignancy due to the gentleman's age, change in bowel habit and haematochezia.
4. I   Ulcerative colitis. In a patient with the same symptoms but aged 60+, the consideration of malignancy would be much higher. This young lady has IBD. Left iliac fossa tenderness would suggest ulcerative colitis rather than Crohn disease, which more often affects the ileum.
5. J   Zollinger–Ellison syndrome. This is characterized by a duodenal or pancreatic gastrin-secreting tumour leading to profuse ulceration.

Altered bowel habit
1. G   Diverticulitis
2. D   Irritable bowel syndrome
3. B   Crohn disease
4. A   Ulcerative colitis
5. C   Colorectal carcinoma

Jaundice
1. D   Pancreatic carcinoma
2. C   Hepatocellular carcinoma
3. I   Chronic pancreatitis
4. E   Gallbladder carcinoma
5. J   Liver abscess

Dysphagia
1. D   Pharyngeal pouch. Pharyngeal pouches occur most commonly in elderly patients (over 70 years) and typical symptoms include dysphagia, regurgitation, chronic cough, aspiration and weight loss. The aetiology remains unknown but theories centre upon a structural or physiological abnormality of the cricopharyngeus.
2. J   Oesophageal web. These webs are thin (2–3 mm) membranes of normal oesophageal tissue consisting of mucosa and submucosa that can partially protrude/obstruct the oesophagus. They are mainly observed in Plummer-Vinson syndrome, which is associated with chronic iron-deficiency anaemia.
3. C   Oesophageal carcinoma. Prominent symptoms usually do not appear until the cancer has infiltrated over 60% of the circumference of the oesophagus. Dysphagia is experienced first with solid foods and later with softer foods and liquids. If the cancer has spread elsewhere, symptoms related to metastatic disease may appear.
4. A   Achalasia. It is characterized by incomplete lower oesophageal sphincter (LES) relaxation, increased LES tone and lack of peristalsis of the oesophagus.
5. I   Retrosternal thyroid. A goitre with a portion of its mass located in the mediastinum causes symptoms of hyperthyroidism and difficulty swallowing.

Biliary disease
1. D   Biliary peritonitis. This patient has initially developed acute cholecystitis, but due to his age and comorbidities, such as ischaemic heart disease and diabetes, he is at increased risk of a perforation of the gallbladder. This happens when he suddenly develops generalized abdominal pain. He has signs of peritonitis, with a tachycardia and generalized abdominal tenderness, particularly on the right side, and absent bowel sounds.

2. C Biliary colic. This patient has a chronic history of pain that occurs intermittently and resolves spontaneously. She has not required admission to hospital as the pain is due to biliary colic, where the gallbladder is trying to contract against an obstruction (i.e., the gallstone). It may last for several hours.

3. B Acute pancreatitis. This patient is known to have gallstones. She has a classic history of acute pancreatitis (i.e., pain radiating through to the back and vomiting). She has signs of localized peritonism and systemic signs of dehydration and a tachycardia.

4. G Empyema of the gallbladder. This is a chronic history which has been going on for several weeks. The patient initially started with an episode of acute cholecystitis, which was probably unrecognized. The gallbladder, however, has remained obstructed and so has become swollen due to retention of fluid within it. This gives the palpable mass. The flu-like symptoms and a swinging pyrexia are consistent with an abscess (i.e., an empyema of the gallbladder).

5. E Cholangiocarcinoma. This patient has painless obstructive jaundice. His confusion may be due to the jaundice, secondary infection or associated renal impairment. He is afebrile and abdominal examination does not show a distended gallbladder, which might be present if his gallbladder was not diseased and was able to distend secondary to obstruction of his bile duct (i.e., Courvoisier's law). In many cases, however, although the bile duct is obstructed, the gallbladder is fibrosed and fails to distend despite the obstruction.

SBA ANSWERS

Question 1

D. Tobacco smoking is the most common cause of COPD. Other factors, such as air pollution and genetics, play a smaller role. Long-term exposure to these irritants causes an inflammatory response in the lungs, which results in the breakdown of lung tissue and narrowing of airways. Diagnosis is based on lung function tests.

Question 2

C. When the patient arrives in hospital, arterial blood gases should be measured and the inspired oxygen concentration noted in all patients with an exacerbation of COPD, so that controlled oxygen therapy can be tailored. These measurements should be repeated regularly, according to the response to treatment.

Question 3

B. Individuals with COPD typically depend on a degree of hypoxia to maintain respiratory drive, so it is best to commence low oxygen concentrations via a Venturi mask. The oxygen saturation and arterial blood gas results should be regularly assessed to determine correct oxygen therapy.

Question 4

D. The diagnosis is obstructive sleep apnoea, caused by a combination of alcohol, which decreases muscle tone, and obesity. All of the listed options can occur in obstructive sleep apnoea but excessive daytime sleepiness is the most common and is the hallmark of the disease.

Question 5

A. A typical presentation of cystic fibrosis. The presence of clubbing suggests a chronic respiratory disease process as opposed to acute infections or inhaled foreign body. It is an autosomal recessive disorder which affects the lungs, pancreas, liver, kidneys and gastrointestinal tract.

Question 6

E. High-resolution CT of the chest is the most frequently used imaging test to establish the diagnosis of bronchiectasis. Other investigations may also need to be performed to determine the underlying cause (e.g., sweat test for cystic fibrosis).

Question 7

D. Exacerbations of pulmonary symptoms in patients with cystic fibrosis must be recognized early and treated vigorously to maintain pulmonary function and relieve symptoms. Antibiotic treatment is prescribed based on new symptoms or worsening of existing symptoms.

Question 8

D. Because of defective chloride channels ((cystic fibrosis transmembrane conductance regulator (CFTR)), the concentration of chloride in sweat is elevated in patients with cystic fibrosis. The sweat test measures the amount of chloride excreted in sweat. A chloride level of greater than or equal to 60 mmol/L means that cystic fibrosis is likely to be diagnosed.

Question 9

C. Farmer's lung is a hypersensitivity pneumonitis induced by the inhalation of biologic dusts coming from hay dust or mould spores or any other agricultural products. Acute farmer's lung starts about 4 to 8 hours after the person breathes in a large amount of dust from mouldy crops, causing breathlessness, cough, nausea and fevers. Symptoms usually decrease after 12 hours, but could be longer.

Question 10

B. The next step in the management plan is to add on a low-dose inhaled steroid. If this is inadequate, then a long-acting β_2 agonist is added. If control of asthma symptoms is still inadequate, then a high-dose inhaled steroid may be added. Add-on therapy (e.g., leukotriene receptor antagonist or theophylline) or oral steroids are for more advanced cases.

Question 11

E. Nebulized salbutamol or terbutaline in addition to oral steroids are the initial treatment of acute severe asthma. Oral steroids are as effective as intravenous steroids. Intravenous magnesium is added in life-threatening exacerbation.

Question 12

A. *S. pneumoniae* is the most common cause of community-acquired pneumonia where a pathogen is isolated, accounting for about 50% of cases. Other bacterial causes include *H. influenzae*, *C. pneumoniae*, *M. pneumoniae* and *S. aureus*.

Question 13

C. The mortality associated with community-acquired pneumonia is dependent on the CURB 65 score as recommended by the British Thoracic Society. A respiratory rate of 30 breaths/min is a key risk factor, not 20. If the score is 1 or less, the patient could potentially be managed at home. If it is a 2, a short stay in hospital is needed. If the score is 3 or more, hospitalization is recommended.

Question 14

D. *M. pneumoniae* causes a form of atypical pneumonia which can cause extra-pulmonary symptoms including erythema multiforme, haemolytic anaemia, Guillain–Barré syndrome, renal failure and pericarditis.

Question 15

A. *C. psittaci* is an intracellular bacterial species found in birds, cattle, pigs, sheep and horses. Transmission is by inhalation, contact or ingestion among birds and then to humans. This type of pneumonia in humans often starts with flu-like symptoms. Tetracyclines and macrolides are used to treat this type of pneumonia.

Question 16

C. Intravenous drug users have a 10-fold increased risk of community-acquired pneumonia compared with the general population. *S. aureus* pneumonia is often seen in intravenous drug abusers, and can result in lung abscess.

Question 17

E. *Legionella* transmission is via inhalation of water droplets from a contaminated source that has allowed the organism to grow and spread (e.g., cooling towers). It usually starts with flu-like symptoms, followed by gastrointestinal tract and central nervous system symptoms, causing diarrhoea, nausea and confusion.

Question 18

A. Mild pneumonia is usually managed at home with treatment from GP. A common regimen is a 5–7-day course of oral amoxicillin 500 mg three times a day.

Question 19

D. CXR is the gold-standard investigation in pneumonia. The X-ray findings of pneumonia are airspace opacity, lobar consolidation/air bronchograms or interstitial opacities. TB, *Klebsiella* and staphylococcal infections can all cause lung abscesses.

Question 20

D. *M. tuberculosis* is often seen in Asian immigrants. Classic symptoms are chronic cough with blood-containing sputum, fever, night sweats and weight loss. In 20% of active cases of TB, the infection has extrapulmonary features (e.g., TB meningitis, Pott disease of the spine and osteomyelitis).

Question 21

B. TB infection begins when mycobacteria reach the pulmonary alveoli, where they invade and replicate within macrophages. Macrophages are responsible for engulfing the bacilli in an attempt to eliminate them by phagocytosis. The bacilli have a resistant mycolic capsule that protects them from toxic substances in the macrophages. They are able to reproduce inside the macrophage and eventually kill the immune cell.

Question 22

B. Multiple sputum cultures are usually taken to look for acid-fast bacilli if the patient is producing sputum. Induced sputum samples can be taken if there is no spontaneous sputum production. Auramine–rhodamine staining (fluorescence microscopy) is more sensitive than Ziehl–Neelsen stain.

Question 23

C. The recommended treatment of new-onset pulmonary TB is 6 months of quadruple therapy consisting of rifampicin, isoniazid, pyrazinamide and ethambutol for the first 2 months, and dual therapy with rifampicin and isoniazid for the last 4 months. Streptomycin is used in patients who have previously been treated for TB as they are more likely to have developed some drug resistance.

Question 24

A. Rifampicin can cause hepatotoxicity, fevers, gastrointestinal disturbances and rashes. It can also cause certain bodily fluids, such as urine, sweat and tears, to become orange-red. This is sometimes used to monitor effective absorption of the drug.

Question 25

E. This patient has a diagnosis of sarcoidosis, which is a systemic inflammatory disease that can affect any organ. Up to 90% of patients complain of eye involvement. Manifestations in the eye include uveitis (commonest), uveoparotitis and retinal inflammation, which can lead to loss of visual acuity.

Question 26

E. Tissue obtained from biopsy can be used to confirm the diagnosis of sarcoidosis and rule out an infective cause. Biopsy shows evidence of noncaseating granulomas. Supporting investigations include CXR showing hilar lymphadenopathy, hypercalcaemia, raised liver function tests and raised serum ACE.

Question 27

D. All the above except D are causes of upper zone fibrosis. Cryptogenic fibrosing alveolitis is a disease of unknown aetiology, which is characterized by a cellular alveolar infiltrate and later by fibrosis of the alveolar walls. It usually presents with progressive dyspnoea, persistent cough and finger clubbing.

Question 28
A. Extrinsic allergic alveolitis is an inflammation of the alveoli within the lung caused by hypersensitivity to a huge variety of inhaled organic dusts. Worldwide, there are differences, but forking mouldy hay (farmer's lung) is the most common cause from the listed options.

Question 29
E. Prolonged inhalation of asbestos fibres can cause serious and fatal illnesses including all of the above. Top at-risk occupations are construction workers, firefighters, industrial workers, power plant workers and shipyard workers. Sufferers with any of the above options are usually able to claim compensation for past exposure.

Question 30
A. Squamous cell carcinoma of the lung is closely correlated with a history of tobacco smoking, and smoking is the most common cause of lung cancer. Although working in a shipyard puts the patient at risk of mesothelioma, this is not as common as SCC of the lung.

Question 31
C. Adenocarcinoma is a type of nonsmall cell lung carcinoma. It is currently the most common type of lung cancer in lifelong nonsmokers. These account for 40% of all lung cancers.

Question 32
E. This patient has clinical features of Cushing syndrome. Because of its high-grade neuroendocrine nature, small cell carcinomas can produce ectopic hormones including adrenocorticotropic hormone (as in this case) and antidiuretic hormone. Lambert–Eaton myasthenic syndrome (LEMS) is a well-known paraneoplastic condition linked to small cell carcinoma.

Question 33
A. All of the above can be found in lung cancers, but clubbing is the most common extrapulmonary feature. It is usually associated with nonsmall cell lung cancer (SCLC) (>50% cases). SCLCs are also associated with various paraneoplastic syndromes.

Question 34
E. Transudate has low protein/albumin levels when compared with exudate. Light criteria are usually applied when trying to determine whether pleural fluid

is a transudate or exudate. Glucose levels are usually lower in infection. Amylase levels may be increased with pancreatitis, oesophageal rupture or malignancy.

Question 35
A. Causes of transudative effusions include heart failure, cirrhosis, hypoalbuminaemia/nephrotic syndrome, hypothyroidism, peritoneal dialysis and Meigs syndrome.

Question 36
A. This patient has a pulmonary embolus best diagnosed by CTPA as it has the best diagnostic accuracy of all the advanced noninvasive imaging methods. If there is a contraindication to CTPA (e.g., contrast allergy/ severe renal failure), then a ventilation–perfusion (V/Q) scan may be performed.

Question 37
C. Ultrasound scan-guided tap is 'diagnostic' and will result in pleural fluid for cultures and Gram stain. Features suggestive of an empyema on thoracic ultrasound include the presence of echogenic fluid, loculations and septations. The use of ultrasound to guide thoracentesis (pleural tap/aspiration) reduces complications. Pleural tap revealed >100,000 neutrophils/μL, bacteria seen on Gram stain and pH <7.2, which may be presumed to be empyema.

Question 38
B. The presence of bubbling in an underwater seal means that there is a consistent air leak, and when it stops bubbling it means that either the air leak has stopped (pneumothorax resolved) or the drain is blocked. Thus the drain can only be removed when it has stopped bubbling, and a CXR is done to demonstrate that there is no re-expansion after the drain is clamped (as a test).

Question 39
C. Common complications include puncture of the lungs resulting in a 'pneumothorax' especially with a subclavian approach (as opposed to via an internal jugular approach).

Question 40
B. The most characteristic findings of a pneumothorax are hyperresonance and decreased breath sounds. A tension pneumothorax may displace the mediastinum to the unaffected side. This is associated with distended neck veins and hypotension. A needle insertion in the second intercostal space in the midclavicular line decompresses the system, is life saving and provides relief to the patient.

Question 41

D. When dyspnoea is accompanied by decreased breath sounds unilaterally and the tracheal deviation, the most likely diagnosis will be pneumothorax. In the case of pneumothorax, there is no orthopnoea or paroxysmal nocturnal dyspnoea and also S3 gallop is not a feature of pneumothorax. Pneumothorax is the collection of air in the thoracic cavity, which presents with diminished breath sounds and tracheal deviation away from the pathological site.

Question 42

C. SCCs are associated with hypercalcaemia (parathyroid hormone-related protein producing). SCLC may be associated with syndrome of inappropriate antidiuretic hormone secretion (SIADH), resulting in hyponatremia. Adenocarcinomas are associated with hypertrophic osteoarthropathy (clubbing). Lung cancer metastasizes to the adrenals, brain, bone, liver and skin.

Question 43

E. SCLC is strongly associated with smoking and, due to its central location, results in recurrent or slowly resolving pneumonia/lung collapse. A bronchoscopy is warranted to view the obstruction and take biopsies.

Question 44

D. The large mass is consistent with an SCC, which is seen mainly in smokers. Mesothelioma is rare; it is characterized by a bulky pleural mass in a person with prior asbestos exposure. *P. carinii* (*jirovecii*) pneumonia is a diffuse process and occurs in immunocompromised patients. Haemoptysis does not occur. Granulomatous inflammation is typical for mycobacterial and fungal infections; though a solitary granuloma may be present, it is usually not larger than 2 to 3 cm in size.

Question 45

B. Extrapulmonary symptoms suggest atypical bacteria, and classically hotels (stagnant water source) are a breeding ground for *Legionella*. *H. influenzae* is normally a community-acquired pneumonia affecting COPD patients and children, via aerosol transmission. The symptoms are more indicative of atypical bacteria however. *M. pneumoniae* is an atypical bacterium; common in teens, mostly causing pharyngitis/ bronchitis only, which is not concordant with the clinical picture in the question.

Question 46

B. Bronchiectasis is an illness of the bronchi and bronchioles involving obstructive and infectious processes that injure airways and cause luminal dilatation. In addition to daily vicious, often purulent sputum production with occasional haemoptysis, wheezing and dyspnoea occurs in 75% of patients. Emphysema and chronic bronchitis, forms of COPD, also cause a decreased FEV_1:FVC ratio, but the baseline sputum is generally mucoid and luminal dilatation of bronchi is not characteristically present.

Question 47

A. CPAP is the most effective treatment for obstructive sleep apnoea in adults. Results with devices that move the tongue or mandible forward are variable and inconsistent. Uvulopalatal surgery often reduces snoring but may not reduce the frequency of apnoeic episodes during sleep.

Question 48

D. Radiation pneumonitis is common after radiotherapy, resulting in a localized pneumonitis, which would result in fibrosis eventually. TB would produce upper lobe cavitation rather than shadowing. Pulmonary lymphoma is extremely rare; it is the involvement of lung parenchyma from lymphoma, and usually bilateral. Tuberculosis presents with nonspecific clinical signs of cough, fever, haemoptysis.

Question 49

C. Pulmonary fibrosis is associated with finger clubbing, hypoxaemia and restrictive PFT picture as it is in this patient. Bronchial asthma is associated with an obstructive PFT picture with reduced peak flows. It would not be associated with finger clubbing. Emphysema would be associated with an obstructive PFT, as well as quiet breath sounds.

Question 50

B. Silicosis is a respiratory disease caused by inhalation of silica dust. The fact that the patient worked as a rock miner is enough evidence that the patient is suffering from silicosis. In such conditions, there is bilateral upper lobe involvement accompanied by hilar lymphadenopathy and eggshell calcification of the lymph nodes. People who are involved in the occupations of mining, quarrying, sand blasting, stone cutting and glass manufacturing fall easy prey to silicosis. The symptoms of this disease include cough, unexplained weight loss and SOB.

Question 51

C. Pneumoconiosis is the general term for lung disease caused by inhalation and deposition of mineral dust, with asbestosis more specifically being pneumoconiosis caused by asbestos inhalation. The term refers to a group of naturally occurring, heat-resistant fibrous silicates. Because the development of asbestosis is dose dependent, symptoms appear only after a latent period of 20 years or longer. This latent period may be shorter after intense exposure. Dyspnoea upon exertion is the most common symptom and worsens as the disease progresses. Patients may have a dry (i.e., nonproductive) cough. A productive cough suggests concomitant bronchitis or a respiratory infection. Patients may report nonspecific chest discomfort, especially in advanced cases.

Question 52

C. Absent breath sounds, decreased wheezing, pulsus paradoxus, cyanosis, diaphoresis with inability to speak in full sentences and increasing levels of CO_2 in blood are all ominous signs of impending respiratory failure in the patients of asthma exacerbation. It is important to be ready with rapid sequence intubation in such patients.

Question 53

A. Asthma is typically associated with an obstructive impairment that is reversible with short-acting bronchodilators. A reduced FEV_1 and FEV_1:FVC ratio indicates airflow obstruction. A reduced FVC_1 with a normal or increased FEV_1:FVC ratio is consistent with a restrictive pattern of lung function.

EMQ ANSWERS

Pneumonia

1. G   A common cause of pneumonia in cystic fibrosis or individuals who are immunocompromised. More than 60% of adults with cystic fibrosis have *Pseudomonas*.
2. E   This is the most common cause of acute exacerbations of COPD. Other common causes include *S. pneumoniae* and *Moraxella catarrhalis*.
3. B   Seen particularly in those in close contact with infected parrots. It often starts with flu-like symptoms. Additional features include high fever and meningism.
4. C   *S. aureus* is a common cause of pneumonia in intravenous drug users or in patients with central venous catheters.
5. D   Likely cause of pneumonia associated with contaminated water systems in hotels.

Respiratory drugs

1. D   This drug also causes pink coloured urine and body secretions.
2. A   Ethambutol is known to result in visual disturbances such as colour blindness and central scotoma formation.

3. H   The diagnosis is *S. aureus* pneumonia most appropriately treated with flucloxacillin.
4. B   Additional side effects include rashes and arthralgia.
5. E   This individual is at risk of aspiration pneumonia; most appropriately treated with metronidazole as infection is commonly due to anaerobes.

Lung cancer

1. E   This is especially associated with nonsmall cell lung carcinoma. These patients get clubbing and increased bone deposition on long bones.
2. G   The growing tumour can cause compression of the brachial plexus and cause pain in the shoulder and inner arm.
3. D   This could be familial or secondary to endocrine conditions (e.g., diabetes mellitus, obesity), drug related (e.g., steroid use) or malignancy as a paraneoplastic syndrome.
4. F   Classic features of Horner syndrome as a result of involvement of the preganglionic sympathetic nerves. In this case it is caused by a Pancoast tumour.
5. A   Symptoms are associated with a defective release of acetylcholine at the neuromuscular junction. About 60% of those with LEMS have an underlying malignancy, most commonly SCLC.

Diseases of the respiratory tract

1. G   Classic definition of emphysema. Severe destruction can lead to development of bullous emphysema.
2. F   A viral infection associated with myalgia, headaches, cough and a sore throat. Management is usually symptomatic relief.
3. E   Features are essentially due to inflammatory oedema involving the larynx.
4. A   Cystic fibrosis is the most common cause of bronchiectasis, which is a permanent dilatation of airways.
5. H   Typical features of acute bronchitis, which is a short-term inflammation of the bronchi causing cough, wheeze, breathlessness, fever and chest discomfort.

Investigative findings

1. I   This condition is associated with a ground-glass appearance progressing to a honeycomb lung on CXR.
2. G   Typical X-ray features of extrinsic allergic alveolitis, an inflammation of the alveoli within the lung caused by hypersensitivity to a large range of inhaled organic dusts.
3. A   Patients with COPD have partially reversible airflow limitation with an increase in FEV_1 of less than 15% on inhalation of a β_2 agonist.

4. J   Typical presentation of pneumonia, with *S. pneumoniae* being the most common bacterial cause.

5. D   This is an autoimmune, systemic, small to medium vessel vasculitis affecting the upper respiratory tract, lungs and kidneys with antineutrophil cytoplasmic antibodies found in over 90% of cases.

Lung diseases

1. D   Tar-stained fingers indicate long-term tobacco use, which results in the development of COPD.

2. J   Pneumothorax. A history of trauma, respiratory distress and unilateral loss of breath sounds suggests a pneumothorax.

3. F   Pleural effusion. Symptoms suggest that this is likely secondary to a lung malignancy.

4. I   Rheumatoid lung. This patient has underlying rheumatoid arthritis. Rheumatoid lung disease includes nodules, pulmonary fibrosis, pulmonary hypertension, pleural effusions and bronchiolitis obliterans.

5. E   Cor pulmonale. The occupational history indicates exposure to metal shards or chemicals, leading to pulmonary fibrosis and subsequent right-sided heart failure.

Shortness of breath

1. B   Aortic stenosis. Patients present with angina, breathlessness and syncope. Causes include degeneration, bicuspid aortic valve and rheumatic fever.

2. I   Right middle lobe pneumonia. The acute history, X-ray findings and raised inflammatory markers all indicate a right-sided pneumonia. The most common bacterial cause is *S. pneumoniae*.

3. F   Pleural effusion. The underlying cause is likely to be lung carcinoma given the significant smoking history. This type of effusion is usually exudative.

4. J   Spontaneous pneumothorax. This occurs in the absence of underlying lung disease and is usually due to the formation of small sacs of air blebs in lung tissue that rupture, causing air to leak into the pleural space. Risk factors include male gender, smoking and a family history of pneumothorax.

5. G   Bronchial carcinoma. This patient's occupation puts her at risk of lung carcinoma. The most common symptoms are cough, haemoptysis, breathlessness, weight loss and chest pains. The majority of cases are caused by long-term tobacco smoking. About 10% of cases occur in nonsmokers but those exposed to carcinogens (e.g., asbestos) or those with genetic factors.

Respiratory infections

1. C   A common gram-negative bacterium that is associated with hospital-acquired infections (e.g., ventilator-associated pneumonia). It is frequently multidrug resistant and is difficult to treat.

2. B   Organisms that cause lung abscesses include *S. aureus*, *Klebsiella*, *Aspergillus* and *Pseudomonas*. Alcoholism is the most common condition predisposing to lung abscesses.

3. E   *Legionella* transmission is via inhalation of water droplets from a contaminated source that has allowed the organism to grow and spread (e.g., cooling towers). It usually starts with flu-like symptoms, followed by gastrointestinal tract and central nervous system symptoms, causing diarrhoea, nausea and confusion.

4. D   *E. coli* is a gram-negative bacterium commonly found in the gastrointestinal tract. Following intraabdominal surgery, it is possible for the bacterium to track up to the lung to cause pneumonia and sepsis.

5. F   This is a classic presentation of community-acquired pneumonia. *S. pneumoniae* is the most common bacterial cause.

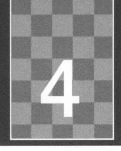

SBA ANSWERS

Question 1

E. The patient has prerenal renal failure. This is diagnosed, in combination with clinical examination, by a urine osmolality greater than 500 mOsm/kg and a urinary sodium of less than 20 mmol/L. Causes of prerenal renal failure include hypovolaemia, decreased cardiac output, renal artery obstruction and liver failure. Acute tubular necrosis is an example of intrinsic renal failure.

Question 2

A. All the options are used in patients with suspected renal failure, but serum urea and electrolytes are the gold-standard initial investigation that can confirm suspected renal failure.

Question 3

A. A potassium of 6.5 mmol/L is a medical emergency, so must be treated as a matter of urgency. This is done by intravenous (IV) administration of calcium gluconate 10% (10 mL) to stabilize the heart, followed by insulin and dextrose infusion to drive potassium into cells. Salbutamol nebulizers can also be used. Cardiac monitoring is important throughout.

Question 4

E. Refer patients for dialysis immediately if any of the following are not responding to medical management: hyperkalaemia, metabolic acidosis, symptoms or complications of uraemia (e.g., pericarditis), encephalopathy, fluid overload and pulmonary oedema. Anaemia is not an indication.

Question 5

B. This can be acute or chronic. Common causes include infection, or reaction to medications, for example, analgesia (NSAIDs), antibiotics (penicillin, cephalexin), proton-pump inhibitors, allopurinol, phenytoin and cimetidine. ACE inhibitors cause ischaemic nephropathy.

Question 6

A. Renal osteodystrophy is the alteration of bone morphology in patients with chronic kidney disease (CKD). There are many radiological findings including osteopenia, salt and pepper skull, subperiosteal erosions, brown tumours, pseudofractures and 'rugger jersey spine' sign. Bamboo spine is a finding seen in ankylosing spondylitis.

Question 7

D. People with estimated glomerular filtration rate less than 30 mL/min per 1.73 m^2, with or without diabetes, should be referred for specialist assessment. Patients should ideally be referred at least 1 year before they might be anticipated to require dialysis. Conservative management including vitamin D analogues, erythropoietin and dietary control is also important but early referral for specialist assessment is the most important step in this patient's management.

Question 8

B. The most common complications from peritoneal dialysis are infections, for example, peritonitis. Noninfectious complications include:
- Catheter related: perforation, haemorrhage, obstruction of flow, leakage
- Related to increased intraabdominal pressure: hernia, hydrothorax, back pain
- Metabolic: hyperglycaemia, hypertriglyceridaemia
- Others: haemoperitoneum, encapsulating peritoneal sclerosis

Question 9

D. PKD can be either autosomal dominant or recessive. Diagnosis is suspected if patient presents with flank pain, haematuria, hypertension, headaches, abdominal pain and positive family history. This patient is likely to have PKD in view of his positive family history and clinical presentation. Renal ultrasound is the most reliable and noninvasive way to diagnose the condition.

Question 10

C. Autosomal dominant PKD is the most common of all the inherited cystic kidney diseases, with an incidence of 1:500 live births. The autosomal recessive form is less common, with an incidence of 1:20,000 live births and typically identified in the first few weeks after birth.

Question 11

B. Renal cell carcinoma originates in the lining of the proximal convoluted tubule. Symptoms include haematuria, flank pain, abdominal mass, weight loss, fevers, hypertension, night sweats and general malaise. The recommended treatment is usually surgical removal of all or part of the affected kidney.

Question 12

B. This man is likely to be suffering from prostatic cancer. PSA is elevated in the condition and should be measured initially, but is not specific, as benign prostate hyperplasia can also cause PSA to be elevated. Transrectal ultrasound and prostate biopsy, and magnetic resonance imaging are subsequently performed for disease confirmation and staging.

Question 13

B. Teratomas are nonseminomatous germ cell tumours. Most of them present with a lump in the testis, which is usually painless, but can be painful or give a dragging sensation. Elevated levels of beta-hCG are almost always found with this type of tumour. Alpha-fetoprotein (AFP) level is usually also raised. These tumour markers are not raised in seminomas.

Question 14

B. Teratomas are nonseminomatous germ cell tumours. Most of them present with a lump in the testis, which is usually painless, but can be painful or give a dragging sensation. Elevated levels of beta-hCG are almost always found with this type of tumour. AFP level is usually also raised. These tumour markers are not raised in seminomas. However, normal marker levels do not exclude testicular cancer.

Question 15

A. The man probably has a seminoma in view of no cystic spaces. It has metastasized to his lungs causing him to be short of breath. Following orchidectomy, seminomas with metastases are best treated by chemotherapy. Metastases below the diaphragm are best treated with radiotherapy.

Question 16

C. Stress incontinence is due to the insufficient strength of the closure of the bladder, resulting in loss of urine when coughing, laughing, sneezing, exercising or any movement that increases intraabdominal pressure. Risk factors in females are pregnancy, childbirth and menopause.

Question 17

B. This patient is likely to suffer from overflow incontinence, which is characterized by the involuntary release of urine from an overfull bladder. It occurs in people with a blockage of the bladder outlet (e.g., from benign prostate hyperplasia or prostate cancer). The gold standard for all urinary incontinence is a urodynamic study.

Question 18

C. This patient has renal colic, commonly caused by kidney stones. The pain is classically loin to groin.

This patient has gout, which is a risk factor for developing kidney stones due to high levels of uric acid. Most stones pass and therefore the most appropriate management is effective analgesia, usually NSAIDs and opiates. Large stones that cannot pass naturally may require interventions, for example, extracorporeal shockwave lithotripsy, ureteroscopy, percutaneous nephrolithotomy or even open surgery, depending on the size and location of the stones.

Question 19

B. This patient has developed renal stones as a result of dehydration. Of the available options, abdominal X-ray is the most appropriate as it may reveal radio-opaque stones, but it may miss small stones or radiolucent stones. A computed tomography KUB is a better imaging modality to investigate for renal stones and is now the investigation of choice for suspected cases.

Question 20

A. *Escherichia coli* is the most common cause of community-acquired UTIs, with a frequency of over 80%. *Staphylococcus saprophyticus* causes 5% to 10% of cases. Catheter-associated UTIs can be caused by *E. coli*, *Klebsiella*, *Pseudomonas*, *Candida*, *Proteus* or *Enterococcus*.

Question 21

A. UTIs are generally rare in young men and may require further investigations including HIV testing and STD screening. Dysuria is the most frequently presenting complaint. Urine microscopy and culture are the first-line investigations.

Question 22

E. This patient is likely to suffer from a severe UTI. IV antibiotics (e.g., gentamicin) is most appropriate. Trimethoprim/nitrofurantoin/amoxicillin are generally for uncomplicated UTIs where the patients are not acutely unwell.

Question 23

A. This child is likely to suffer from nephrotic syndrome. Patients present with a triad of significant proteinuria, hypoalbuminaemia and oedema. In children, the most common cause is minimal change disease. A 24-hour urine collection and serum albumin measurement will confirm the diagnosis. A renal biopsy may be indicated to investigate the underlying cause. Treatment is usually with a course of oral corticosteroids.

Question 24

C. Minimal change disease is by far the most common cause of nephrotic syndrome in children aged between 1 and 7. The hallmarks of the disease are diffuse loss of podocyte foot processes, vacuolation and the appearance of microvilli on histology.

Question 25

B. Dalteparin. This patient has nephrotic syndrome, which causes a hypercoagulable state due to loss of antithrombin III in the urine. This patient has developed a renal vein thrombosis. This presents with loin pain, haematuria, a palpable kidney and sudden deterioration of renal function. This requires treatment with low-molecular-weight heparin such as dalteparin. Following this, warfarin should be given for at least 3 months.

Question 26

B. This patient has developed nephrotic syndrome as a result of focal segmental glomerulosclerosis, which is associated with both HIV and heroin use, but can also be idiopathic.

Question 27

D. This patient has developed pericarditis as a result of uraemia, which is an indication for haemodialysis, which would remove urea and therefore relieve this patient's symptoms.

Question 28

A. Normally in CKD, patients become anaemic due to reduced production of erythropoietin. However, in PKD there is production of erythropoietin from the multiple cysts that form in the kidneys. Therefore these patients are less likely to become anaemic.

Question 29

C. Ramipril. This patent has developed proteinuria as a result of nephrotic syndrome. Proteinuria is best treated with an ACE inhibitor or an angiotensin II receptor blocker. Human albumin solution would not reduce loss of albumin via the kidneys.

Question 30

A. This patient has developed rhabdomyolysis as a result of his prolonged muscular crush injury. The skeletal muscle breakdown leads to myoglobin being released into the bloodstream, which is nephrotoxic. First-line treatment is IV fluid rehydration to prevent AKI. Haemodialysis may be required, but fluid rehydration would occur first.

Question 31

A. Churg–Strauss syndrome is a small vessel P-ANCA-positive (myeloperoxidase (MPO)-positive) vasculitis. It can cause pulmonary–renal syndrome, which presents with haemoptysis and haematuria. This patient has developed nephritic syndrome and AKI as a result of a rapidly progressive glomerulonephritis.

Question 32

C. In bilateral renal artery stenosis, use of an ACE inhibitor can cause AKI and lead to flash pulmonary oedema, which is what this patient has presented with. It presents with cough, dyspnoea, orthopnoea and bilateral fine inspiratory crackles. Other causes of flash pulmonary oedema include acute myocardial infarction, acute respiratory distress syndrome, heroin and cocaine use.

Question 33

C. The build-up of urine has caused hydronephrosis, which presents with enlarged kidneys, bladder and renal failure. Any cause of obstruction can lead to hydronephrosis. Causes include renal calculi, benign prostatic hyperplasia, malignancy (bladder cancer, prostate cancer and urethral cancer), urethral stenosis and retroperitoneal fibrosis.

Question 34

E. ECG findings associated with hyperkalaemia include prolonged PR interval, tall T waves, widened QRS complexes, absent P waves and eventually sinusoidal waves (severe hyperkalaemia).

Question 35

E. On the contrary, hypercoagulability state is present in nephrotic syndrome. Venous thrombosis and pulmonary embolism are well-known complications of the nephrotic syndrome. Hypercoagulability in these cases appears to derive from urinary loss of anticoagulant proteins, such as antithrombin III and plasminogen, along with the simultaneous increase in clotting factors, especially factors I, VII, VIII and X.

Question 36

A. Carpal tunnel syndrome is the tingling and pain of the hands due to impingement of the median nerve in the carpal tunnel of the hand. In dialysis patients, it is secondary to dialysis-related amyloidosis due to deposition of β_2-microglobulin.

EMQ ANSWERS

Renal disease

1. H Typical presentation includes renal colic and haematuria. Diagnosis is usually made by excretion urography.
2. G Typical features include acute loin pain, haematuria and abdominal discomfort. Individuals are at risk of developing hypertension.
3. A The offending organism is typically β-haemolytic streptococci. Additional features include hypertension and oedema of the legs and sacrum.

4. B   Management typically involves high-dose prednisolone.

5. D   NSAIDs are a common cause of tubulointerstitial nephritis.

Complications of renal failure

1. D   Essentially osteosclerosis is an increase in bone density. If present in the vertebrae it can give rise to a 'rugger jersey' spine.

2. E   Congo red staining or tissue biopsy are the gold-standard methods of diagnosing amyloidosis.

3. A   In this case, decreased erythropoietin formation results in reduced red blood cell formation and subsequent anaemia.

4. F   This is commonly due to uraemia. Dialysis is essential in such cases.

5. B   Classic description of osteomalacia. Renal failure results in phosphate retention and impaired production of vitamin D.

Clinical features of renal disease

1. B   Classic presentation of nephrotic syndrome.

2. G   Additional features include neurological and cardiovascular abnormalities.

3. I   Patients may also experience notable weight loss and bone or chest pain due to metastases.

4. E   The patient has gout, which may be associated with uric acid stone formation.

5. A   Classic presentation of nephritic syndrome.

Investigations

1. D   Renal failure may be precipitated by ACE inhibitors in patients with renal artery stenosis (pressured atheromations in this case). Magnetic resonance angiography is the gold standard for the diagnosis of renal artery stenosis.

2. E   The diagnosis is renal colic, which may be diagnosed by abdominal X-ray of the kidneys, ureters and bladder.

3. F   The diagnosis is urinary tract obstruction, which is most appropriately investigated by renal ultrasound in the first instance.

4. C   This patient has a UTI. A urine dipstick, together with urine microscopy and culture, is essential.

5. J   This patient has stress incontinence, which is most appropriately diagnosed by urodynamic investigations.

Management of renal disease

1. D   This patient is likely to have benign prostatic hypertrophy. Alpha-blockers would help to relax the smooth muscle in the bladder neck and prostate.

2. F   The diagnosis is renal colic. Analgesia is the mainstay form of management.

3. E   This patient is likely to be suffering from a UTI and would require antibiotic therapy.

4. G   The diagnosis is nephrotic syndrome most appropriately treated with steroid therapy.

5. C   The diagnosis is renal cell carcinoma most appropriately managed by surgical intervention.

Disease of the tubules and interstitium

1. E   UTI. Common in pregnancy due to high levels of progesterone and smooth muscle relaxation.

2. K   Acute pyelonephritis. The ascending infection causes the systemic signs.

3. J   Ischaemic acute tubular necrosis. The blood loss following the trauma causes hypoperfusion and ischaemia.

4. D   Urate nephropathy. In tumour lysis syndrome, the sudden breakdown of tumour cells releases large quantities of uric acid. This can lead to AKI.

5. G   Chronic pyelonephritis. Infection (usually in early childhood) results in chronic scarring and can lead to hypertension and chronic renal failure. This is a T-cell-mediated inflammatory response.

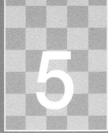

SBA ANSWERS

Question 1

A. The diagnosis is myasthenia gravis (MG), which is initially investigated by demonstrating the presence of acetylcholine receptor antibodies. Single-fibre EMG is more sensitive for diagnosis than acetylcholine receptor antibodies but is less widely available.

Question 2

E. The patient is demonstrating myotonia: a delay in muscle relaxation (prolonged contraction) after voluntary contraction or electrical stimulation. Causes include myotonic dystrophy, myotonia congenita and paramyotonia congenita.

Question 3

C. Typical presentation of the X-linked recessive condition Duchenne muscular dystrophy. Symptoms of muscle weakness usually present around the age of 4 in boys and progress quickly. Muscle loss occurs first in the upper legs and pelvis resulting in difficulty standing up. Becker muscular dystrophy usually presents later but may have similar clinical features.

Question 4

B. Alcoholics are often at risk of thiamine (vitamin B_1) deficiency, which can lead to neurological abnormalities such as ataxia, nystagmus and ophthalmoplegia (Wernicke encephalopathy). Long term, there is a risk of brain damage and memory loss (Korsakoff syndrome).

Question 5

E. The diagnosis is Guillain–Barré syndrome, which is an autoimmune disorder that causes rapid-onset muscle weakness starting from extremities and spreading to respiratory muscles. Over 50% of patients with Guillain–Barré syndrome have experienced an infection before the onset of the condition, for example, gastroenteritis (*Campylobacter jejuni*) or respiratory tract infection.

Question 6

C. Typical presentation of median nerve damage, which results in lack of ability to abduct and oppose the thumb due to paralysis of thenar muscles, weakness in forearm pronation and wrist and finger flexion, sensory loss in the thumb, index finger, middle finger and radial aspect of the ring finger.

Question 7

E. Motor neurone disease is a clinical diagnosis and needs no investigative involvement. Investigations are usually performed only to rule out other neurological problems with a similar presentation.

Question 8

B. Classic presentation of Friedreich ataxia, which is an autosomal recessive condition. Additional features include pes cavus, scoliosis, diabetes and cardiac conditions (e.g., atrial fibrillation and hypertrophic cardiomyopathy).

Question 9

A. The likely diagnosis is syringomyelia, which is a disorder in which a cyst/cavity called a 'syrinx' forms within the spinal cord that can elongate over time. It leads to a cape-like bilateral loss of pain and temperature sensation along the back and arms, and also causes paralysis and weakness. The investigation of choice is spinal MRI studies.

Question 10

B. This patient has spinal cord compression, which is a medical emergency requiring prompt diagnosis and treatment to prevent irreversible spinal cord injury. The patient should be referred to the neurosurgical team for surgical decompression.

Question 11

C. Typical presentation of a cluster headache. The cause is unknown but risk factors include exposure to tobacco smoking and family history. Additional autonomic features include rhinorrhoea and ptosis.

Question 12

B. Giant-cell arteritis is a form of vasculitis affecting large and medium vessels. Visual loss is due to occlusion of the ciliary and central retinal arteries. Prompt diagnosis is required as a delay could cause irreversible ischaemia and blindness. Treatment, if clinically suspected, is with glucocorticoids.

Question 13

E. The diagnosis is giant-cell arteritis. High-dose steroids (prednisolone) should be the first choice of management in this case, which can reduce inflammation and prevent vascular occlusion. The dose of prednisolone is then slowly tapered over a course of months to years.

Question 14

A. The diagnosis is giant-cell arteritis. This condition leads to visual loss due to central retinal artery occlusion. As a result, the retina appears white with a cherry red spot on the macula.

Question 15

D. Typical presentation of a migraine. This typically starts with a prodrome phase (e.g., altered mood and craving for certain foods). This is followed by an aura phase, which can be visual, sensory or motor in nature. The pain phase follows, which is classically a unilateral, throbbing severe headache lasting hours. The pain accompanies vomiting and photosensitivity. The attack ends with a postdrome, which is like a 'hung over' sensation.

Question 16

A. The diagnosis is a migraine. This is believed to be a neurovascular disorder but many neurotransmitters, such as serotonin, appear to play a role in the disease.

Question 17

D. Because of his past medical history, ergotamine and sumatriptan are contraindicated. The most appropriate management would be analgesia and antiemetics. Pizotifen and methysergide are only useful if attacks are frequent in nature.

Question 18

C. The frontal lobe plays a role in higher mental functions (e.g., motivation, planning, social behaviour and speech production). Symptoms include movement disorders (e.g., tremor and clumsiness), emotional disorders (e.g., disinhibition and depression), behavioural disorders (e.g., compulsive eating) and language disorders (e.g., aphasia).

Question 19

B. Owing to distortion of normal structures at a distance from the expanding tumour, a third and sixth nerve palsy are common additional findings.

Question 20

A. In adults, *Neisseria meningitidis* and *Streptococcus pneumoniae* together cause 80% of bacterial meningitis cases. In premature babies and newborns, group B streptococci is common. Risk of infection with *Listeria monocytogenes* is higher in elderly individuals.

Question 21

B. Clinical findings are suggestive of meningococcal septicaemia, which requires immediate use of cefotaxime or ceftriaxone as recommended by the Meningitis Research Foundation.

Question 22

B. LP is the appropriate investigation in suspected meningitis. However, LP is contraindicated if there is a space-occupying lesion or raised intracranial pressure as this may lead to brain herniation, so a CT is recommended prior to LP in these patients.

Question 23

E. Acute bacterial: low glucose, high protein, neutrophil predominant; acute viral: normal glucose, normal or high protein, lymphocyte predominant; tuberculosis: low glucose, high protein, lymphocyte predominant.

Question 24

E. The diagnosis is multiple sclerosis (MS). The main characteristics are the formation of plaques in the central nervous system, inflammation and destruction of myelin sheaths of neurons. The peripheral nervous system is rarely involved.

Question 25

A. The most likely diagnosis here is MS. History and examination alone may be sufficient to diagnose MS but investigations may be required. This usually begins with brain MRI, which may show areas of demyelination.

Question 26

E. Testing of CSF obtained from an LP can provide evidence of chronic inflammation in the central nervous system. CSF is tested for oligoclonal bands of immunoglobulin G (IgG) on electrophoresis, which are inflammatory markers found in over 70% patients with MS.

Question 27

D. This is the most common movement disorder. Over half of cases are found to be autosomal dominant. The tremor characteristically improves with alcohol and propranolol and is made worse by any sort of physical/mental stress.

Question 28

A. Chorea is an abnormal involuntary movement disorder, characterized by brief, semidirected, irregular movements that are not repetitive or rhythmic, but appear to flow from one muscle to the next. This patient is most likely to be taking levodopa for his Parkinson's, which is known to cause chorea as a side effect.

Question 29

C. Myoclonus is a brief, involuntary twitching of a muscle or a group of muscles. The most common circumstance under which they occur is while falling asleep. It is seen in healthy people when it occurs occasionally, but persistent myoclonus can be seen in a wide variety of diseases (e.g., Parkinson disease, Alzheimer disease (AD) and Creutzfeldt--Jakob disease (CJD)).

Question 30

D. Dystonia is a neurological movement disorder whereby sustained or repetitive muscle contractions result in twisting and repetitive movements or abnormal fixed postures. Causes include hereditary, physical trauma, infection, lead poisoning and reaction to neuroleptics. Botulinum helps to inhibit the release of acetylcholine from nerve endings into muscle.

Question 31

E. The diagnosis is Parkinson disease and this patient is suffering from motor symptoms of the disease, which is the result of reduced dopamine production in the basal ganglia. Levodopa is the initial treatment of choice, which can pass through the blood–brain barrier where it is readily converted to dopamine. However, long-term use of levodopa leads to development of dyskinesias and fluctuations in the effectiveness of the medication.

Question 32

A. This patient has Parkinson disease. The pathogenesis of this condition is primarily the result of depletion of dopamine-containing neurones in the substantia nigra and basal ganglia.

Question 33

C. Parkinson plus syndromes are a group of neurodegenerative diseases featuring the classical features of Parkinson disease with additional features that distinguish them from simple idiopathic Parkinson disease. This patient is likely to suffer from progressive supranuclear palsy.

Question 34

A. Tonic-clonic seizure is a type of generalized seizure that affects the entire brain, consisting of a tonic phase (tense skeletal muscles), clonic phase (violent shaking, eyes rolling back, tongue biting, jaw contractions, peripheral cyanosis, urinary incontinence) and postictal phase (drowsiness, confusion, total amnesia).

Question 35

B. Also commonly known as a petit mal seizure. This is characterized by a brief loss and return of consciousness, without a postictal state. These absences can be easily induced by hyperventilation in most cases.

Question 36

C. The presentation is that of a Jacksonian seizure, where a simple partial seizure spreads from the distal part of the limb to the rest of the ipsilateral side of body. It can lead to paralysis of involved limbs for several hours.

Question 37

D. The diagnosis is a temporal lobe seizure due to experience of olfactory hallucinations. Visual hallucinations and experience of déjà vu are also common.

Question 38

D. Sodium valproate commonly causes nausea, vomiting, drowsiness, dizziness and weakness. It has a black box warning for hepatotoxicity, pancreatitis and teratogenicity.

Question 39

A. Common side effects include nausea, loss of appetite, increased hair growth, gingival hyperplasia. Other side effects include folate deficiency leading to megaloblastic anaemia, cerebellar features (nystagmus, ataxia, tremor), vitamin D deficiency and osteomalacia. This is done by the induction of enzymes in the liver that metabolize vitamin D.

Question 40

C. Ethosuximide is used in the treatment of absence seizures. Common side effects include abdominal pain, fatigue and loss of appetite. Serious side effects include pancytopenia, suicidal thoughts, night terrors, paranoid psychosis, systemic lupus erythematosus and Stevens–Johnson syndrome.

Question 41

E. Diazepam given rectally is a useful alternative if intravenous access is difficult.

Question 42

D. Blood glucose measurement should be taken immediately to ensure the patient is not hypoglycaemic. A CT scan should then be arranged to ensure there is no evidence of an intracranial haemorrhage.

Question 43

A. The most likely diagnosis is a subarachnoid haemorrhage with features of raised intracranial pressure. An urgent CT head scan is the initial investigation.

Question 44

B. A yellow-coloured supernatant is diagnostic of a subarachnoid haemorrhage and is due to lysis of red blood cells.

Question 45

C. Subdural haematoma is usually associated with traumatic brain injury, causing tears in bridging veins that cross the subdural space. Onset is slower than other brain haemorrhages. They are often seen in elderly or alcoholic patients who have cerebral atrophy. This is because the length the bridging veins have to traverse between the two meningeal layers is longer, therefore increasing the likelihood of shearing forces causing a tear.

Question 46

E. The diagnosis is most likely to be an extradural haemorrhage due to temporal bone fracture and subsequent rupture of the middle meningeal artery.

Question 47

D. Such neurological symptoms that improve within 24 hours are indicative of TIAs. The risk of stroke occurring after a TIA can be predicted using the ABCD2 score.

Question 48

E. Transient global amnesia is associated with the vertebrobasilar vasculature and not the carotids.

Question 49

B. The most likely diagnosis is a cerebral hemisphere infarct caused by occlusion of the middle cerebral artery.

Question 50

D. The diagnosis is lateral medullary syndrome caused by occlusion of the PICA. Additional features may include palatal paralysis, nystagmus and Horner syndrome.

Question 51

A. The most likely diagnosis is an ischaemic stroke. A head CT scan is the initial investigation to exclude a haemorrhage, although an infarct may not be shown in the early stages. In the case of an infarct, carotid dopplers would then be performed as the bruit is indicative of stenosis and there is a potential for carotid endarterectomy depending on the degree of stenosis.

Question 52

E. High-dose aspirin is the first-line management following a cerebral infarct. He has presented too late to be considered for thrombolysis.

Question 53

D. Opening eyes spontaneously = 4, Confused speech = 4, Withdrawing to pain = 4.

Question 54

A. A scotoma is an area of depressed vision within the visual field. Such a finding is seen in lesions of the optic nerve which are commonly associated with demyelination, as is the case with MS.

Question 55

A. The nerve also supplies the levator palpebrae superioris (responsible for upper eyelid) and sphincter pupillae (responsible to pupil constriction). Therefore third nerve palsy results in pupillary dilatation.

Question 56

D. The diagnosis is a third nerve palsy. Aneurysms of the posterior communicating artery are the third most common circle of Willis aneurysm and this can lead to oculomotor nerve palsy.

Question 57

C. Ramsay Hunt syndrome is the reactivation of herpes zoster in the geniculate ganglion. It results in a lower motor neurone facial palsy, deafness, vertigo and pain. The triad of ipsilateral facial paralysis, ear pain, and vesicles on the face/ear/in the ears is the typical presentation.

Question 58

B. This patient is experiencing vertigo as a result of gentamicin toxicity to the vestibular apparatus. Vertigo indicates a disturbance of the inner ear, eight cranial nerve or brainstem.

Question 59

E. Pseudobulbar palsy is the result of damage of motor fibres travelling from the cerebral cortex to the lower brainstem. Patients suffer from slow and indistinct speech, dysphagia, brisk jaw jerk, dysarthria. In pseudobulbar palsy, the tongue is small and spastic. There are no notable fasciculations. Causes include progressive supranuclear palsy, amyotrophic lateral sclerosis, MS and various motor neuron disease.

Question 60

B. As MS may affect the cerebellum, horizontal nystagmus is typically seen. Vertical nystagmus is seen in syringobulbia and Budd–Chiari malformation.

Question 61

B. The clinical manifestations presented in this case study are indicative of fat embolism. Fat embolism is a common accompaniment of fractures of long bones and is usually asymptomatic. It mainly affects the lungs and brain and is characterized by dyspnoea, tachycardia and changes in the mental state of the individual. In rare cases, this condition can lead to death. Fat embolism in the lungs can be histologically visualized. Presence of multifocal petechiae in the white matter of the brain region represents the most profound pathological change.

Question 62

C. NPH is not a disease but a clinical symptom characterized by abnormal gait, urinary incontinence and dementia. This occurs due to impaired reabsorption of CSF at the arachnoid villi. Often, NPH is misdiagnosed as AD or Parkinson disease due to the nature of the symptoms and the chronic nature of the disease. NPH is a reversible condition and can be easily cured with treatment. One of the treatment modes include insertion of a ventricular shaft to drain off the excess CSF. There have been some pieces of evidence suggesting the development of NPH several years after sustaining a subarachnoid haemorrhage, head injury, cranial surgery or central nervous system infection.

Question 63

C. Seizures originating in one area of the brain that affect consciousness are labelled as complex partial seizures. In most patients, complex partial seizures represent underlying temporal lobe epilepsy. The predominant symptoms occurring during a seizure event determine the seizure type. Symptoms start with aura (a simple partial seizure), which is a subjective sensation and is the initial part during which the patient is aware. Typically, it is of brief duration, rarely lasting longer than seconds. Followed by impaired consciousness, this implies decreased responsiveness and awareness of one's self and surroundings. Usually, during a complex partial seizure, a patient is unresponsive and does not remember events that occurred. Automatisms are nonpurposeful, stereotyped and repetitive behaviours that commonly accompany complex partial seizures. The most common automatisms, at least in temporal lobe epilepsy, are oral (e.g., lip smacking, chewing, swallowing) and manual (e.g., picking, fumbling, patting). A typical complex focal seizure lasts about

60–90 seconds and is followed by brief postictal confusion. However, generalized weakness, asthenia and fatigue may last for a few days.

Question 64

E. The frontal lobe is the area of the brain most closely associated with personality. Patients who develop a neoplasm in this area often present with profound disturbances in their personality; loved ones will mention a distinct change and uncharacteristic behaviour.

Question 65

A. CJD is a degenerative disorder of the central nervous system that is caused by accumulation of abnormally folded protein (PrPsc) particles termed 'prions'. Normal prion protein is termed PrPc (cellular), whereas an abnormal, pathogenic isoform of the prion protein is designated PrPsc. It usually presents in late middle age (50–75 years), with rapidly progressive dementia, ataxia, dysarthria, myoclonic fasciculations, somnolence and eventually death, usually following pneumonia, within a year of onset. MRI typically shows bilateral areas of increased intensity, predominantly in the caudate and putamen. On light microscopy, the pathologic hallmarks of CJD are spongiform degeneration, astrogliosis and the lack of an inflammatory response. Spongiform changes occur in the putamen, caudate nucleus, cerebral cortex, thalamus and cerebellum. The amyloid plaques that are seen in about 10% of cases are histologically different from those seen in scrapie or Kuru. There is no known effective therapy for treating or preventing CJD, with the exception of the prevention of iatrogenic cases.

Question 66

D. AD is initially associated with memory impairment that progressively worsens. Vascular dementia results in a stepwise deterioration. Repetitive statements or movement and occasional muscle twitches are features of the moderate presentation of AD. Agnosia means failure to identify or recognize objects despite intact sensory function. It is one of the criteria in cognitive disturbances.

Question 67

A. Migraine is a chronic neurological disorder characterized by recurrent moderate to severe headaches often in association with a number of autonomic nervous system symptoms. Typically, the headache is unilateral (affecting one-half of the head) and pulsating in nature, lasting from 2 to 72 hours. In more than 40% of cases, however, the pain may be bilateral, and neck pain is commonly associated. Associated symptoms may include nausea, vomiting, photophobia (increased sensitivity to light), phonophobia (increased sensitivity to sound) and the pain is generally aggravated by physical activity. Up to two-thirds of people with migraine headaches perceive no aura.

Question 68

A. Cluster headache is a rare form of primary headache. It occurs in recurrent bouts of deep pain, usually retro-orbital and often excruciating in intensity, nonfluctuating and explosive in quality. Episodes occur more frequently during the night. The typical cluster headache patient has daily bouts of one to two attacks of relatively short-duration, unilateral pain for a dozen weeks a year; this is usually followed by a pain-free interval that averages a little less than 1 year. Patients are generally perfectly well between episodes. Patients with cluster headache tend to move about during attacks, pacing, rocking or rubbing their head for relief; some may even become aggressive during attacks.

Question 69

E. Viral labyrinthitis (vestibular neuronitis) can present suddenly, with a prodrome of viral symptoms as is in this case. The vomiting is as a cause of the vertigo symptoms. Tertiary syphilis (late symptomatic syphilis) consists of end-organ damage (neurosyphilis, cardiovascular syphilis, gummatous syphilis). Neurosyphilis can result in damage of the dorsal columns of the spinal cord (tabes dorsalis). Features include ataxia, incontinence, Argyll Robertson pupils and dorsal column loss (loss of proprioception and vibration). Brain involvement can result in personality changes, memory impairment, seizures and confusion.

Question 70

C. The accessory nerve is a motor nerve. It consists of a small cranial root that is distributed through the branches of the vagus nerve to the muscles of the soft palate, pharynx and larynx, and a large spinal root that innervates the sternocleidomastoid and trapezius muscles. There are many causes for injury to the accessory nerve or its spinal branch including lymph node biopsy in the posterior triangle of the neck, radical neck dissection and penetrating injuries. Shoulder pain is the most common presenting symptom, and limited or loss of sustained abduction of the shoulder is the most common sign. The ipsilateral shoulder may droop (trapezius causes elevation of the whole shoulder girdle) and scapular winging or prominence of the medial border of the scapula and protraction may be found.

Question 71

C. The radial nerve is usually injured due to compression in the spiral groove of proximal humerus as it winds in the groove due to improper positioning of the arm for long periods. The symptoms of compression are wrist drop, inability to extend fingers, thumb abduction and sensory loss in dorsal web between the thumb and index finger.

Question 72

D. MG is a disease of the motor endplate, most often affecting the cranial nerves, especially the oculomotor nerves and the eyelids. The disease begins with weakness and fatigue but can progress over days to months. Confirmatory testing consists of acetylcholine receptor antibody testing or EMG when the situation is not urgent. When the diagnosis must be made promptly, the old-fashioned Tensilon test gives immediate and dramatic results.

Question 73

A. MG is an autoimmune disease. Antibodies bind to the nicotinic receptor located at the postsynaptic neuromuscular junction. Patients usually progress with progressive muscular weakness. Over 80% of patients with MG have thymic abnormalities, with 15% having a thymoma or thymic malignancy. Expansion of thymic tissues results in a widened mediastinum.

EMQ ANSWERS

Delirium

1. B   Diabetic ketoacidosis. This is a classic first presentation of diabetes, with children more likely to complain of abdominal pain.
2. E   Hypercalcaemia. This is a medical emergency, the mainstay of treatment being rehydration and bisphosphonates.
3. F   Hypercapnia. Respiration in this situation is driven by hypoxia, highlighting the potential dangers of oxygen therapy.
4. K   Subdural haematoma. A classic presentation which is common in elderly individuals and alcoholics; often insidious in onset, and easily missed.
5. C   Encephalitis. Herpes simplex is the commonest cause of viral encephalitis in the UK, but insect-borne causes are important in other parts of the world.

Cranial nerve lesions

1. C   Characteristic features of a third nerve palsy.
2. G   Additional features include undue sensitivity to sound.
3. D   Typical presentation of damage to the trochlear nerve.

4. B This visual loss is commonly known as a scotoma, which may occur centrally or paracentrally.

5. E Such lesions may also be associated with jaw deviation to the side of the lesion.

Diseases of the peripheral nerves

1. F Also seen in patients with hypothyroidism. Carpal tunnel syndrome may also be associated with sensory loss of the palm and radial three and a half fingers.

2. D Hereditary (duplication at chromosome 17) motor and sensory neuropathies of the peripheral nervous system.

3. E Autoimmune disorder that causes rapid-onset muscle weakness beginning distally and spreading proximally, affecting respiratory muscles.

4. B Chronic thiamine deficiency can lead to Wernicke encephalopathy and Korsakoff syndrome.

5. A Isoniazid is associated with vitamin B_6 (pyridoxine) deficiency, which can lead to skin rashes, atrophic glossitis with ulceration and sensory neuropathy.

Diseases of the muscle

1. J Duchenne muscular dystrophy is an X-linked recessive condition caused by a mutation on chromosome 21. Onset is usually 4 years of age and death is common in the late teens.

2. C Additional features include fatigability of extraocular muscles and muscles of facial expression.

3. D Additional features include cardiomyopathy, glucose intolerance and hypogonadism.

4. E Either autosomal dominant or recessive. The myotonia is often made worse by periods of inactivity.

5. A An autosomal recessive condition that can progress to severe disability within 20 years.

Epilepsy

1. A Tonic-clonic seizures are also frequently associated with jaw claudication and tongue biting and urinary incontinence.

2. B Absence seizures cause a brief loss and return of consciousness, usually without an obvious postictal state.

3. D A simple partial seizure that can lead to paralysis of the involved limb(s) for several hours.

4. A Carbamazepine or sodium valproate are also useful agents.

5. E Additional features include olfactory and visual hallucinations/distortions.

Extrapyramidal diseases

1. D This is progressive supranuclear palsy, which is a Parkinson plus syndrome. There is often a poor response to levodopa in these cases.

2. H This is usually caused by infarction or haemorrhage in the contralateral subthalamic nucleus.

3. G An autosomal dominant condition where typical features include chorea, personality change and dementia.

4. J Sudden, repetitive, nonrhythmic motor movement/ vocalization involving discrete muscle groups. Common tics including eye blinking and throat clearing.

5. B Sites typically affected include the optic nerves, the brainstem, the cerebellum and the cervical spinal cord.

Headache 1

1. H Subarachnoid haemorrhage. This type of headache is often described as 'the worst type of pain ever felt' or as 'feeling like you have been hit over the back of the head by a cricket bat'.

2. J Tension headache. Commonest type of primary headache. The lack of associated symptoms and stable nature of the headache suggest this benign type of headache. The headaches usually respond well to simple analgesia.

3. C Giant-cell arteritis. Medium to large vessel vasculitis usually in elderly patients causing headache, jaw claudication and tenderness on the scalp. It may lead to visual loss if treatment with high-dose steroids is delayed.

4. E Meningitis. Most infections are caused by viruses (enteroviruses, herpes simplex virus, Varicella zoster virus), followed by bacterial (*Streptococcus pneumoniae*, *N. meningitidis*) and fungal (*Cryptococcus neoformans*) agents. The absence of neck stiffness does not alter the working diagnosis.

Nerves of the upper limb

1. C Lower brachial plexus. This boy has arrested his fall with an outstretched arm and there has been stretching of the lower brachial plexus. This may be a neuropraxia which will hopefully resolve.

2. E Median nerve. This lady describes a classical carpal tunnel syndrome. Symptoms may be worse at night due to fluid redistribution (especially in pregnancy) and flexion of the wrist.

3. H Radial nerve. This injury is associated with fractures of the proximal humerus. This gentleman has both motor and sensory loss.

4. A Axillary nerve. This injury is also associated with fractures of the proximal third of the humerus. The anaesthesia over the regimental patch can vary considerably.

5. B Long thoracic nerve of Bell. The long thoracic nerve passes through the axilla and innervates serratus anterior which, when injured, causes winging of the scapula.

Headache 2

1. B Benign intracranial hypertension. Headache worsens with activities that further increase intracranial pressure (e.g., coughing and sneezing). This is often described as affecting young obese women; the underlying cause is unknown.
2. F Giant-cell arteritis. This is a vasculitic disorder affecting the temporal artery and classically causes thick pulseless temporal arteries. Diagnosis is confirmed by biopsy, though sampling error is common as the vasculitis does not affect the whole vessel. Treatment is with high-dose steroids and should not be delayed, tapering down over months to weeks.
3. E Cluster headache. These are migrainous headaches that occur in clusters, which may be separated by months or years. The patient describes fortification spectra preattack. It is often accompanied by eye watering, eye swelling and nasal congestion.
4. J Tension headache. This gentleman is suffering from tension headaches, or muscle contraction headaches as they are also known. This seems to be brought on by stress in his current post, although other causes should be excluded. Treatment with simple analgesia is usually effective.
5. A Bacterial meningitis. This is more common among those living in crowded conditions (such as students). Kernig sign, headache and photophobia should always be treated as meningitis until proven otherwise. The CSF findings here are consistent with bacterial cause.

Strokes

1. G TACS. This man has the required three features to make up a total anterior circulation syndrome.
2. A Lacunar infarct. Caused by occlusion of a single deep penetrating artery that supplies the brain's deep structures (e.g., internal capsule, pons, corona radiata, basal ganglia and thalamus).
3. F PICA occlusion. Also known as the lateral medullary syndrome or Wallenberg syndrome, a very specific constellation of symptoms makes up this syndrome.
4. H TIA. This lady has an episode of focal neurology, of presumed vascular origin, that lasted less than 24 hours. She requires a full work up and treatment of her vascular risk factors.
5. B PACI. This man has two of the three factors for diagnosis of a total anterior syndrome, and a CT scan demonstrating an infarct makes this a PACI rather than a PACS.

Headache 3

1. F Extradural haematoma. Between the dura mater and the skull; usually with lucid interval immediately following the trauma before symptoms occur. About 20% of cases are fatal.
2. K Viral encephalitis. Clinical presentation may be similar to bacterial meningitis; hence CSF sampling must be obtained to differentiate the two. Common viruses include enteroviruses, herpes simplex and varicella zoster virus.
3. J Idiopathic intracranial hypertension. Cause unknown but more common in obese females. If uncontrolled, can lead to visual loss. Treatment is mainly via reduction of CSF pressure (e.g., by LP) and lifestyle modification (e.g., weight loss).
4. E Subdural haematoma (chronic). More common in alcoholics and elderly individuals. Onset can be gradual and progressive because the lower pressure bridging veins bleed at a slower rate than arteries.
5. D Tension headache. Commonest type of primary headache; no pathology on CT; caused by stress, sleep deprivation and eye strain. Treatment with simple analgesia is usually effective.
6. H Cerebral infarct. This patient has a history of angina and peripheral vascular disease; hence she is a high risk for developing a stroke. Lesions in the internal capsule cause contralateral hemiparesis/hemiplegia.

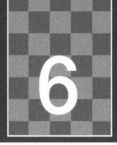

Rheumatology 6

SBA ANSWERS

Question 1
B. Osteoarthritis is a degenerative joint disease that commonly affects the following: DIP joints and first carpometacarpal joints of the hand, cervical and lumbar spine, knee and hip joints.

Question 2
D. The likely diagnosis is osteoarthritis. Stiffness is often worse in the morning and typically lasts less than 30 minutes. The most useful investigation is an X-ray of the knee, which may demonstrate the following typical osteoarthritic changes: joint space narrowing, subchondral sclerosis, subchondral cysts and osteophytes.

Question 3
E. Osteoarthritis can result in the formation of hard, bony outgrowths on the PIP joints (Bouchard nodes) or DIP joints (Heberden nodes) of the hands. Lifestyle changes, exercise, physiotherapy and analgesia are the mainstay of treatment. Paracetamol is the first line of treatment in terms of analgesia as it is the simplest and safest. NSAIDs are the next step in treatment if pain is not controlled by paracetamol. Heat and hydrotherapy may be used in conjunction with analgesia. Surgery and steroids would only be considered if the aforementioned modalities fail to control symptoms.

Question 4
C. This is a case of rheumatoid arthritis. It commonly affects younger women, and primarily presents with pain, stiffness and swelling of the PIP joints and wrist joints symmetrically. It can also affect multiple organs in the body, such as the skin causing rheumatoid nodules over the elbows and heels. RF and anticyclic citrullinated peptide antibodies are the best investigations, but up to 25% of cases can be seronegative.

Question 5
A. Rheumatoid arthritis is a multiorgan disease. Common signs in the joints include swelling of the PIP joints, ulnar deviation, swan neck deformity, boutonniere deformity and Z thumb. Anaemia is a common extraarticular manifestation of the condition, where chronic inflammation results in anaemia of chronic disease.

Question 6
E. Methotrexate is a disease-modifying antirheumatic drug (DMARD), which helps to minimize symptoms, prevent irreversible joint damage and maintain activities of daily living. NSAIDs and COX-2 inhibitors have no disease-modifying effect and are used to manage pain. Tumour necrosis factor-α blockers are monoclonal antibodies, which are also DMARDs, but they are not first-line treatment. Surgery is confined to very severe situations.

Question 7
A. Ankylosing spondylitis is an autoimmune disease primarily affecting the joints of the spine. Onset is usually <40 years of age. It initially presents with pain and stiffness of the lower back. As disease progresses, patients experience loss of mobility in the spine and chest expansion, resulting in a kyphotic posture. Extraarticular manifestations include uveitis, aortic valve incompetence and pulmonary fibrosis.

Question 8
D. Reactive arthritis, also known as Reiter syndrome, is a type of inflammatory arthritis that develops following an infection, commonly urinary tract infection. The triad of symptoms consists of arthritis of large joints, urethritis and conjunctivitis/uveitis.

Question 9
B. Psoriatic arthritis is a chronic inflammatory arthritis in patients with psoriasis. There are five main types of the disease depending on the joints involved: oligoarticular, polyarticular (rheumatoid arthritis-like), DIP joint predominant, spondyloarthritis and arthritis mutilans. Psoriasis can also cause nail changes (e.g., pitting and onycholysis).

Question 10
E. This is a case of septic arthritis and is a medical emergency. The joint inflammation is caused by invasion of an infectious agent. The most common cause in adults (as in this case) is *Staphylococcus aureus*. Prompt diagnosis is required and treatment with antibiotics should be initiated if clinically suspected.

Question 11
B. The patient is probably suffering from SLE. Up to 70% of patients have skin manifestations including malar rash, discoid lupus and photosensitivity. ANAs are the mainstay of serological testing.

Question 12

C. The woman is suffering from scleroderma, which is an autoimmune disease of the connective tissue. The limited form is called CREST syndrome, which consists of calcinosis, Raynaud phenomenon, oesophageal dysfunction, sclerodactyly and telangiectasia. The diffuse form also affects the gastrointestinal tract, kidneys, heart and lungs. Diagnosis is usually achieved by clinical examination and the presence of autoantibodies in the blood, specifically anticentromere antibodies and antitopoisomerase antibodies.

Question 13

A. Dermatomyositis is a chronic autoimmune inflammatory disorder of the muscles. It presents with a periorbital heliotrope rash around the eyes and proximal myopathy. Other features include erythematous plaques over the fingers and knuckles called Gottron papule, arthritis and respiratory disorders.

Question 14

E. Polymyositis causes proximal muscle weakness and myalgia. There is no skin involvement in polymyositis (as opposed to dermatomyositis). Systemic features include conduction abnormalities of the heart, interstitial lung disease and increased risk of malignancy. Diagnosis is by history and clinical examination, combined with creatine kinase levels and EMG. Confirmation of disease is by muscle biopsy, which demonstrates inflammation of the endomysium of muscle.

Question 15

A. This patient is likely to suffer from Sjögren syndrome, a chronic autoimmune disorder affecting primarily sweat and tear glands, resulting in dry eyes and dry mouth. Anti-Ro and anti-La antibodies are present in 60% to 70% of patients.

Question 16

B. Henoch–Schönlein purpura is a type of systemic vasculitis. The classic triad of symptoms are arthritis, purpura and abdominal pain. The purpuric rash is often on the legs and buttocks. About 40% will also present with haematuria. The condition is more common in children, and usually follows an upper respiratory tract infection.

Question 17

D. This man is suffering from acute gout, which is an inflammatory arthritis commonly affecting the metatarsal phalangeal joint of the big toe, but any joint may be affected. Risk factors include the metabolic syndrome, alcohol consumption, renal failure, medications such as thiazide use. The treatment of choice is with NSAIDs or colchicine if NSAIDs are contraindicated.

Question 18

D. This woman has pseudogout secondary to haemochromatosis. It is a form of inflammatory arthritis formed from the deposition of calcium pyrophosphate crystals in and around the joint. The presentation is similar to gout, but in pseudogout joint fluid microscopy would demonstrate brick-shaped crystals, which would be positively birefringent under polarized light.

Question 19

D. This woman suffers from osteomalacia, which is a form of metabolic bone disease caused from an inadequate mineralization of bones in the body. This is due to a deficiency in calcium, vitamin D or phosphate, or increased calcium resorption. Symptoms include generalized arthralgia and bony pains, muscle weakness (especially the proximal muscles), causing a difficulty in climbing stairs or rising up from squatting position, and a waddling gait.

Question 20

D. Lifestyle changes such as smoking cessation and increasing weight-bearing exercise are very important in the management of osteoporosis, but bisphosphonates are the most appropriate step in the management of this patient as they act to decrease the risk of further fractures in those who have already sustained a fracture secondary to osteoporosis.

Question 21

B. Paget disease of the bone is a type of metabolic bone disease, where there is excessive breakdown and disorganized remodelling of the bone. The most common symptom is bony pain. Diagnosis is achieved by an elevated level of serum ALP in the presence of normal calcium, phosphate and alanine aminotransferase levels. Plain X-rays show characteristic changes, which can be analyzed in more detail by performing a full body skeletal survey.

EMQ ANSWERS

Limp

1. D   Fractured neck of femur. This is a classic presentation and must always be considered in an elderly patient who has pain or mobility problems after a fall, however trivial.

2. E   Gout. Thiazide (loop) diuretics cause hyperuricaemia, which in turn can lead to gout. It can also cause hyperglycaemia and hypokalaemia.

3. I Slipped upper femoral epiphysis. This is a fracture through the growth plate, resulting in a slippage of the overlying end of the femur. It causes groin pain on the affected side and/or knee or thigh pain with a painful limp. Avoid the pitfall of labelling such presentation as 'growing pains'.
4. B Compartment syndrome. Also known as 'shin splints', this is due to increased pressure in the anterior tibial compartment as a result of swelling or bleeding from a muscle tear.
5. F Osteoarthritis of hip. Another classic presentation with referred pain from the hip to the knee. The patient's knee would be normal on examination (unless he also had osteoarthritis in that joint!).

Finger clubbing

1. G Pulmonary abscess. This pus-filled cavity is usually caused by aspiration. It is a progressive disease and patients are typically cachectic on presentation.
2. B Crohn disease. The terminal ileum and right side of the colon are the sites most frequently affected by the disease, and malabsorption is a key feature.
3. E Fibrosing alveolitis. This is an insidious, progressive disease, and for good reason labelled 'cryptogenic'.
4. F Infective endocarditis. An increasingly common presentation with a wide range of potential causative agents. Intravenous drug users commonly introduce S. aureus into the right-sided valves.
5. D Familial clubbing. There is no direct association between asthma and clubbing.

The painful joint

1. A Ankylosing spondylitis. The majority of affected persons carry the HLA-B27 antigen, with a male:female ratio of 4:1. Extraarticular manifestations include uveitis/iritis, aortic valve incompetence and pulmonary fibrosis.
2. J SLE. Up to 70% patients have skin manifestations including malar rash, discoid lupus and photosensitivity. SLE can also affect other organs (e.g., lungs, kidneys, heart and brain).
3. G Reiter syndrome. There is a strong association with the HLA-B27 antigen, as there is for ankylosing spondylitis. The classical triad of symptoms consists of arthritis of large joints, urethritis and conjunctivitis/uveitis.
4. D Osteoarthritis. Osteoarthritis is by far the most common form of arthritis, shows a strong association with ageing and is a major cause of pain and disability in the elderly.
5. C Gout. Gout is a crystal arthropathy with a strong (over 10:1) male:female predominance. Loop diuretics (e.g., thiazides) are known to be a risk factor for developing gout.

Arthritis

1. F Additional features include involvement of the first metatarsophalangeal joint of the foot, bony swellings at the DIP joints (Heberden nodes) and at the PIP joints (Bouchard nodes).
2. H Additional features include ulnar deviation, hyperextension of the PIP joint (swan neck deformity), flexion of the PIP joint (boutonniere deformity) and Z thumb.
3. G There are five main types of the disease depending on the joints involved: oligoarticular, polyarticular (rheumatoid arthritis-like) DIP joint predominant, spondyloarthritis and arthritis mutilans. Psoriasis can also cause nail changes (e.g., pitting and onycholysis).
4. E This inflammatory arthritis develops following an infection, commonly urinary tract infection. The triad of symptoms consists of arthritis of large joints, urethritis and conjunctivitis/uveitis.
5. A Ankylosing spondylitis is linked to the development of inflammatory bowel disease, psoriasis and uveitis.

Connective tissue

1. C Features include discoid rash, malar rash, photosensitivity, arthritis, pleural effusions, neurological abnormalities, pericarditis, renal failure, anaemia and antiphospholipid syndrome.
2. D Discoid lupus is a chronic photosensitive skin eruption characterized by persistent scaly, disc-like plaques on the scalp, face and ears that may cause scarring and alopecia.
3. A Additional features include an increased risk of deep vein thrombosis, stroke and myocardial infarction, thrombocytopenia and livedo reticularis.
4. F Dermatomyositis causes a periorbital heliotrope rash around the eyes and proximal myopathy. Other features include erythematous plaques over the fingers and knuckles called Gottron papule, arthritis and respiratory disorders.
5. B The limited form is called CREST syndrome, which consists of calcinosis, Raynaud phenomenon, oesophageal dysfunction, sclerodactyly and telangiectasia. The diffuse form also affects the gastrointestinal tract, kidneys, heart and lungs.

Vasculitis

1. A Polymyalgia rheumatica causes pain and stiffness in the shoulders/pelvic girdle, fatigue and loss of appetite. Associated with temporal arteritis. Treatment is with corticosteroids.
2. B Temporal arteritis causes headaches, scalp tenderness, jaw claudication and visual loss. It is associated with an increased risk of stroke.

3. H Additional features may include mononeuritis multiplex, hypertension and weight loss. There is a strong link with hepatitis B antigen with regard to pathogenesis. Small aneurysms are strung like the beads of a rosary (rosary sign).

4. J A small-vessel vasculitis that causes systemic symptoms and renal failure. Rapidly progressive glomerulonephritis may occur. Management typically involves prednisolone and cyclophosphamide.

5. I Typical features include painful mouth and genital ulcers, inflammatory eye disease, arthritis and erythema nodosum.

Drugs

1. B Additional side effects include muscle weakness, double vision and a yellow discolouration of the skin.

2. E Hydroxychloroquine is specifically associated with retinopathy.

3. F A well-recognized side effect of auranofin.

4. D Additional side effects include blood dyscrasias, gastrointestinal disturbances and central nervous system reactions.

5. G Additional side effects include thrombocytopenia and hepatoxicity.

Back pain

1. G A medical emergency that requires urgent neurosurgical input. Main features are saddle anaesthesia, severe lower back pain, bowel and bladder dysfunction, sexual dysfunction.

2. C Most common forms are cervical and lumbar spinal stenosis. Main cause is ageing. Most appropriate investigation is MRI.

3. A Treatment typically involves bed rest, analgesia and physiotherapy.

4. B This is commonly due to the slipping of one vertebra on another, most commonly L4/L5.

5. D Additional features include loss of lumbar lordosis, kyphosis and reduced chest expansion.

Joint pain

1. E Pseudogout. Deposition of calcium pyrophosphate dihydrate crystals in joints, commonly the knee joint. Common in older patients. Fluid microscopy demonstrates brick-shaped crystals, which are positively birefringent under polarized light.

2. G Septic joint. A medical emergency that requires prompt diagnosis and treatment with antibiotics if clinically suspected.

3. A Rheumatoid arthritis. About 30% of cases are seronegative.

4. B Psoriatic arthritis. There are five patterns of joint involvement: oligoarticular, polyarticular (rheumatoid arthritis-like), DIP joint predominant, spondyloarthritis and arthritis mutilans.

5. J SLE. Multiorgan involvement. The arthritis is nonerosive, unlike in rheumatoid arthritis.

6. F Gout. Loop diuretics (e.g., thiazides) are known to cause gout.

7. E Pseudogout. This patient has an underlying diagnosis of haemochromatosis, which is known to precipitate pseudogout.

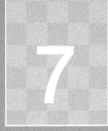

Endocrine and diabetes

SBA ANSWERS

Question 1

C. Pituitary tumours typically cause a bitemporal hemianopia due to compression of the optic nerve by the tumour at the optic chiasm. The temporal visual field on both sides becomes affected.

Question 2

A. FSH and LH are usually affected first, with TSH and ACTH affected last. Causes of hypopituitarism include tumours (e.g., pituitary adenomas), infections (e.g., meningitis), radiation, Empty sella syndrome and pituitary apoplexy.

Question 3

E. The most common cause of hypopituitarism is a tumour in over 70% of cases. Most pituitary tumours are adenomas, which are usually benign in nature. Pituitary tumours account for 8% of all brain tumours.

Question 4

C. Glossitis. This is inflammation of the tongue. It may occur in anaemia and certain other deficiency states, most notably vitamin B_{12} deficiency. The most common symptoms are difficulty with chewing and swallowing foods, tender tongue, smooth tongue swelling and a change in colour (is paler if caused by pernicious anaemia).

Question 5

A. Most pituitary hormones can be replaced indirectly by administering the products of the effector glands orally. Levothyroxine is used for hypothyroidism; hydrocortisone is used for adrenal insufficiency; testosterone for male hypogonadism; oestradiol for female hypogonadism. Cortisol is essential for life and therefore should be replaced first. From the list above, thyroid hormone replacement is next important. It is important that ACTH deficiency is diagnosed and treated appropriately prior to starting levothyroxine in order not to provoke an Addisonian crisis.

Question 6

D. Galactorrhoea in a man is due to hyperprolactinaemia either due to increased secretion or decreased elimination (renal or hepatic disease). The first step in diagnosis is always to measure serum prolactin concentrations (at least three times). The neurological

symptoms in this case suggest a prolactinoma and an MRI of the pituitary will then be necessary.

Question 7

B. The diagnosis is acromegaly. The majority of cases are due to an overproduction of growth hormone by a pituitary adenoma. IGF-1 is the most sensitive test for diagnosis of the condition. This is followed by a growth hormone suppression test following an oral glucose bolus, which confirms the diagnosis following a positive screening test for IGF-1. MRI of the pituitary will confirm the size and location of the tumour.

Question 8

E. Iodine deficiency is the most common cause of primary hypothyroidism and endemic goitre in developing countries. Hashimoto thyroiditis is the most common cause in countries with sufficient dietary iodine. It is an autoimmune condition where there is infiltration of thyroid gland with T lymphocytes and autoantibodies against thyroid peroxidase, thyroglobulin and TSH receptor.

Question 9

B. Anaemia in individuals who are hypothyroid is typically normocytic or macrocytic. Other causes of macrocytic anaemia include B_{12} deficiency, pernicious anaemia and alcoholism.

Question 10

D. Cortisol is essential for life and therefore replacement is of critical importance. This patient has a background of hypopituitarism and should be treated promptly with IV hydrocortisone in the first instance. Stress dosing with hydrocortisone is always mandatory during major surgery, trauma or severe illness.

Question 11

D. Graves disease is the most common cause of hyperthyroidism worldwide. It is an autoimmune disease where thyroid-stimulating immunoglobulin (IgG antibodies with similar effect to TSH) binds to TSH receptor and causes overproduction of thyroid hormones.

Question 12

E. Ophthalmoplegia is associated with Graves disease. Additional features include exophthalmos, thyroid acropathy and pretibial myxoedema. All the other features listed in the question can occur with any cause of thyrotoxicosis.

Question 13

D. Anti-TSH receptor antibodies are present in almost all cases of Graves disease and are diagnostic of the disorder. Thyroid growth immunoglobulins and thyrotropin binding-inhibiting immunoglobulins are also recognized autoantibodies to the TSH receptor.

Question 14

A. Carbimazole takes approximately 120 days to take effect. Propranolol will help to provide symptomatic control and will relieve symptoms of tachycardia/palpitations almost immediately.

Question 15

A. The most common side effect is a rash, which is often treated with antihistamines. The most serious side effect is bone marrow suppression leading to neutropenia and agranulocytosis.

Question 16

C. Pregnancy is an absolute contraindication for radioactive iodine treatment as it is teratogenic. Surgery is possible but unlikely to be necessary in a pregnant patient.

Question 17

E. The diagnosis is thyroid crisis following radioactive iodine. This is much less common now that patients are adequately prepared. As the patient is severely dehydrated, IV fluids would be the first most appropriate step in management.

Question 18

E. One should aim to normalize thyroid status. Hypothyroidism should be avoided as this may exacerbate visual disturbance.

Question 19

D. An ultrasound is performed in the first instance to confirm the presence of a thyroid nodule and to assess the rest of the thyroid gland. To obtain a definitive diagnosis, a fine-need aspiration for cytology is performed.

Question 20

D. Medullary cell thyroid cancers originate from parafollicular cells (C cells) which are responsible for the production of calcitonin, which results in hypercalcaemia. It is the third most common of all thyroid cancers and 25% are genetic in nature.

Question 21

A. Anaplastic carcinomas are associated with a poor prognosis due to their aggressive behaviour and resistance to cancer treatment. Surgical resection is indicated for the few cases that are confined to the thyroid gland. Treatment is generally palliative, consisting of radiation therapy combined with chemotherapy.

Question 22

E. High cortisol levels in Cushing syndrome cause a suppression of innate immune and T-cell responses, resulting in lymphopenia, and increasing the patient's risk of severe viral and opportunistic infections.

Question 23

D. The diagnosis is Addison disease. In suspected cases, demonstration of low adrenal hormone levels using the ACTH stimulation test (synacthen test) is used to confirm the diagnosis. The synthetic pituitary ACTH called tetracosactide is used for this investigation.

Question 24

A. Autoimmune adrenalitis is the most common cause of adrenal insufficiency (90% of all cases). The destruction of the adrenal cortex is caused by an immune reaction against the enzyme 21-hydroxylase.

Question 25

C. The diagnosis here is Addisonian crisis, which is a medical emergency and potentially life-threatening. It may be the result of a previously undiagnosed or untreated Addison disease, suddenly stopping glucocorticoids or an intercurrent infection/trauma. The first-line management is IV hydrocortisone administered with fluid support immediately after taking a blood sample for random cortisol. Intramuscular hydrocortisone can be used if there is no venous access.

Question 26

E. The diagnosis here is secondary hypoadrenalism as a result of long-term steroid use. Use of high-dose steroids for more than 1 week begins to suppress adrenal glands because the exogenous glucocorticoids suppress hypothalamic corticotropin-releasing hormone and ACTH. This is best diagnosed with a long tetracosactide test.

Question 27

D. This woman has Cushing syndrome. Of the given options, the most common cause is a pituitary adenoma which secretes ACTH. This is also called Cushing disease, which is responsible for 70% of endogenous Cushing syndrome.

Question 28

D. The raised ACTH suggests that the high cortisol level is not of adrenal origin. Suppression of plasma cortisol following dexamethasone confirms a pituitary-dependent aetiology, typically an adenoma.

Question 29

E. Surgical treatment is the best approach for pituitary tumours, most commonly via a transsphenoidal approach. Most patients require postoperative steroid replacement in the interim, as long-term suppression of pituitary ACTH and normal adrenal tissue does not recover immediately.

Question 30

C. The criteria for diagnosis include a low serum sodium, low plasma osmolality, a urine osmolality higher than plasma osmolality and an elevated urinary sodium.

Question 31

E. The diagnosis here is SIADH and is treated initially with fluid restriction, usually starting at 500 mL/day of water with adjustments based on serum sodium levels. Long-term fluid restriction of 1200–1800 mL/day may maintain a symptom-free state.

Question 32

E. A side effect of lithium is diabetes insipidus. This patient is likely to have hypernatraemia, dilute urine with low specific gravity and low urine osmolarity. Diagnosis is obtained with water deprivation test with desmopressin.

Question 33

B. Secondary hyperparathyroidism is a physiological response to hypocalcaemia, which in this case is due to a low vitamin D. This condition is seen especially in patients with chronic renal failure.

Question 34

B. Hypercalcaemia, if untreated, can lead to arrhythmias and cardiac arrest. It is treated with IV saline as the first-line management. Bisphosphonates are then used. These are taken up by osteoclasts and inhibit osteoclastic bone resorption.

Question 35

E. Hypocalcaemia causes numbness, muscle spasms, seizures, confusion or cardiac arrest. A diagnosis of hypocalcaemia is most commonly due to renal failure. From the given list, renal failure is the most common cause of hypocalcaemia from hypoparathyroidism.

Question 36

A. A high aldosterone-to-renin ratio confirms the diagnosis of primary hyperaldosteronism, where renin is suppressed and aldosterone is increased. If a diagnosis is confirmed, imaging is then used to look for underlying tumour.

Question 37

D. This is a typical presentation of a phaeochromocytoma and the suspected diagnosis is confirmed by a measurement of 24-hour urinary catecholamines and metanephrines, the breakdown product of adrenaline.

Question 38

A. This is type 2 diabetes mellitus. Of the listed options, diet therapy is always the first-line management, particularly in elderly individuals. However, metformin is the first-line pharmacological agent and is usually used as well.

Question 39

B. Metformin is particularly useful in obese individuals as it does not increase appetite and result in weight gain. The most common side effect is gastrointestinal symptoms (e.g., diarrhoea and abdominal cramps). The most serious side effect is lactic acidosis.

Question 40

E. The most common side effect is gastrointestinal symptoms (e.g., diarrhoea, abdominal cramps, nausea and vomiting). The most serious side effect is lactic acidosis.

Question 41

C. This patient is likely to have type I diabetes mellitus. Many patients present with diabetic ketoacidosis (DKA), as in this case. Patients with type I diabetes always need treatment with insulin, in additional to diet modification.

Question 42

C. Hypoglycaemia in diabetic patients is usually due to overmedication. In an unconscious patient it is always treated with IV dextrose initially. Intramuscular glucagon is used if venous access is not possible.

Question 43

A. The diagnosis is DKA, which is a medical emergency as it is a potentially life-threatening complication of diabetes. The most important initial therapeutic intervention in DKA is appropriate fluid replacement followed by fixed-rate IV insulin administration. The main aims for fluid replacement are restoration of circulatory volume, clearance of ketones and correction of electrolyte imbalance.

Question 44

C. Preproliferative retinopathy describes increasing ischaemia superimposed on background diabetic retinopathy. Cotton wool spots are soft exudates that represent microinfarcts in the nerve fibre layer. Close monitoring is required even if the patient is asymptomatic due to the high risk of neovascularization.

Question 45

E. Symmetrical sensory neuropathy affects the toes and soles of the feet initially. Involvement of the hands does occur, which results in sensory loss in a characteristic 'glove and stocking' distribution.

Question 46

E. Diabetes in pregnancy can lead to neonatal hypoglycaemia not hyperglycaemia due to hypersecretion of insulin from foetal islets cells.

Question 47

A. This patient has a pancreatic insulinoma. These are rare neuroendocrine tumours arising from the Islet cells. They are usually benign in nature. The definitive treatment is surgical removal of the tumour, which may involve part of the pancreas as well.

Question 48

E. Pituitary apoplexy is caused by impaired blood supply of the pituitary gland. This is usually in the presence of a pituitary tumour. Diagnosis is achieved with MRI of the pituitary gland. Treatment is by correction of hormone deficiencies, and in many cases surgical decompression is required.

Question 49

D. Conn syndrome (primary hyperaldosteronism) is the excess production of aldosterone by the adrenal glands, usually by an adrenal adenoma. This is a benign tumour of the adrenal cortex.

Question 50

B. Cushing disease is a cause of Cushing syndrome characterized by increased secretion of ACTH from a pituitary adenoma. The first line of treatment is surgical resection of the tumour via transsphenoidal surgery.

Question 51

D. Neurogenic diabetes insipidus is due to a lack of ADH production in the brain. Causes include tumours, infections (e.g., encephalitis), trauma or neurosurgery. About 25% of cases are of unknown aetiology. Treatment is with ADH analogues (e.g., desmopressin).

Question 52

C. SIADH is characterized by excessive insuppressible release of ADH either from the posterior pituitary gland or from a nonpituitary source. The following criteria should be fulfilled for a diagnosis of SIADH to be made:
- plasma sodium concentration <135 mmol/L
- plasma osmolality <280 mOsmol/kg
- urine osmolality >100 mOsmol/kg
- urinary sodium concentration >30 mmol/L
- patient clinically euvolaemic
- absence of clinical or biochemical features of adrenal and thyroid dysfunction
- no diuretic use (recent or past)

Question 53

E. This patient has a diagnosis of osteoporosis but with no previous fractures. Diet supplementation with calcium and vitamin D is intended to prevent osteoporosis and reduce the incidence of fracture. Bisphosphonates reduce risk of fracture in patients with prior fragility fractures.

Question 54

D. In patients with diabetes symptoms (e.g., polyuria, polydipsia) diagnosis of type 2 diabetes mellitus can be obtained from:
- a random venous plasma glucose concentration ≥11.1 mmol/L or
- a fasting plasma glucose concentration ≥7.0 mmol/L (whole blood ≥6.1 mmol/L) or
- 2-hour plasma glucose concentration ≥11.1 mmol/L two hours after 75 g anhydrous glucose in an oral glucose tolerance test.

As this patient is confused, a random blood glucose is the most appropriate investigation.

Question 55

B. About half of the patients with carcinoid syndrome develop cardiac abnormalities, classically a secondary restrictive cardiomyopathy caused by serotonin-induced fibrosis of the valvular endocardium, notably tricuspid and pulmonary valves. This is usually tricuspid insufficiency and pulmonary stenosis.

Question 56

A. PCOS develops when the ovaries are stimulated to produce excessive amounts of androgenic hormones, especially testosterone, by the release of excessive LH by the anterior pituitary or through high levels of insulin in the blood.

Question 57

B. During acute intercurrent illnesses, patients will have higher need for insulin. In general patients already on insulin will need to have regular insulin, or to increase their dosages to prevent hyperosmolar hyperglycaemic state (HHS) or DKA.

Metformin can cause lactic acidosis, especially in dehydrated patients, and so should be avoided. Short-acting insulin should be given if their original oral antihypoglycaemics do not control the high blood sugar levels (BMS), not starting an oral sulphonylurea.

Question 58
B. National Institute for Health and Care Excellence (NICE) guidelines suggest that type 2 diabetes mellitus should be aimed for <130/80 mm/Hg if any sign of vascular damage is noted (i.e., diabetic retinopathy); otherwise, blood pressure targets should be 140/80 mm/Hg.

Question 59
A. No clear evidence for prevention of macrovascular disease, but there is evidence of long-term prevention of microvascular complications of type 2 diabetes. Sulphonylureas act on the membranes of beta cells, causing closure of ATP-sensitive potassium channels. When the potassium channels are closed, it results in opening of calcium channels and exocytosis of insulin.

Question 60
D. Vitamin C deficiency causes scurvy (typically presents with ecchymosis, petechiae, bleeding gums, impaired wound healing) as it is in this patient. Gingivitis is inflammation of the gingiva. The majority of cases are related to bacteria-induced inflammation caused by the dental plaque causing inflammation of the gingiva and bleeding on tooth-brushing.

Question 61
E. This patient has the triad of signs consistent with hyperaldosteronism: hypertension, hypokalaemia and metabolic alkalosis. In this patient, the primary aldosteronism is caused by bilateral adrenal hyperplasia (bilateral adrenal enlargement in the CT scan). The treatment of choice in patients with primary hyperaldosteronism and bilateral adrenal hyperplasia is an aldosterone receptor antagonist such as spironolactone/eplerenone. Even though other antihypertensive agents can also be used to control the blood pressure in these patients, it is believed that the effect of high aldosterone itself is harmful in the long term. Blocking its effect using an aldosterone receptor antagonist therefore would be the treatment of choice. For patients with unilateral adenoma causing hyperaldosteronism, removal of the adrenal gland on that side is the preferred treatment. This patient has bilateral adrenal hyperplasia, however, and therefore medical therapy is the treatment of choice.

Question 62
D. Hypercalcaemia can be treated with IV saline and furosemide. Fluid replacement with IV saline and forced diuresis with saline and a loop diuretic, such as furosemide, is a rapid and safe way to lower serum calcium and should be the initial approach to therapy. This patient has lung cancer and is probably exhibiting a paraneoplastic secretion of parathyroid-related hormone, which is making her hypercalcaemic.

Question 63
C. Vitamin E is fat soluble and may become deficient in the setting of cholestasis. Tremor and hyporeflexia are classical findings in the setting of vitamin E deficiency. All patients with cystic fibrosis must receive supplementation with fat-soluble vitamins (A, D, E and K). B vitamins are water soluble and cholestasis is not a risk factor for deficiency. B-vitamin deficiency may cause ataxia, memory problems and paraesthesia. Tremor and hyporeflexia are not common findings.

Question 64
A. Beta cells secrete insulin in response to increases in blood glucose. The resulting increase in insulin acts to lower blood glucose back to normal levels at which point further secretion of insulin is stopped. By contrast, the secretion of insulin by insulinomas is not properly regulated by glucose and the tumours will continue to secrete insulin, causing glucose levels to fall further than normal. Patients with insulinomas present with symptoms of hypoglycaemia, such as tremulousness, shakiness, sweating, which are improved by eating. The diagnosis of an insulinoma is usually made biochemically with low blood glucose, elevated insulin, proinsulin and C-peptide levels and confirmed by localizing the tumour with medical imaging or angiography. Surgery is the most appropriate treatment.

Question 65
C. Hyponatraemia and hyperkalaemia unresponsive to IV rehydration should lead the clinician to think about Addison disease (primary adrenal insufficiency). A low serum cortisol and markedly elevated ACTH level confirm the diagnosis. DHEA production starts to increase in midchildhood around the onset of adrenarche. In an adult or adolescent, a normal DHEA level suggests a functional adrenal gland but the test is very unreliable in a young child prior to the onset of adrenarche.

Question 66
D. Hypercalcaemia of malignancy should be treated initially with aggressive rehydration, followed

by diuresis with furosemide, phosphorus replacement if hypophosphataemia is present and IV bisphosphonates. Adjunctive therapies include dialysis, glucocorticoids, calcitonin, plicamycin and gallium nitrate.

Question 67

A. Diagnosis achieved by excluding other aetiologies such as pregnancy, lactation, hypothyroidism and medications before starting the work-up for hyperprolactinemia. If basal fasting morning prolactin levels fall between >100–200 mg/L in nonpregnant woman such as in our presenting patient, that will indicate MRI of the pituitary. Prolactin level more than 100 ng/mL suggests probable pituitary adenoma, and hence the MRI indication.

Question 68

A. Graves disease, also known as toxic diffuse goitre is an autoimmune disease that affects the thyroid. It frequently results in hyperthyroidism and an enlarged thyroid. Signs and symptoms of hyperthyroidism may include irritability, muscle weakness, sleeping problems, fast heartbeat, heat intolerance, diarrhoea and weight loss. Other symptoms may include thickening of the skin on the shins, known as pretibial myxoedema, and eye problems such as bulging, a condition known as Graves ophthalmopathy. About 25% to 80% of people develop eye problems. This presentation might be confused with postpartum thyroiditis but the presence of bruit is significant for Graves disease but not for postpartum thyroiditis.

Question 69

A. Thyroid malignancy presents with solid cold nodules in the thyroid glands. Treatment involves removal of the nodules through surgery. Surgery would be effective when the cancer has not spread to other body parts. These nodules can be felt in the neck. The nodules present a significant degree of concern when diagnosed in individuals under the age of 20 years. The solid cold nodules are diagnosed during physical examination and the patient is then referred to an endocrinologist for further examination. The symptoms include difficulty in swallowing, pain in the neck, vocal changes and swollen lymph nodes. It has been estimated that women have a three times greater risk of developing thyroid cancer as compared with men.

Question 70

E. It remains controversial whether development of these changes in thyroid metabolism reflects a protective mechanism or a maladaptive process during illness. According to current data, thyroid hormone replacement therapy has not been shown to be of benefit in the vast majority of these patients.

EMQ ANSWERS

Pituitary disease

1. D   Kallmann syndrome is associated with gonadotrophin deficiency with absent sense of smell (anosmia), colour blindness and renal impairment.
2. B   This condition is associated with pituitary infarction following postpartum haemorrhage.
3. A   Infarction or haemorrhage into a pituitary tumour. Headaches and visual loss are typical symptoms.
4. C   The sella turcica appears devoid of pituitary tissue on radiological imaging, and the area is filled with cerebrospinal fluid instead.
5. E   Classic presentation of acromegaly, which is almost always due to a pituitary tumour-secreting growth hormone.

Thyroid disease

1. G   Inflammation of the thyroid gland due to a viral infection. Often associated with fever, neck pain and malaise.
2. E   Graves disease is associated with the binding of autoimmune IgG antibodies to the TSH receptor, causing the overproduction of thyroid hormones, resulting in symptoms of hyperthyroidism.
3. A   Hashimoto thyroiditis is an autoimmune disease that is a common cause of hypothyroidism where autoantibodies against thyroid peroxidase, thyroglobulin and TSH receptors are developed.
4. H   Likely to represent a thyroid cancer, specifically medullary cell carcinoma. The increased calcium in these tumours is due to coexisting increased parathyroid hormone and some cases are part of multiple endocrine neoplasia type 2 (MEN-2).
5. I   A rare complication associated with deterioration of hyperthyroidism following intercurrent infection, stress or radioactive iodine therapy.

Diabetic complications

1. E   Additional features include numbness, tingling and pain particularly at night.
2. C   In addition to background diabetic retinopathy (dot and blot haemorrhages, microaneurysms, hard exudates), the retina also develops multiple cotton wool spots. The patient is at risk of developing proliferative retinopathy.
3. A   Patients are usually asymptomatic at this stage.

4. I More common in type 2 diabetes. Symptoms include pain in buttocks, hips, thighs or legs, muscle weakness, fasciculations and diminished knee reflexes.

5. G Symptoms are typically worse at night and are best treated with tricyclic antidepressants.

Drugs

1. D Typical side effects of acarbose. It inhibits alpha-glucosidase, an intestinal enzyme that releases glucose from larger carbohydrates.

2. C Typical side effects of metformin. Its main effect is to decrease liver glucose production (gluconeogenesis).

3. C Used in obese individuals as it does not increase appetite or cause weight loss.

4. A A sulphonylurea that acts via closure of K^+ ATP channels, leading to calcium influx and insulin release. Unlike tolbutamide, it is long acting and therefore avoided in the elderly due to the risk of hypoglycaemia.

5. F An insulin-releasing agent, which helps to lower postprandial hyperglycaemia.

Investigation

1. B The diagnosis is acromegaly. IGF-1 and growth hormone suppression test following an oral glucose load are used to diagnose the condition.

2. G The diagnosis is Cushing syndrome. This test will help confirm the raised cortisol.

3. J Presentation of a phaeochromocytoma diagnosed by measurement of urinary catecholamines and their breakdown products.

4. E This is Addison disease and is usually diagnosed via the short synacthen test.

5. H This is likely to be diabetes insipidus. This is usually first investigated by measurement of urine and plasma osmolality, to look for psychogenic polydipsia, but will need a supervised water deprivation test to confirm the diagnosis.

Diabetes

1. B Diabetes insipidus. This can be confused with diabetes mellitus due to the polydipsia and polyuria. The normal blood glucose and reduced serum osmolarity should point towards the diagnosis.

2. F Hyperosmolar nonketotic coma. This gentleman has presented in hyperosmolar nonketotic coma brought on by his choice of sugary fluid to rehydrate himself. He requires rehydration and cautious correction of his blood sugar.

3. C DKA. This boy has presented in DKA, which may have been precipitated by his chest infection. He requires fluid resuscitation, insulin and replacement of potassium.

4. H Random serum glucose >7.1 mmol/L but below 12 mmol/L. These are the levels for impaired glucose tolerance. Sugars should be monitored as the patient may go on to develop full-blown diabetes.

5. I Type I diabetes mellitus. This most commonly presents in the young and is characterized by absolute insulin deficiency. Type II usually presents in the older population (middle aged onwards) and is more characterized by relative insulin lack or resistance.

The pancreas and diabetes

1. A Type 2 diabetes mellitus is due to insufficient insulin production and insulin resistance. Treatment is with lifestyle modification and oral hypoglycaemic agents in the first instance. Insulin is only used in the advanced stages of disease.

2. F MODY describes hereditary forms of diabetes mellitus due to ineffective insulin production or release by pancreatic beta cells. Defects are mutations of transcription factor genes (e.g., glucokinase gene).

3. E This consists of central obesity, hypertension, hyperglycaemia/insulin resistance and hypercholesterolaemia. It is associated with development of cardiovascular disease and type 2 diabetes mellitus.

4. D Type 1 diabetes usually presents with DKA, which is a medical emergency requiring prompt treatment with fluid rehydration and insulin and potassium replacement.

5. B This is especially common during the third trimester of pregnancy. Infants born to mothers with gestational diabetes are at risk of macrosomia, intrauterine growth restriction, polyhydramnios, neonatal hypoglycaemia and respiratory distress syndrome.

The adrenal glands

1. F Primary adrenal insufficiency; the most common cause is autoimmune adrenalitis.

2. B Primary hyperaldosteronism caused by adrenal adenoma.

3. A A neuroendocrine tumour that secretes high amounts of catecholamines.

4. D The most common cause of Cushing syndrome is the long-term use of glucocorticoids, as in this case (iatrogenic Cushing).

5. E The most common type of congenital adrenal hyperplasia involves the gene for 21-hydroxylase.

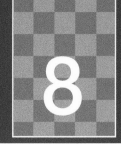
SBA ANSWERS

Question 1
A. In this case, the INR is 7.2 and the patient does not report of any bleeding. In situations when blood INR is between 5 and 9 and bleeding is absent, then warfarin should be stopped with immediate effect.

Question 2
D. Pro-inflammatory cytokines cause thrombocytosis whereas all else cause low platelets

Question 3
D. The diagnosis is polycythaemia vera based on the blood count, splenomegaly and raised red cell volume. This is usually managed via venesection in the first instance. There is no absolute cure.

Question 4
C. 'Tear drop'-shaped red cells are found in myelofibrosis and can also be found in other myeloproliferative disorders, pernicious anaemia, thalassaemia, myeloid metaplasia and some haemolytic anaemias.

Question 5
D. Determination of full blood count is the first essential test. The hallmark of immune thrombocytopaenic purpura (ITP) is isolated thrombocytopaenia. Careful examination of the peripheral smear is essential in a patient with thrombocytopaenia. Peripheral blood smear would show that the morphology of red blood cells (RBCs) and leukocytes is normal, and that of platelets is typically normal, with varying numbers of large platelets. Some persons with acute ITP may have megathrombocytes or stress platelets, reflecting the early release of megakaryocytic fragments into the circulation. In addition, careful examination of the smear is essential to exclude thrombotic thrombocytopaenic purpura (TTP) and rare instances of acute leukaemia presenting as thrombocytopaenia. In TTP, a striking degree of RBC fragmentation is seen in addition to thrombocytopaenia.

Question 6
A. This patient is experiencing an anaphylactic reaction best managed with 0.5-mg adrenaline intramuscularly.

Question 7
C. MCV is very sensitive for alcohol intake. There will be thrombocytopaenia due to splenic sequestration and liver failure; however, it is a very late sign. White cell count is inversely associated with alcohol intake. However, it is very nonspecific. A blood film may show thrombocytopaenia, macrocytosis and haemolysis, but they are nonspecific. Erythrocyte sedimentation rate does not increase with alcohol intake.

Question 8
D. Factor VII initiates the clotting process following tissue damage.

Question 9
A. This patient is likely to be suffering from autoimmune thrombocytopaenic purpura. Platelet count is the first-line investigation.

Question 10
C. Multiple myeloma often has plasma cell infiltrates >10%, with rouleaux formations (stacks of RBCs) and lytic lesions on skeletal survey. International Myeloma Working group states that MGUS bone marrow biopsy should reveal <10% plasma cells and asymptomatic MGUS may have a chance of developing into multiple myeloma, and so monitoring is required.

Question 11
D. This patient is suffering from haemophilia A, which is due to deficiency of factor VIII. The history suggests mild haemophilia and the treatment in this case is replacement of factor VIII for bleeding episodes.

Question 12
E. Vitamin K is necessary for the activity of prothrombin II, VII, IX and X. Absorption of vitamin K and other fat-soluble vitamins will be impaired by cholestasis and hence lead to impaired coagulation by altering activity of these factors.

Question 13
A. The diagnosis is a probable deep vein thrombosis. Doppler ultrasound is useful for iliofemoral thrombosis. Calf vein thrombosis is best assessed by venography.

Question 14

C. The endemic form of Burkitt lymphoma is associated with Epstein–Barr virus. Facial involvement in 50% of patients. Immunodeficiency-associated Burkitt lymphoma rarely involves facial masses. HTLV-1 is thought to be associated with adult T-cell lymphoma/leukaemia.

Question 15

C. APTT is used for monitoring of unfractionated heparin. PT and INR are utilized for warfarin monitoring.

Question 16

A. CLL is a disease of the elderly presenting with enlarged, 'rubbery', nontender lymph nodes. Hodgkin lymphoma commonly affects young adults presenting with night sweats, weight loss, fevers (B symptoms); it also presents with anaemia, splenomegaly and multiple lymph node enlargements. Histology shows Reed–Sternberg cells.

Question 17

D. The warfarin should be stopped and reinstituted when the INR has fallen within the therapeutic range. Other measures are usually only necessary if the INR is very high (>9) or if there is bleeding.

Question 18

C. Auer rods are characteristic of acute myeloid leukaemia.

Question 19

E. Hyponatraemia does not occur in acute tumour lysis syndrome.

Question 20

B. IgA. The defences of the small intestine are in the most part due to T and B lymphocytes. The main type of antibody produced by intestinal B cells is IgA, the major Ig of external secretions. IgA prevents microorganisms from entering the gut lumen as it binds and neutralizes them directly without the need for other effector systems. A much smaller amount of IgM is also secreted by the intestinal B cells.

Question 21

D. All-*trans* retinoic acid is proven to induce remission in this form of leukaemia.

Question 22

A. The Philadelphia chromosome is invariably present in chronic myeloid leukaemia but can occasionally occur in acute lymphoblastic leukaemia.

Question 23

E. Target cells are due to disproportional cell membrane surface area-to-volume ratio. Can also be due to an increase in cell surface membrane (liver disease) or decreased haemoglobin content (thalassaemias). Schistocytes are red cell fragments and are an indicator of mechanical, heat, toxin damage to RBCs.

Question 24

C. In addition to the central nervous system, this form of leukaemia may affect the testes in males.

Question 25

C. Tyrosine kinase inhibitors such as imatinib are the initial treatment of choice for chronic myeloid leukaemia and has better outcomes than alpha-interferon plus cytarabine, which was the previous standard of care.

Question 26

D. Smear cells are characteristic of CLL. They reflect fragility and distortion of B-CLL cells while the film is being made.

Question 27

E. This patient is likely to be suffering from Hodgkin disease, which is most appropriately diagnosed by lymph node biopsy and histology.

Question 28

C. SCD is characterized by RBCs that assume an abnormal, rigid, sickle shape. Sickling decreases the cells' flexibility and results in a risk of various life-threatening complications. SCD usually manifests early in childhood. The most common clinical manifestation of SCD is vasoocclusive crisis. A vasoocclusive crisis occurs when the microcirculation is obstructed by sickled RBCs, causing ischemic injury to the organ supplied and resultant pain. Pain crises constitute the most distinguishing clinical feature of SCD and are the leading cause of emergency department visits and hospitalizations for affected patients.

Question 29

D. Characteristic presentation of Hodgkin disease.

Question 30

C. Iron tablets. The low haemoglobin and low MCV suggest microcytic anaemia. In females of menstrual age, the most common cause of this is iron-deficiency anaemia caused by menorrhagia, sometimes on a background of an iron-deficient diet. Patients should have further blood samples sent off for iron studies to confirm the diagnosis, and then be started on iron tablets, such as ferrous sulphate, if appropriate. If patients had either vitamin B_{12} or folate deficiency, then the MCV should be high.

Question 31
B. Sternberg–Reed cells are malignant B lymphocytes and are diagnostic of Hodgkin disease.

Question 32
E. Additional 'B' symptoms include fever and weight loss.

Question 33
C. Age is not an important factor when determining treatment in the vast majority of cases.

Question 34
E. The gastrointestinal tract may be affected but not in all cases.

Question 35
C. Pernicious anaemia. The low haemoglobin and high MCV are indicative of macrocytic anaemia. Pernicious anaemia is the only answer given here that is a cause of macrocytic anaemia. Iron-deficient anaemia and thalassaemia are both causes of microcytic anaemia, whereas anaemia of chronic disease and haemolytic anaemia are causes of normocytic anaemia.

Question 36
D. MALT lymphoma typically affects the stomach.

Question 37
C. Burkitt lymphoma typically affects African children and can result in jaw tumours.

Question 38
B. Key features of multiple myeloma. Additional features include gangrene and bleeding.

Question 39
D. The initial test is protein electrophoresis, which will reveal the presence of a monoclonal protein ('M' bands). A bone marrow examination showing 10% or more clonal bone marrow plasma cells will be necessary to make the diagnosis.

Question 40
C. Heavy menstruation is known to cause iron-deficiency anaemia.

Question 41
B. This patient has iron-deficiency anaemia in view of her low ferritin. The blood film will show all except macrocytosis.

Question 42
A. This is commonly seen in chronic illnesses, such as Crohn disease, renal failure and tuberculosis. Laboratory findings include a low serum iron, low serum iron-binding capacity and an increased or normal serum ferritin. Treatment is of the underlying cause.

Question 43
C. Vitamin B_{12} deficiency is commonly seen in vegans who do not consume animal products.

Question 44
E. In view of her autoimmune thyroid disease, age and microcytosis, the most likely diagnosis is pernicious anaemia, an autoimmune disease. She will be vitamin B_{12} deficient but the key to the diagnosis is the presence of intrinsic factor antibodies, which are more specific for the disease than parietal cell autoantibodies.

Question 45
C. All of these could cause vitamin B_{12} deficiency but the history makes coeliac disease the most likely.

Question 46
C. Megaloblastic anaemia is seen in vitamin B_{12} and folate deficiency. In this case the cause is not clear, so replacement with both vitamin B_{12} and folate is given pending the results for measurement of vitamin B_{12} and serum folate. Folate alone has been shown to worsen the neurological complications of vitamin B_{12} deficiency.

Question 47
C. The reticulocyte count is increased in haemolytic anaemia.

Question 48
D. The clinical features are characteristic of beta thalassaemia major.

Question 49
B. This patient is experiencing a sickle cell crisis. As her oxygen saturation is currently within normal range, analgesia would be the most suitable management step.

Question 50
A. Systemic lupus erythematosus is associated with autoimmune haemolytic anaemia. Coombs test is diagnostic in this form of anaemia.

Question 51
D. The diagnosis is cold antibody haemolysis, which is best managed by avoidance of cold exposure.

Question 52

D. Stage 3B disease (lymph node areas on both sides of the diaphragm) and constitutional symptoms.

Question 53

A. Warm antibody haemolytic anaemia is characterized by IgG antibodies. Cold antibody haemolytic anaemia is characterized by IgM antibodies.

Question 54

A. Cold autoimmune haemolytic anaemia involves IgM autoantibodies that are most active at 4°C to 6°C, resulting in transient ischemia of Raynaud phenomenon in cold weather. Mycoplasma pneumonia is often associated with cold agglutinins.

Question 55

C. Atrophic gastritis is often followed by pernicious anaemia. Megaloblastic changes result in hypersegmented neutrophils (5+ lobes)

Question 56

D. The PTT or APTT is a performance indicator measuring the efficacy of both the intrinsic and the common coagulation pathways. Apart from detecting abnormalities in blood clotting, it is also used to monitor the treatment effects with heparin, a major anticoagulant. It is used in conjunction with the PT, which measures the extrinsic pathway. It is significantly prolonged in severe haemophilia, but may be normal in mild or even moderate haemophilia. The diagnosis is suggested by an elevated APTT level in a male patient with a positive family history. Laboratory studies for suspected haemophilia include a complete blood cell count, coagulation studies and a factor VIII assay.

EMQ ANSWERS

Anaemia

1. C Such a form of anaemia is best treated supportively with red cell and platelet transfusion in addition to antibiotic use for infections associated with neutropenia.

2. I Common in Northern Europe, this form of anaemia can result in splenomegaly and leg ulcers. Treatment is usually a splenectomy.

3. J Cigar-shaped RBCs are characteristic of hereditary elliptocytosis. Treatment is usually not required.

4. F Haemolysis is the result of oxidant red cell damage. In addition to fava beans, drugs such as sulphonamides may precipitate haemolysis.

5. D This condition may eventually progress to myelodysplasia and leukaemia.

Lymphadenopathy

1. A Epstein–Barr virus is typically transmitted in saliva. In rare cases, there may be splenic rupture, myocarditis and meningitis.

2. F The virus may be transmitted sexually or via contaminated blood products in the main. HIV is an RNA virus which binds to CD4 cells via gp120 to cause cellular damage.

3. C Characteristic description of a lymphoma.

4. D Genetic factors such as the Philadelphia chromosome are responsible for the majority of chronic myeloid leukaemia cases. Environmental factors include radiation exposure and drugs such as chemotherapy.

5. B Additional features may include retinitis, loss of visual acuity and orbital pain.

Splenomegaly

1. A This is characteristic of schistosomiasis, which is most prevalent in Africa.

2. H Characteristic features of kala-azar. Additional features include pyrexia, sweats, a burning sensation in the feet and joint pain.

3. D Four main malarial parasites exist. These include *Plasmodium falciparum*, *P. vivax*, *P. ovale* and *P. malariae*. Clinical features of falciparum malaria include impaired consciousness, uraemia, respiratory distress syndrome and splenic rupture.

4. G A classic description of Gaucher disease of which there exists three types. Type 2 and type 3 have a propensity to involve the central nervous system.

5. J Additional features may include epistaxis and bruising. Ciprofloxacin is the mainstay form of treatment.

SURGERY ANSWERS

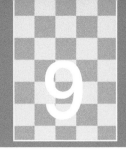
SBA ANSWERS

Question 1
D. Classic hemisection of the spinal cord. A rare occurrence but resulting in ipsilateral power and proprioceptive loss below the lesion with contralateral loss of pain and temperature sensation.

Question 2
E. For children under the age of 6, an intraosseous needle in the proximal tibia is a useful emergency route for fluid administration in times of difficult access.

Question 3
C. Echocardiogram is the diagnostic test of choice, and earliest finding is usually collapse of right atrium and ventricle. ECG shows electrical alternans (swinging QRS complexes) as the heart moves in the fluid-filled pericardial sac. However, this is a late and nonsensitive sign.

Question 4
C. McBurney point is the name given to the point over the right side of the abdomen that is one-third of the distance from the anterior superior iliac spine to the umbilicus (navel). This point roughly corresponds to the most common location of the base of the appendix where it is attached to the cecum.

Question 5
B. An open pneumothorax allows air to be sucked into the pleural cavity on inspiration and forced out on expiration. Immediate management is to close the defect with occlusive dressing.

Question 6
D. Rovsing sign is a sign of appendicitis. If palpation of the left lower quadrant of a person's abdomen increases the pain felt in the right lower quadrant, the patient is said to have a positive Rovsing sign and may have appendicitis.

Question 7
A. The diagnosis is acute appendicitis. Abdominal CT scan or ultrasound is the most preferred investigative tools. Abdominal X-ray is of no diagnostic benefit.

Question 8
A. Extradural haematomas are often associated with a head injury and are classically depicted by a brief period of unconsciousness followed by a lucid interval of recovery. A CT head is the gold-standard investigation.

Question 9
A. The 'drip and suck' technique. Patients are severely dehydrated and require IV saline for adequate fluid resuscitation.

Question 10
E. This is simply a life or death situation. When there is a clinical suspicion of abdominal aortic aneurysm (AAA) you should proceed ahead straight to theatres; unoperated upon, AAA rupture results in 100% mortality.

Question 11
A. This patient is likely to have acute pancreatitis best diagnosed by an abdominal CT scan.

Question 12
C. A massive haemothorax is associated with the accumulation of over 1500 mL of blood in the chest. The chest is notably dull to percussion and breath sounds are absent.

Question 13
B. Cullen sign is superficial oedema and bruising in the subcutaneous fatty tissue around the umbilicus. This sign takes 24 to 48 hours to appear and can predict acute pancreatitis, with mortality rising from 8–10% to 40%. It may be accompanied by Grey Turner sign (bruising of the flank), which may then be indicative of pancreatic necrosis with retroperitoneal or intraabdominal bleeding.

Question 14
B. Subdural haematomas are commonly seen in elderly, alcoholic individuals. These individuals are more susceptible on the background of their atrophic brains, which make the connecting veins more likely to rupture.

Question 15
E. The diagnosis is renal colic, which is best assessed by an IV urogram.

Question 16

B. This patient is demonstrating evidence of gall bladder disease best diagnosed by abdominal ultrasound in the first instance.

Question 17

D. The fall has resulted in a flail chest. This occurs when one or more ribs are fractured in more than one place. The broken segment of chest wall moves independently from the rest of the chest resulting in a paradoxical motion. The underlying lung is often severely contused as a result.

Question 18

E. Presentation of a ruptured AAA. Surgery is the most appropriate intervention.

Question 19

C. Presentation of lower limb ischaemia on the background of atrial fibrillation. In view of her satisfactory blood pressure and oxygen saturation, an emergency embolectomy would be the next most appropriate management step.

Question 20

A. The diagnosis is acute diverticulitis. Additional features would include rectal bleeding and altered bowel habit. Such a condition is best diagnosed by abdominal CT scan.

Question 21

D. The diagnosis is cholecystitis in view of his right upper quadrant pain, pyrexia and elevated inflammatory markers. The mainstay form of treatment is regular analgesia and antibiotic use.

Question 22

C. Additional features may include menstrual cycle irregularities and micturition abnormalities.

Question 23

E. Additional features would include swelling of the testicle and no relief of pain upon elevation of the scrotum. This is unlike epididymitis where elevation may help improve the pain.

Question 24

A. Classical presentation of epididymitis. Antibiotics and analgesia are the mainstay form of treatment.

Question 25

A. A tension pneumothorax occurs when the pleura is breached, allowing air to escape into the pleural cavity. Immediate management involves passing a large-bore IV cannula into the pleural cavity through the midclavicular line second intercostal space.

EMQ ANSWERS

Trauma

1. K Tension pneumothorax. This develops if the communication between the pleura and lung is small and acts as a one-way valve, allowing air to enter the pleural space during inspiration, but preventing it from escaping.
2. F Open pneumothorax. This occurs when the communication between the lung and pleural space does not seal and allows air to transfer freely between the two.
3. C Flail chest. This is a clinical syndrome resulting from major trauma to the chest walls, sufficient to cause fracture of several ribs in at least two places, resulting in paradoxical movement of part of the chest on respiration.
4. A Airway obstruction. An inhaled foreign body is more likely to enter the right main bronchus.
5. L Traumatic aortic rupture. Similar radiological findings in association with severe chest pain radiating to the back are found in aortic dissection.

Acute abdomen 1

1. H A classic presentation of bowel obstruction.
2. J Free gas on an erect chest X-ray is diagnostic of a perforation.
3. C Typical presentation of renal colic.
4. B An abnormal amylase together with abdominal tenderness is a key feature of pancreatitis.
5. F The diagnosis is a dissecting aortic aneurysm in view of symptomatology and a widened mediastinum.

Glasgow Coma Scale

1. J Obeys commands = 6, normal speech = 5, spontaneous eye movement = 4.
2. A Flexes to pain = 3, incomprehensible sounds = 2, no eye movement = 1.
3. D Withdraws to pain = 4, confused speech = 4, eyes open to pain = 2.
4. D No motor response = 1, normal speech = 5, spontaneous eye movement = 4.
5. G Inappropriate speech = 3, obeys commands = 6, eyes opening on command = 3.

Acute abdomen 2

1. A Acute pancreatitis. This is consistent with the abdominal pain experienced by the patient, as well as dehydration, nausea, vomiting and the implied excess alcohol consumption that often accompanies holidays.

2. I Small bowel obstruction. This lady has absolute constipation, nausea, vomiting and high-pitched bowel sounds, all consistent with small bowel obstruction. This is a surgical emergency.

3. F Perforated peptic ulcer. This is suggested by the left upper quadrant pain and recent nonsteroidal antiinflammatory drug use. He is also peritonitic.

4. B Acute pyelonephritis. This is suggested by the flank pain radiating to the groin and associated rigors.

5. E Perforated appendix. This young man has features of peritonism related to a right iliac fossa tenderness. Other causes of right iliac fossa pain and peritonism would be unusual in a boy of this age.

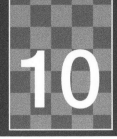
SBA ANSWERS

Question 1
C. This patient has notable features of sepsis, namely pyrexia, an elevated white cell count and CRP. The patient could have concurrent hypovolaemic shock due to sepsis and postoperative timeline, but with a fever and elevated inflammatory markers, sepsis is the most urgent diagnosis.

Question 2
C. Contrast used for radiological investigations/ procedures is notorious for adversely affecting renal function as the contrast is nephrotoxic. Precontrast (and postcontrast) hydration with normal saline is used; some centres use sodium bicarbonate as well. Nephrotoxics should be stopped pre- and postcontrast injection for a few days until the creatinine resolves.

Question 3
E. According to current National Institute of Health and Clinical Excellence (NICE) guidelines, none of the listed investigations are recommended prior to surgery.

Question 4
B. According to the NICE, an ECG is highly recommended. If he had not had a prior chest X-ray, then that would be warranted too.

Question 5
E. According to the World Health Organization (WHO) analgesic ladder, diclofenac would be the next recommended choice of drug.

EMQ ANSWERS

Postoperative complications
1. J Wound infection. This wound discomfort is due to infection rather than a simple haematoma. A haematoma would have been apparent immediately postoperatively. A wound infection, however, takes several days to develop. Infection may have been precipitated by the presence of a haematoma, as it is a good culture medium.
2. H Pseudo-obstruction. This patient has been immobilized in bed following orthopaedic surgery. He has developed a postoperative ileus, with vomiting and constipation. The appearance of a grossly distended abdomen that is tympanitic and nontender is associated with pseudo-obstruction. If he had just been constipated, the rectum would have been loaded and the distension would not have been as significant. He has probably not passed urine for 8 hours because of dehydration.
3. A Atelectasis. This patient has had emergency upper abdominal surgery. She is probably not breathing satisfactorily because of postoperative pain. She therefore has a reduced oxygen saturation. At this stage (i.e., less than 24 hours postoperatively), the alveoli have collapsed because of inadequate ventilation. At the present time, she has not developed secondary infection but, if she receives good pain relief and physiotherapy, one should be able to avoid secondary infection of the collapsed alveoli.
4. B Anastomotic dehiscence. The history of sudden-onset severe abdominal pain 4 days postoperatively suggests peritonitis. The patient is showing signs of septicaemia (i.e., a temperature of 38°C and hypotension). The most likely cause is an anastomotic dehiscence. This is a significant risk after a low anterior resection if the blood supply to the anastomosis is inadequate or there has been poor operative technique.
5. D Deep vein thrombosis. Patients who are having surgery for malignancy and pelvic surgery are at increased risk of deep vein thrombosis. Poor mobility and low albumin and protein levels postoperatively may cause bilateral ankle oedema. The presence of a pyrexia and tenderness in the right calf suggests a deep vein thrombosis.

Preoperative investigations
1. G Echocardiogram. Examination of the patient suggests a diagnosis of aortic stenosis. This needs to be confirmed by an echocardiogram so that the anaesthetist is aware and maintains a good blood pressure throughout the operation.
2. J Spirometry. This patient needs assessment of her respiratory function, rather than just a chest X-ray.
3. E Clotting screen. This patient is to undergo an invasive procedure of which one complication is internal bleeding. As she has been jaundiced,

her clotting may be abnormal because of failure to absorb vitamin K and produce some clotting factors, such as II, VII, IX and X. Before the procedure, her clotting should be normal or corrected appropriately.

4. C Carotid Doppler scan. The history is suggestive of transient ischaemic attacks, secondary to carotid artery stenosis. This needs to be known about before coronary artery surgery as hypotension may precipitate a further event.

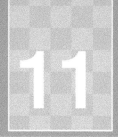

Question 1

B. Meckel diverticulum. Meckel diverticulum is the remnant of the vitelline duct present in embryonic life. It connects the developing embryo with the yolk sac. It is often asymptomatic; however, acute inflammation of the diverticulum may occur, mimicking acute appendicitis. The mucosa at the mouth of the diverticulum may become inflamed and lead to intussusceptions and obstruction, or the diverticulum may perforate and cause peritonitis. More common in males.

Question 2

E. Ischaemic bowel. Ischaemic bowel is difficult to diagnose and commonly missed. It usually presents as abdominal pain out of proportion to clinical findings and investigations, and is often a diagnosis of exclusion; however, the presence of metabolic acidosis helps. It rarely occurs in patients less than 60 years old.

Question 3

C. Intussusception. Intussusception occurs when one segment of the bowel slides inside the adjacent segment, like a telescope. The most common site is at the ileocaecal valve. Patients typically present aged 5–12 months of age, with periods of screaming, vomiting, blood in the faeces (redcurrant jelly) and drawing up of the legs. The child is pale and a sausage-shaped mass may be felt on palpation of the abdomen.

Question 4

C. IV fluids. There is clinical evidence of shock with the patient being tachycardic and hypotensive, so the initial management should be resuscitation with IV fluids. All of the other investigations are relevant, and should be done once the patient is haemodynamically stable.

Question 5

E. Cholangitis. The triad of symptoms which includes fever, abdominal pain and jaundice is typical in cholangitis. Cholangitis occurs when gallstones become impacted in the bile duct; the bile, which is unable to escape, becomes concentrated and infected, resulting in acute cholecystitis. This causes a rise in the liver function test results, particularly bilirubin and alkaline phosphatase. The other diseases do not cause jaundice with pain.

Question 6

B. Dukes B. Dukes classification is most widely used to stage and predict the prognosis of colorectal carcinoma. Dukes stages are as follows: stage A, invaded submucosa and muscle layer of the bowel, but confined to the wall; stage B, breached the muscle layer and bowel wall, but no involvement of lymph nodes; stage C1, spread to immediately draining pericolic lymph nodes; stage C2, spread to higher mesenteric lymph nodes; stage D, distant visceral metastases.

Question 7

A. Mesenteric ischaemia. The key to diagnosis here is in the history. The neck ultrasound scan is likely to be a carotid Doppler scan, suggesting that there may be a history of ischaemia. Smoking is also considered a risk factor for this. Mesenteric ischaemia generally only affects people over 50 years of age and is associated with conditions causing arterial emboli and thrombosis. It presents as a colicky poorly localized pain with minimal tenderness in the early stages, leading eventually to signs and symptoms of peritonitis.

Question 8

A. Pyloric stenosis. Pyloric stenosis, or narrowing, occurs in about 1 in 150 male infants and 1 in 750 female infants. Stenosis is caused by hypertrophy of the circular muscles of the pylorus, obstructing the pyloric canal and the flow of contents from the stomach into the duodenum. Typically, it presents 4 to 6 weeks after birth with projectile vomiting within half an hour of a feed. Note that there is no bile in the vomit because the obstruction is proximal to the ampulla of Vater. Peristaltic waves are visible in the child, a sausage-shaped mass (the enlarged pylorus) can be felt in the right upper quadrant and the hypertrophied pyloric muscle can be observed using ultrasonography. Treatment is surgical.

Question 9

B. Direct inguinal hernia. A hernia is the protrusion of any organ or tissue through its coverings and outside its normal body cavity. If reducible, hernias can be pushed back into the compartment from which they came. Inguinal hernias are the most common and may be direct (protruding through the posterior wall of the inguinal canal), or indirect (passing through the inguinal canal). Indirect hernias are much more common, and lie lateral to the inferior epigastric vessels. Direct inguinal hernias are less common, and lie medial to the inferior epigastric vessels.

Question 10

E. Colonoscopy. This history of a change in bowel habit for greater than 6 weeks with rectal (PR) bleeding is one of the criteria of the National Institute for Health and Care Excellence (NICE) guidelines for an urgent 2-week referral for patients of any age. This should include an urgent colonoscopy and review by a colorectal surgeon.

Question 11

D. Squamous cell carcinoma. Achalasia is a known risk factor for the development of squamous cell carcinoma of the oesophagus. This is thought to be caused by chronic inflammation and stasis within the oesophagus. Other risk factors for the development of squamous cell carcinoma are smoking, alcohol, tylosis and Plummer–Vinson syndrome.

Question 12

C. The most likely diagnosis is acute diverticulitis. Abdominal and pelvic CT scan is the most appropriate investigation. Ultrasound would be poorly tolerated and would not be specific.

Question 13

C. The staging investigations suggest Dukes stage C cancer. Surgery in addition to postoperative chemotherapy is the most effective form of management.

Question 14

E. The clinical diagnosis is acute cholecystitis most appropriately investigated by abdominal ultrasound scan. Blood tests would show an inflammatory response but would not be specific.

Question 15

A. A classic presentation of an indirect inguinal hernia. Such hernias pass through the internal ring lateral to the inferior epigastric artery, along the canal to emerge at the external ring above the pubic crest and tubercle.

Question 16

B. A description of a direct inguinal hernia. Such hernias bulge through the posterior wall of the canal, medial to

the inferior epigastric artery. They do not protrude into the scrotum.

Question 17

C. Femoral hernias are four times more common in women and present below and lateral to the pubic tubercle.

Question 18

A. A classic description of an umbilical hernia. Such hernias are at great risk of strangulation.

Question 19

A. Epigastric hernias typically present in the midline and are often tender and irreducible.

Question 20

C. Spigelian hernias present as lumps at the lateral margin of the rectus sheath. Strangulation or obstruction often occurs.

Question 21

B. Obturator hernias are typically seen in elderly women. The hernia occurs through the obturator canal within the pelvis, so the patient often presents with small bowel obstruction. There may also be pain along the medial aspect of the thigh due to pressure on the obturator nerve.

Question 22

C. Left-sided abdominal pain and dark red rectal bleeding are diagnostic features of ischaemic colitis. Except in the most severe cases, ischemic colitis is treated with supportive care.

Question 23

B. This is the most definitive step in the treatment for sigmoid volvulus. Caecal volvulus requires immediate surgery.

Question 24

E. The diagnosis is haemorrhoids. Injection sclerotherapy is the preferred management option in such a condition, with an overall success rate of up to 85%.

Question 25

A. Classic presentation of a perianal haematoma. There is often a history of straining prior to the perianal pain.

Question 26

D. Glyceryl trinitrate is regarded as the first-line form of management in those with a chronic anal fissure. It helps to relax the internal anal sphincter, allowing fissure healing and thus relieving the pain. For more acute anal fissures, managing constipation is first line.

Question 27

C. Such studies help to measure internal and external sphincter pressures and assess integrity of the sphincter complex using endoanal ultrasound, hence confirming such a diagnosis.

Question 28

D. Classic presentation of an anal fistula. Diagnosis may be aided by performing a fistulogram, proctoscopy and/or sigmoidoscopy.

Question 29

B. The diagnosis is an oesophageal perforation in view of the presence of crepitus in the suprasternal notch. This is best investigated by a chest X-ray in the first instance.

Question 30

A. The diagnosis is corrosive oesophagitis which involves an urgent endoscopy in the first instance to assess extent of damage.

Question 31

C. The diagnosis is achalasia. The most effective management plan is a Heller myotomy, which involves division of the muscles of the lower oesophageal sphincter.

Question 32

C. This patient has evidence of jaundice. An abdominal ultrasound is of key importance in such cases to assess evidence of bile duct dilatation.

Question 33

E. The diagnosis most likely is liver cancer. Serum alpha-fetoprotein is highly sensitive and specific for such cancers.

Question 34

D. The diagnosis in this case is acute cholecystitis. Patients may often demonstrate Boas sign, which is hyperaesthesia below the right scapula.

Question 35

B. Taking into account evidence of distant metastases, the mainstay form of management would be palliative. Resection of such a tumour with the hope for cure is less than 15%.

Question 36

C. The diagnosis is gastric cancer, most appropriately investigated by endoscopy and biopsy.

Question 37

B. Dukes stage B cancers extend into the muscularis or into or through the serosa. The latter is referred to as stage B2 and the former B1.

Gastrointestinal bleeding

1. B Colonic carcinoma. The prognosis is good if detected early, so prompt referral is necessary.
2. E Duodenal ulcer. Altered blood almost always comes from haemorrhage in the upper GI tract.
3. G Haemorrhoids. Haemorrhoids commonly follow, or are exacerbated by, childbirth but often resolve spontaneously.
4. I Mallory–Weiss tear. Another classic presentation due to tearing at the gastro-oesophageal junction as a result of excess vomiting.
5. J Oesophageal varices. Oesophageal varices are associated with portal hypertension caused, in turn, by hepatic cirrhosis.

Hernia

1. G Richter. A partially obstructed hernia which can lead to bowel perforation through ischaemia.
2. J Diaphragmatic. Such hernias occur when part of the stomach or intestine protrude into the chest cavity through a defect in the diaphragm.
3. I Spigelian. Such hernias are often difficult to distinguish from inguinal hernias and may lead to strangulation or obstruction.
4. B Pantaloon. Such hernias are essentially a combination of an indirect and direct hernia.
5. A Inguinal. A classic description of a direct inguinal hernia.

Upper gastrointestinal disorders

1. D Zollinger–Ellison syndrome. Management typically involves the use of high-dose proton-pump inhibitors or surgery.
2. G Adenocarcinoma. Squamous cell carcinomas usually affect the middle third of the oesophagus and are due to a high intake of alcohol, smoking and salted fish consumption.
3. A Achalasia. Chest X-ray features may show evidence of a fluid level behind the heart. Management typically involves surgical division of the lower oesophageal sphincter.
4. F Duodenal ulcer. Characteristic features of a duodenal ulcer. Gastric ulcers typically result in pain after food.
5. I Plummer–Vinson syndrome. Such swallowing difficulties are due to a web-like formation in the upper part of the oesophagus.

Lower gastrointestinal disorders

1. B Intussusception. Classic presentation of intussusception. Additional features may include a mass in the right iliac fossa. Management typically involves surgery.

2. C   Perianal haematoma. Classic presentation of a perianal haematoma.
3. F   Angiodysplasia. In addition to colonoscopy, a diagnosis of angiodysplasia is often made following arteriography.
4. E   Crohn disease. Additional macroscopic features include the presence of skip lesions.
5. J   Ischaemic colitis. Complications include gangrene, perforation and stricture formation.

Hepatobiliary disorders

1. G   Biliary colic. Classic presentation of biliary colic. The pain is often quite severe in nature and associated with episodes of vomiting.
2. D   Cholangiocarcinoma. Such tumours carry a poor prognosis with a 5-year survival rate of approximately 35% following surgery.
3. F   Cholecystitis. Such a finding is known as Boas sign and is characteristic of acute cholecystitis.
4. A   Cholangitis. This triad of features is known as Charcot triad and is characteristic of cholangitis.
5. E   Hepatoma. Other predisposing factors may include hepatitis or haemochromatosis. Treatment often involves surgical resection.

Abdominal pain

1. A   Acute appendicitis. The pelvic symptoms suggest a pelvic appendicitis causing an unusual presentation, as it irritates the rectum and bladder. However, the causes of such a history in a young, previously well man are limited, as is right iliac fossa pain in such people.
2. I   Ulcerative colitis. The age is suggestive of ulcerative colitis, which is associated with sacroiliitis.
3. G   Renal colic. It can present as testicular or labial pain; haematuria makes the diagnosis more likely. Torsion is uncommon after the age of 20.
4. E   Familial adenomatous polyposis. The family history and previous colonoscopy make this more likely.
5. B   Acute diverticulitis. A diverticular bleed is likely.

Hernias

1. D   Incarcerated hernia. This gentleman has an irreducible hernia that has no signs of strangulation.
2. E   Incisional hernia. These are not uncommon after abdominal surgery (≈2%).
3. G   Obturator hernia. These are uncommon but do occur in thin women and can present with features of bowel obstruction.
4. F   Inguinal hernia. This is more common in those with a family history. Differentiating between direct and indirect hernias clinically can be attempted, but is not evidence based.

5. K   Umbilical hernia. These hernias usually resolve within 2 years of birth but leave a weak spot; they can reappear in the elderly and in postpartum females.

Acute abdominal pain

1. H   Perforated sigmoid diverticular disease. This can occur acutely but is often proceeded by left iliac fossa pain and constipation due to oedema of the sigmoid colon. Constant pain implies diverticulitis with localized inflammation. A sudden change and increase in severity of the pain with associated hypotension and tachycardia imply perforation causing generalized peritonitis.
2. B   Acute cholecystitis. Gallbladder disease is common in overweight women. The symptoms are not those of biliary colic because she has signs of inflammation with pyrexia and a positive Murphy sign, which is due to localized peritonism in the right hypochondrium.
3. A   Acute appendicitis. The symptoms and signs are typical of acute appendicitis. The symptoms of dysuria and frequency are not uncommon with appendicitis, as the appendix can be irritating the bladder.
4. F   Large bowel obstruction. The symptoms are of increasing constipation and colicky lower abdominal pain, so that the patient has now developed absolute constipation. This is due to large bowel obstruction rather than small bowel obstruction, because the abdomen is grossly distended and tympanitic, and there is no history of vomiting.
5. D   Acute pancreatitis. This patient describes sudden onset of epigastric pain. This history may suggest a perforated duodenal ulcer. An erect chest X-ray which does not show gas under the diaphragm does not rule this out, as 30% of perforated duodenal ulcers do not give free gas. If, however, the diagnosis was that of perforation, the patient would have been cold, clammy and hypotensive, with generalized guarding and rigidity of the abdomen. Diagnosis is therefore that of alcohol-induced pancreatitis.

Intestinal obstruction

1. B   Carcinoma caecum. This history of abdominal distension, pain and feculent vomiting suggests small bowel obstruction. Examination reveals abdominal distension, with visible peristalsis, suggestive of small bowel obstruction. The most likely diagnosis in someone aged 80 years, with a history of malaise and weight loss, is caecal carcinoma.
2. E   Gallstone ileus. Small bowel obstruction is suggested by the history. This could be due to

adhesions from previous abdominal surgery, but the abdominal X-ray shows air in the biliary tree. This implies the presence of a cholecystoduodenal fistula, which is due to a gallstone eroding into the duodenum and causing small bowel obstruction when it lodges in the ileum.

3. G   Pseudo-obstruction. Immobilized patients often develop an ileus, particularly after orthopaedic surgery. This is usually painless and may be associated with decreased potassium levels. The abdominal X-ray shows a grossly distended colon with no cut-off to imply obstruction.

4. I   Strangulated femoral hernia. This patient has symptoms of small bowel obstruction. There is a mass in the right groin, which in a man is usually due to irreducible inguinal hernia, but men can also develop femoral hernias, and this is implied by the fact that swelling is below and lateral to the pubic tubercle.

5. H   Sigmoid volvulus. This is an elderly patient with dementia who often suffers with chronic constipation. In view of the dementia, she is not able to give a good history, but is just unwell with malaise and is obviously in some discomfort. The presence of a very distended tympanitic abdomen is usually indicative of sigmoid volvulus and this is compatible with the abdominal X-ray appearance.

Gastrointestinal bleeding

1. G   Posterior duodenal ulcer. This is an elderly person who is on nonsteroidal antiinflammatory drugs and therefore is at increased risk of developing an ulcer. Ulcers that bleed are usually in the posterior part of the duodenum because the bleeding is from the erosion of the gastroduodenal artery.

2. A   Angiodysplasia. The differential diagnosis is diverticular disease or angiodysplasia. Both can produce a significant GI blood loss, which is painless. By contrast, a sigmoid carcinoma would not usually bleed enough to require a transfusion, but would be associated with chronic blood loss causing anaemia. Angiodysplasia is only diagnosed by colonoscopy. Diverticulae would be seen on a barium enema.

3. C   Caecal carcinoma. This patient has presented with anaemia, which suggests chronic blood loss. The most likely diagnosis is that of a caecal carcinoma, which is associated with a mass in the right iliac fossa and weight loss. Hepatomegaly implies metastatic disease.

4. F   Oesophageal varices. An alcoholic person with haematemesis and melaena could have a duodenal ulcer, gastritis or oesophageal varices. The presence of splenomegaly, however, suggests that he probably has portal hypertension, and

oesophageal varices are a possibility. Drowsiness implies hepatic encephalopathy precipitated by the bleeding.

5. I   Sigmoid carcinoma. The history suggests a perforated sigmoid carcinoma. The anaemia is due to chronic blood loss from the sigmoid carcinoma. This has also caused a recent change of bowel habit with an increase in constipation. The presence of pyrexia and localized peritonism in the left iliac fossa suggests the presence of inflammation. This diagnosis could be diverticular disease, but a localized perforation of the obstructed carcinoma would fit with the iron-deficiency anaemia.

Oesophagogastric disorders

1. B   Duodenal ulcer disease. This patient's symptoms are typical of a duodenal ulcer. He has increased weight because of drinking milk and eating to relieve his epigastric pain.

2. A   Achalasia. This diagnosis is suspected as the patient is only 19 years old and has had symptoms over the last few months. The recurrent chest infections are due to aspiration pneumonias, as food and fluid collect in a dilated oesophagus above a 'rat-tail' stricture of the lower oesophagus.

3. J   Pyloric stenosis. This man has a long history of peptic ulceration which has been left untreated. It has therefore healed with scarring, to cause pyloric stenosis. He is dehydrated because of vomiting. The succussion splash is suggestive of it. The classic biochemical abnormality is hypochloraemic alkalosis.

4. H   Oesophageal adenocarcinoma. This man has a history of reflux that has been self-treated with antacids. This does put him at risk of developing a benign oesophageal stricture secondary to his oesophagitis. He is also at increased risk of oesophageal carcinoma, particularly in a Barrett oesophagus which is related to reflux. However, the presence of an iron-deficiency anaemia and cachexia is more compatible with oesophageal adenocarcinoma. This is also related to the fact that he has progressive dysphagia and weight loss, whereas with a benign oesophageal stricture, the dysphagia may not be so progressive.

5. G   Mallory–Weiss tear. This man has had haematemesis, which could be due to gastritis, peptic ulcer disease or oesophageal varices. He has been drinking heavily and has subsequently vomited. The haematemesis developed after the vomiting, which suggests it is due to trauma caused from the vomiting that has caused a minor tear in the lower oesophagus.

Foregut investigations

1. A Abdominal ultrasound. The history is suggestive of gallstones, and the simplest test to make this diagnosis is an abdominal ultrasound scan.
2. G Endoscopic ultrasonography. This patient has an oesophageal carcinoma. It could be staged by doing a CT scan, which will show liver metastases, but a more accurate way of assessing whether the carcinoma has spread to the local structures, including the thoracic aorta, is by using an endoscopic ultrasound.
3. E CT scan. The history is suggestive of pancreatic carcinoma. An ultrasound scan has shown a dilated common bowel duct. The possible diagnosis is carcinoma of the head of the pancreas. A CT scan would be the best way of staging this. This would show the evidence of liver metastases and whether the pancreatic carcinoma involves the superior mesenteric vessels.
4. C Barium swallow. The history is suggestive of a pharyngeal pouch. It is not appropriate to do an endoscopy because of the risk of perforation. A barium meal looks at the stomach and duodenum, not the oesophagus. A barium swallow is therefore the most appropriate investigation, and will show the function and anatomy of the oesophagus.
5. I Laparoscopy. This man has carcinoma of the stomach. A CT scan shows no evidence of liver metastases and an endoscopy shows a localized lesion in the antrum of the stomach. A CT scan suggests operability, but is not appropriate for diagnosing peritoneal metastases as they may not be evident on CT. A laparoscopy is, therefore, the appropriate way forward.

Abdominal mass

1. B Caecal carcinoma. This often presents insidiously with fatigue due to anaemia before there are any bowel symptoms. The colicky abdominal pain and vomiting imply obstruction developing. The age of the patient makes the diagnosis more likely to be caecal carcinoma, rather than Crohn disease. The gynaecological pathologies are not likely to present with obstruction.
2. J Sigmoid carcinoma. This patient has symptoms of a change of bowel habit of gradual onset. She also has anaemia consistent with malignancy. The mass is nontender but a diverticular mass is usually tender and not associated with anaemia.
3. C Crohn disease. Although this woman has an acute presentation, this is on a chronic history of malaise and weight loss, which fits with a localized

perforation of Crohn disease. The differential is an appendix mass, when the history is usually a few days to 10 days. On examination, the patients are usually fairly well, with a slightly tender mass in the right iliac fossa.
4. G Mucocoele of the gallbladder. This man has a history of biliary pain. The gallstone has become stuck in the neck of the gallbladder, causing obstruction and then the gallbladder distends. The jaundice is due to partial obstruction of the common bile duct by the distended gallbladder. It is not an empyema as he would have a pyrexia.
5. L Uterine fibroids. These are often associated with menorrhagia, causing anaemia and therefore tiredness. The ovarian cyst and carcinoma are less likely to be associated with anaemia. The mass arising suprapubically is consistent with a uterine mass.

Groin lump

1. C Femoral hernia. This patient has symptoms of obstruction due to a strangulated hernia. It is a femoral hernia because of its classic position, below and lateral to the pubic tubercle. An obturator hernia is internal and is not seen externally.
2. D Inguinal hernia. This is because it is above and medial to pubic tubercle. It goes away when she rests. A saphena varix is below and lateral to pubic tubercle, is compressible and has a cough impulse.
3. G Malignant lymphadenopathy. Although the patient presents with an acute pretibial laceration, the lump has been present for a few weeks. She has had a previous melanoma excised which is likely to recur. It is an irregular lump which is more likely to be malignant rather than reactive nodes.
4. A False aneurysm. This woman has had a radiological intervention to investigate the cause of her leg ulcer. Damage has been caused to the artery by the procedure, so a false aneurysm has developed. This is more likely than a femoral artery aneurysm.

Rectal bleeding

1. J Rectal villous adenoma. The history of rectal bleeding, diarrhoea and tenesmus could be due to a rectal carcinoma, but a villous adenoma produces mucus and causes potassium depletion.
2. A Anal carcinoma. Fresh rectal bleeding can be due to haemorrhoids, anal fissure or rectal carcinoma, but only anal carcinoma causes an indurated,

perianal ulcer. Anal carcinomas are also thought to be linked aetiologically with CIN.

3. B   Anal fissure. Chronic constipation and straining are causes of an anal fissure. It can occur at all ages and can cause some rectal bleeding. Haemorrhoids could also cause rectal bleeding but not likely in a 5-year-old child.

4. D   Angiodysplasia. This is more common in elderly people and can be associated with significant bleeding to cause hypotension. Diverticulosis can also cause spontaneous bleeding but patients usually have a history of some bowel symptoms. This man was previously fit and well and this relates to the fact that he is on no medication, which could predispose to peptic ulceration.

Cardiothoracics and vascular surgery 12

Question 1

C. Clinical opinion also holds that eccentric or saccular aneurysms represent greater rupture risk than more diffuse, cylindrical aneurysms. Using computer modelling, Wall stress is substantially increased by an asymmetric bulge in AAA.

Question 2

B. Cilostazol is a phosphodiesterase inhibitor with therapeutic focus on cyclic adenosine monophosphate. It inhibits platelet aggregation and is a direct arterial vasodilator. Its main effects are dilatation of the arteries supplying blood to the legs and decreasing platelet coagulation. A meta-analysis of eight randomized, placebo-controlled trials of cilostazol for moderate to severe claudication found that 100 mg of the drug twice daily increased maximal and pain-free walking distances by 50% and 67%, respectively.

Question 3

E. Smoking is the number one risk factor for peripheral arterial disease (PAD), and smoking even a few cigarettes a day can interfere with PAD treatment. Smoking increases the risk for PAD by 2–25 times, with the danger being higher when other risk factors are present. Between 80% and 90% of patients with PAD are current or former smokers. Progression to a more critical state of illness is likely for patients who continue to smoke.

Question 4

A. Back pain is characteristic of a thoracic aortic aneurysm. Swallowing impairment is typical due to compression of the cervical oesophagus. This is, however, rare.

Question 5

E. This artery is commonly damaged in AAA repair and is most likely responsible for paraplegia postoperatively.

Question 6

B. Aortoiliac occlusive disease. This patient has developed Leriche syndrome, which is caused by peripheral artery disease affecting the abdominal aorta or the common iliac arteries. It presents with a triad of features: claudication in the buttocks and thighs, absent or decreased femoral pulses and erectile dysfunction in males. PAD affecting both femoral arteries would cause claudication in the thighs, but not the buttocks.

Question 7

E. The mural thrombus is usually located in the abdominal aorta, but, albeit infrequently, it can occur in the thoracic aorta. Generally, thromboembolic events are associated with advanced age, with the thrombus arising from complex and ulcerated atherosclerotic plaques. Fat embolism syndrome typically presents 24 to 72 hours after the initial injury. Patients present with a classic triad: respiratory changes, neurological abnormalities and petechial rash.

Question 8

B. The first most appropriate investigation is ultrasound. CT scanning is only useful later to determine whether endovascular or open repair is appropriate.

Question 9

D. Typical presentation of a mycotic aneurysm. Such aneurysms arise from infection within the vessel wall.

Question 10

A. Annual abdominal ultrasound scans. All males at the age of 65 will have an abdominal ultrasound. If this shows evidence of an AAA, then it will be confirmed using a CT scan of the abdomen. If the AAA is between 3 cm and 4.4 cm, then they will have an annual ultrasound. If it is between 4.5 cm and 5.4 cm, then they will have three-monthly ultrasound scans; however, if it is 5.5 cm or bigger, then patients are considered for surgery.

Question 11

E. Such aneurysms occur when an artery has been damaged. In this case, the femoral artery has been punctured for an angiogram but has failed to seal.

Question 12

B. The diagnosis is intermittent claudication which is most likely investigated via measurement of ankle brachial pressure index. This is often reduced by approximately 60%–70%.

Question 13

D. Risk factor modification is always the first-line management of intermittent claudication, in this case, hypertension. Drug therapy and surgery are rarely common practice in the first instance.

Question 14

E. The hypoglossal nerve may be damaged as it crosses the internal carotid artery.

Question 15

D. This patent has a symptomatic AAA and needs a CT scan of the abdomen. If asymptomatic, then an abdominal ultrasound could be used; however, even if this test is positive, patients are still sent for a CT scan of the abdomen to confirm the diagnosis as CTs are more sensitive for diagnosis of smaller-sized AAAs. An abdominal X-ray would often be normal; however, sometimes if an aneurysm is chronic, there may be evidence of calcification around the walls of the aneurysm.

Question 16

A. Handheld Doppler helps to confirm sapheno-femoral and sapheno-popliteal incompetence. Other useful tests include venography and plethysmography, but these are rarely needed.

Question 17

D. Compression stockings are the initial choice of management. Surgery is a useful second option. Laser therapy and radio frequency ablation are considered if the above options have failed.

Question 18

B. The diagnosis here is most likely to be lymphoedema with treatment being in the form of compression stockings in the main.

Question 19

E. This is mesenteric ischaemia. This should be suspected in any patient who has AF and presents with abdominal pain (due to systemic emboli). Diagnosis can be confirmed by arteriography or MR angiography, but most are made during a laparotomy, which reveals areas of necrotic bowel.

EMQ ANSWERS

Vascular disorders

1. E Also known as Buerger disease. This condition is characterized by segmental thrombotic occlusions of small- and medium-sized vessels in both upper and lower limbs.
2. F Treatment typically involves avoidance of cold and stopping smoking. Medical treatment includes the use of nifedipine.
3. I This is essentially recurrent episodes of superficial thrombophlebitis which may also precede clinical manifestations of malignancy.
4. A Typical features of an AAA. Surgery is typically indicated for aneurysms which are symptomatic or those which are asymptomatic but greater than 5 cm.
5. C Diagnosis is often confirmed via chest X-ray which typically shows a widened mediastinum. Management involves surgery and urgent blood pressure control.

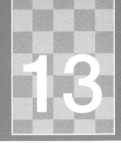
SBA ANSWERS

Question 1

C. Osgood–Schlatter disease is encountered in patients between ages 10 and 15. These patients are often active in sports that involve a lot of jumping. It is thought to be secondary to repetitive microtrauma and traction apophysitis of the tibial tuberosity. This condition is usually self-limited, and most patients are able to return to full activity within 2 to 3 weeks. Treatment includes rest, ice, antiinflammatory medications, a rehabilitation program and an infrapatellar strap during activities.

Question 2

D. Likely diagnosis of acute osteomyelitis most commonly due to *S. aureus* in over 80% of cases.

Question 3

A. MRI has become the gold-standard investigation but may need sedation at this age. Plain limb X-rays may be normal for up to 10 days.

Question 4

E. A tumour derived from osteoblasts. The 'sunray'-like appearance is due to the formation of bony spicules.

Question 5

E. In a patient who has nontraumatic hip pain and is on chronic steroid therapy for a disease such as SLE, one of the major complications is avascular necrosis (AVN). In the setting of AVN, MRI is the most sensitive imaging modality and the diagnostic method of choice when clinical suspicion is high. MRI results will show marked bone marrow oedema even when the X-ray is totally normal and is the only objective test to rule out the disease in this early stage.

Question 6

B. Classic presentation of acromioclavicular osteoarthritis. Excision of the outer end of the clavicle may help to relieve symptoms.

Question 7

A. This is a common problem to affect the shoulder best treated with NSAIDs or steroid injections. The pain is often worsened by shoulder overhead movement and may occur at night, especially if the patient is lying on the affected shoulder.

Question 8

E. Rest improves the pain of osteoarthritis, and increasing muscle strength improves joint stability and reduces pain.

Question 9

C. Typical presentation of a rotator cuff tear. Usually associated with traumatic injury or dislocation. Management is usually through surgery in the young.

Question 10

C. The diagnosis is tennis elbow or lateral epicondylitis best treated with NSAIDs initially. With lateral epicondylitis, there is degeneration of the tendon's attachment, weakening the anchor site and placing greater stress on the area. This can lead to pain associated with activities in which this muscle is active, such as lifting, gripping and/or grasping. Sports such as tennis are commonly associated with this, but the problem can occur with many different activities.

Question 11

B. Neck of femur fracture, which can be intracapsular (subcapital, transcervical, basicervical) or extracapsular (intertrochanteric, subtrochanteric); common in osteoporotic elderly after a fall; affected limb is shortened and externally rotated.

Question 12

B. Usual features of ulnar nerve neuropathy. If the median nerve is damaged, the ability to abduct and oppose the thumb may be lost due to paralysis of the thenar muscles.

Question 13

A. SUFE: overweight boy with pain in groin, front of thigh or knee and limping. Normally ages 10–14 and <10 years associated with hypothyroidism. Pain comes on with movement. Affected leg is shorter and turns outwards. X-ray shows widened growth plates which are denser/lucent.

Question 14

A. The radial nerve may be damaged anywhere in its course. It is most commonly affected in the upper arm where it winds round the humerus and in the extensor muscle compartment of the forearm affecting the posterior interosseous branch. Finger and wrist drop are common, their severity depending upon the site of the lesion.

Question 15

B. This condition is typically due to thickening and shortening of the palmar fascia which becomes adherent to the skin. As a result, the ring and little finger develop a fixed flexion deformity.

Question 16

E. Results from localized thickening of the flexor tendon with associated sheath narrowing causing the finger to catch as it is flexed.

Question 17

C. The diagnosis is most likely to be cauda equina syndrome. MRI is the gold-standard investigation in such cases.

Question 18

B. Meniscal tear. This is a common sporting injury, which classically occurs while performing a sharp turn. It presents with pain and swelling of the knee. Patients complain of locking of the knee joint and a reduced range of movement. On examination an effusion may be present and McMurray test may be positive. During an anterior cruciate ligament tear, patients often state that they hear a 'pop' as the ligament ruptured. It causes pain, swelling and instability. On examination the anterior draw test is positive. Patella tendon rupture is a less common injury. This would lead to an upward displacement of the patella, and an inability to extend the knee joint and inability to 'straight leg raise'.

Question 19

A. Plain X-ray is the best-choice investigation from the listed options.

Question 20

C. Anterior cruciate ligament rupture is the most likely cause in approximately 40% of cases. Symptoms include pain, a popping sound during injury, instability of the knee and joint swelling. Swelling generally appears within a couple of hours.

Question 21

D. Osteosarcoma is the most common primary malignant bone tumour. It mainly occurs in adolescents, and a common site is around the knee. X-ray would show bone destruction and new bone formation (known as 'sunray spicules'), along with uplifting of the periosteum (known as Codman triangle). Ewing sarcoma is a rare primary bone tumour that occurs in children and forms from the round cells of the long bones. Giant-cell tumours are also known as osteoclastomas and are rare tumours that are characterized by multinucleate giant cells. They mainly occur in patients aged between 20 and 45 and form around the epiphysis of the bones. The knee is a common site for them to form. These tumours often progress slowly, and X-rays of the area would show osteolysis and may show pathological fractures.

Question 22

C. Typical presentation of an anterior cruciate ligament injury. It is usually detected in approximately 70% of cases.

Question 23

E. Here the tibia has been forced posteriorly resulting in such an injury.

Question 24

C. The patient has lumbar spinal stenosis. MRI of the lumbar region is the only test to diagnose lumbar spinal stenosis. Lumbar spinal stenosis is characterized by narrowing of the spinal canal, leading to pressure on the spinal cord which results in pain occurring when the back is in extension. The characteristic features of pain in lumbar spinal stenosis include pain while walking, radiating into the buttocks and thighs bilaterally. Pain gets worse when walking downhill and better when sitting. Unsteady gait as well as leg weakness while walking may also result. Pedal pulses and ankle/brachial index are normal and about quarter of the patients have diminished lower extremity reflexes. Pain is much less with activities that involve leaning forward of the patients (e.g., cycling).

Question 25

D. As the child is over 6 months, this is the most suitable management. Before 6 months, a splint is typically used.

Question 26

B. Typical presentation of Perthes disease. A childhood hip disorder initiated by a disruption of blood flow to the femoral head causing osteonecrosis and restricts growth. Over time, healing occurs by new blood vessels infiltrating the dead bone and removing the necrotic bone which leads to a loss of bone mass and a weakening of the femoral head.

Question 27

C. Usual findings of a SUFE best treated with surgery. SUFE refers to a fracture through the physis, which results in slippage of the overlying end of the femur (epiphysis).

Question 28

B. The axillary nerve passes around the neck of the humerus, so any displacement of the proximal humerus can lead to damage to the axillary nerve. In any patient who has dislocated the shoulder, it is important to check sensation over the C5 dermatome.

EMQ ANSWERS

Fractures

1. E Classic history of a distal radius fracture. Associated with a backward angulation and displacement producing a dinner fork wrist.
2. C Radial nerve injury may lead to a wrist drop. Immobilization is the mainstay form of treatment.
3. H This occurs just below the femoral head.
4. D Scaphoid fractures result in tenderness on direct pressure approximately 2 cm distal to the Lister tubercle of the radius and on proximal pressure on the extended thumb. If one suspects this fracture, an additional oblique scaphoid view should be requested.
5. H Presents with external rotation and shortening of the leg. Medial femoral circumflex artery involvement may lead to ischaemic necrosis of the femoral head.

Fracture complications

1. I Hip fractures are commonly associated with the development of pneumonia. The severity of such a condition is based on the CURB-65 score, which assesses the presence of confusion, serum urea, respiratory rate, blood pressure and age.
2. H Classic features of a fat embolism.
3. D Nonunion is commoner in cortical bone rather than in cancellous bone. Predisposing factors include malignancy and infection.
4. B This complication is associated with fluid loss and acute tubular necrosis as a result of myoglobin release. An urgent fasciotomy may be required.
5. E Classic description of malunion. The resulting deformity may be of length, angulation or rotation.

Orthopaedic clinical examination

1. F Tests for laxity of the anterior cruciate ligament. 'Give' of more than 1 cm is considered abnormal.
2. D Tests for a fixed flexion deformity of the hip. This can be a difficult test to explain to the patient and so good communication skills and practice are required.
3. J Tests for weak ipsilateral hip abductor muscles. If the patient is unsteady on the left foot and falls to the right side, the problem is with the left hip.
4. E Tests for a fixed flexion deformity of the lumbar spine. This is a relatively simple test but should be practised as it can seem complex.
5. I Tests for an unstable shoulder girdle. This tests for an unstable shoulder following a prior dislocation. Do not push too far or the shoulder will redislocate.
6. F Tests for laxity of the anterior cruciate ligament. An alternative to the anterior draw test, though it is slightly harder to perform.
7. G Tests for torn medial menisci. Uncommonly asked for in an objective structured clinical examination (OSCE), as if positive, it is painful for the patient.

Knee injuries

1. B Bucket handle tear of meniscus. Meniscal injuries are common in sportsmen and women; the history of locking suggests that there is a meniscal fragment being trapped in the joint.
2. C Dislocation of the knee. This is exceedingly rare but does happen; in this case, the pulses and ligaments should all be checked as the patient may require emergency surgery to repair the vascular supply.
3. J Tibial plateau fracture. These are common and occur with trauma to the knee in which the femoral condyles impact upon the tibia. Schatzker refers to a grading system for these types of fracture.
4. A Anterior cruciate ligament rupture. This is demonstrated by the anterior draw test; other ligaments may be injured at the same time.
5. G Patella fracture. Falling onto the knee may fracture the patella; this is supported by the inability to straight leg raise.

Skin, joint and bone infections

1. E Approximately 20% of all bursitis cases are caused by bacterial infections; rarely, bursitis is caused by fungi and algae. *S. aureus/S. epidermidis* as the offending organism in 90% of cases and *Streptococcus* species in 9% of cases.
2. D Necrotizing fasciitis causes include group A *Streptococcus* (group A strep), *Klebsiella*, *Clostridium*, *E. coli*, *S. aureus*, *Aeromonas hydrophila* and others. Group A strep is considered the most common cause of necrotizing fasciitis.
3. E Prosthetic joint infections (PJIs) occur in 1.5% to 2.5% of all hip arthroplasties. Pain is the most consistent symptom. *Staphylococcus* species are the most common organisms isolated from PJI sites.
4. G *P. multocida* infection in humans is often associated with an animal bite, scratch or lick, but infection without epidemiologic evidence of animal contact may occur.
5. B Puncture wounds of the foot can frequently become infected with *Pseudomonas* species and the patient will present with drainage with a sweet, fruity-smelling discharge. Cellulitis and osteomyelitis are common complications.

SBA ANSWERS

Question 1

D. A perilymphatic fistula between the middle and inner ear may be caused by barotrauma from scuba diving, as well as by direct blows, heavy weightbearing and excessive straining (e.g., with sneezing or bowel movements). This patient's recent trip involved two of these potential factors.

Question 2

B. Presentation is usually during the second or third decade of life. Surgery is the mainstay form of management.

Question 3

C. This cyst is typically smooth and mobile. Diagnosis is often by fine-needle aspiration which produces a creamy-coloured fluid.

Question 4

C. In patients with a sinus infection, acute bacterial rhinosinusitis should be diagnosed and treated with antibiotics only if symptoms have not improved after 10 days.

Question 5

B. Otitis externa, or infection of the external ear canal, can be caused by a variety of organisms, notably including *E. coli*, *P. aeruginosa*, *P. vulgaris* and *S. aureus*. There is, however, a severe subtype of otitis externa, malignant otitis externa, of which you should be aware. This form is specifically caused by *P. aeruginosa*, and tends to affect elderly diabetics and acquired immunodeficiency syndrome (AIDS) patients, causing the findings illustrated in the question stem. *E. coli* can cause both otitis externa and acute otitis media, but does not usually cause malignant otitis externa.

Question 6

D. Auscultation may often reveal a bruit. Surgical excision is the preferred treatment option.

Question 7

C. A plain XR may help to reveal a stone in the parotid duct. Treatment is with mouth care, rehydration and antibiotics.

Question 8

B. Pleomorphic adenoma is a common benign salivary gland neoplasm characterized by neoplastic proliferation of parenchymatous glandular cells along with myoepithelial components, having a malignant potentiality. It is the most common type of salivary gland tumour and the most common tumour of the parotid gland.

Question 9

B. Frey syndrome is a condition that occurs following trauma to the parotid gland. The auriculo-temporal branch of the trigeminal nerve sends parasympathetic fibres to the parotid gland, and sympathetic fibres to the facial sweat glands. Trauma to this area means that these nerves must then regrow, and often they switch places. This results in gustatory sweating, meaning that when the patient eats, the sweat glands on the cheek become stimulated, resulting in sweating and erythema.

Question 10

E. This is a benign tumour which may occur bilaterally in approximately 10% of cases. Warthin tumour primarily affects older individuals (age 60–70 years). There is a slight male predilection according to recent studies. The tumour is slow growing, painless and usually appears in the tail of the parotid gland near the angle of the mandible. In 5% to 14% of cases, Warthin tumour is bilateral, but the two masses usually are at different times. Warthin tumour is highly unlikely to become malignant.

Question 11

A. Typical presentation of otitis externa. Management involves acetic acid topically in mild cases to antibiotic drops in moderate to severe cases.

Question 12

B. Rare after the age of 5. *H. influenzae* is the main organism responsible for such a condition in approximately 40% of cases. Complications include effusion or scarring of the tympanic membrane.

Question 13

E. This child has otitis media. Antibiotics are typically administered for a 7- to 10-day period due to fever. If patient is afebrile, then conservative management is indicated.

Question 14

D. Glue ear is essentially otitis media with effusion and typically occurs between the age of 2 and 6. In over 90% of cases, the effusion resolves spontaneously.

Question 15

C. This condition results in unilateral sensorineural hearing loss and tinnitus. Surgery is the mainstay form of treatment. When nerve deafness is present, then the note is audible at the external meatus, as air and bone conduction are reduced equally, so that the air conduction is better (as is normal) than bone conduction: this is termed 'Rinne positive'.

Question 16

A. Tinnitus, hearing loss and vertigo are associated with Ménière disease. Antihistamines have been shown to decrease middle ear labyrinth excitability and block conduction in the middle ear vestibular cerebellar pathways which primarily aid in reducing vertigo.

Question 17

D. In view of his haemodynamic instability and ongoing blood loss, intravenous access for urgent fluid resuscitation (in this case with blood) is the initial step in management.

Question 18

E. Oral antihistamines may be added following steroid usage. Surgery is often the last resort.

Question 19

D. Pharyngeal pouches are also associated with repeated chest infections and regurgitation of food. Management is typically surgical.

Question 20

B. Smoking and alcohol are the most common risk factors in the development of such a condition, but there is an association with EBV.

Question 21

A. A branchial cyst is a congenital cyst that arises due to either failure to obliterate the second branchial cleft or failure of the fusion of the second and third branchial clefts. It presents with a fluctuant lump on the side of the neck, at the level where the upper third of the sternocleidomastoid muscle meets the middle third of sternocleidomastoid muscle. A dermoid cyst is a midline lump which often occurs in young patients, and when excised, contains dermal structures, such as teeth or hair. A chondroma is a benign cartilaginous tumour, which can form a hard lump in the midline of the neck.

EMQ ANSWERS

Neck swellings

1. E   Additional features include a lack of saliva production. Management is usually symptomatic.
2. H   Salivary gland malignancies are typically carcinomas and usually affect middle- to older-aged people.
3. C   Such tumours are highly vascular and hence their propensity to pulsate.
4. B   Management is typically surgical.
5. J   Such swellings are typically large and thick walled in nature. They may lead to stridor and cyanosis in certain cases.

Neck lumps

1. H   Thyroglossal cyst. Midline, moves on swallowing and tongue protrusion: These are the classic features of a thyroglossal cyst. It has been present since birth, which confirms its congenital nature.
2. F   Lymph nodes. There are multiple small lumps, and their presence in the axilla also confirms the likelihood of lymph nodes; you should check the entire neck, axilla and groin, as well as suggesting a breast examination in a woman (for lumps).
3. A   Branchial cyst. These typically affect young men, and appear in this characteristic location.
4. G   Pharyngeal pouch. A new-onset history of dysphagia with a new neck lump in a previously well elderly man suggests this; the lump should not move on swallowing or tongue protrusion as it is not attached to the thyroid (if it does, reconsider the diagnosis!).
5. I   Thyroid goitre. The features of the lump suggest a multinodular thyroid (it is large and has an irregular surface). Furthermore, the patient has signs of systemic hyperthyroidism, which should be clearly mentioned for extra marks!

Neck swellings

1. H   Submandibular calculus. This is a typical history of a submandibular stone. On eating, the salivary glands are stimulated to produce saliva. As there is a calculus present in the duct, the gland swells because it is obstructed. This occurs most commonly in the submandibular gland. The stone may be palpable in the floor of the mouth.
2. A   Anaplastic carcinoma of the thyroid. This is a very short history of 2 months. The rapid increase in size suggests malignancy. The other features that are compatible with this are the hoarse voice due to involvement of the recurrent laryngeal nerve; the audible wheeze will also be due to pressure on the trachea and paralysis of the recurrent laryngeal

nerve will also have effects on the vocal cord. The hard mass in the lower anterior part of the neck is suggestive of anaplastic carcinoma. Riedel thyroiditis would also produce a hard, irregular swelling of the thyroid gland, but would have a longer history.

3. G   Solitary thyroid nodule. This swelling is benign, as is it oval and smooth. It is obviously connected with the thyroid because it moves on swallowing. It is not a thyroglossal cyst because it is to the left of the midline. It is not a branchial cyst because it moves on swallowing.

4. C   Branchial cyst. This usually presents in young people. It may not be apparent until an infection develops, and the classic position is at the anterior aspect of the upper third of the sternomastoid muscle.

5. J   Virchow node. The history is suggestive of gastric carcinoma at the cardia with secondaries in the supraclavicular nodes (i.e., Virchow node). The dysphagia, weight loss and vomiting would be compatible with a pharyngeal pouch, but this would produce a soft swelling of variable size in the left side of the neck.

SBA ANSWERS

Question 1

D. This patient has epididymo-orchitis. This condition is most often caused by coliform bacteria in men over the age of 35. Non-sexually transmitted epididymitis is usually caused by enteric organisms and is often associated with recent urinary tract instrumentation, systemic disease or immunosuppression. These organisms are effectively treated with ofloxacin. Those less than 35 years with this condition have a higher chance of having a sexually transmitted disease (STD) and would benefit from intramuscular ceftriaxone and oral doxycycline. However, these medications would not adequately cover coliform bacteria. Clindamycin and famciclovir would also be ineffective. Testicular torsion is another possible cause of testicular pain with a quick onset, and would require urgent urology surgery consultation. However, in cases of torsion, the examination usually reveals an elevated testicle and testicular ultrasonography would show decreased or absent blood flow on the affected side.

Question 2

A. Uric acid stone formation can be prevented by alkalinizing the urine with citrate.

Question 3

A. Urinalysis and culture are essential here. The patient has a urinary tract infection as noted by his urinary symptoms and associated pyrexia.

Question 4

A. BPH is a condition characterized by enlargement of the prostate gland that makes urination difficult in males. α-Adrenergic antagonists block the receptors in the bladder neck and prostrate and work by reducing the smooth muscle tone. This improves the urine flow rate and reduces the symptoms associated with the disease.

Question 5

B. This is a severe urinary tract infection with associated pyrexia. Intravenous antibiotics such as cefuroxime or gentamicin may be of use.

Question 6

E. A non-painful testicular mass that does not transilluminate is most likely testicular cancer and a full evaluation must be performed for proper diagnosis and staging. Testicular cancer is the most common cancer in men between 20 and 40 years of age. Lifetime incidence is 0.4% for white males and 0.08% in black males. Cryptoorchidism is the biggest risk factor for testicular cancer and it increases the risk about fourfold. Nearly 95% of all malignant testicular cancers are of the germ cell type that are divided into the seminoma and nonseminoma. Various tumour markers can help distinguish between the two types of germ cell tumours (e.g., β-HCG and AFP).

Question 7

D. Urinary symptoms and suprapubic tenderness are key features of acute cystitis.

Question 8

C. Calcium oxalate containing stones account for approximately 60% of all kidney stones. These stones are radio-opaque, (visible on X-ray). Hypercalciuria is the direct precursor to most calcium stone formations. This increase of calcium levels in the urine can occur from increased intestinal absorption, decreased renal absorption, or increased bone resorption. The patient in this case has no medical problems and his urine is not suggestive of any infection. His stone is visible on x-ray and is most likely to be 'calcium oxalate'.

Question 9

B. Urinary symptoms with a sterile culture is diagnostic of interstitial cystitis. Referral onwards to urology is indicated for consideration of cystoscopy.

Question 10

C. Prostatitis manifests as urinary frequency and dysuria in addition to prostatic tenderness. It is commonly caused by *Escherichia coli* or *Staphylococcus aureus*.

Question 11

A. The clinical presentation is that of renal stones, and the most common stone are calcium oxalate stones. Risk factors include low urine volume, hypercalciuria, hyperuricosuria, hyperoxaluria and hypocitraturia. Reducing dietary calcium is NOT an effective method of prevention; low dietary calcium leads to increased gastrointestinal oxalate absorption and higher urine levels of calcium oxalate

Question 12

B. PSA is sensitive and specific for prostate cells, but not specific to the prostate cancer cells.

Question 13

E. Epididymo-orchitis is commonly seen in young sexually active males. The offending organism is commonly *Chlamydia*.

Question 14

D. Squamous cell carcinoma. Squamous cells appear in your bladder in response to infection and irritation. Over time they can become cancerous. Squamous cell bladder cancer is rare (5%–7%). It is more common in the parts of the world where a certain parasitic infection (schistosomiasis) is a prevalent cause of bladder infections. The species, *Schistosoma haematobium* (SH), is the type that causes urinary bladder infestation, and the most distinguishing symptom is painless haematuria, more common in children who play barefoot in the marshes where SH is endemic.

Question 15

B. A CT scan is the most useful here in diagnosing a possible renal tumour.

Question 16

E. A secondary varicocele is due to compression of the venous drainage of the testicle. A pelvic or abdominal malignancy is a definite concern when a right-sided varicocele is newly diagnosed in a patient older than 40 years of age. The most common cause is renal cell carcinoma, followed by retroperitoneal fibrosis or adhesions.

Question 17

D. The only curative treatment is a nephrectomy.

Question 18

E. Most stones pass spontaneously. Stones greater than 5 mm require treatment.

Question 19

A. This is a classic presentation of ureteric colic. Analgesia is of huge importance in helping to relieve the patient's symptoms.

Question 20

B. Bladder stones can be asymptomatic but can cause irritation to the bladder wall or neck, resulting in suprapubic pain (can be referred to the tip of penis, scrotum, perineum), dysuria, urinary frequency, urgency, nocturia and haematuria. Pain is often aggravated by sudden movements or exercise.

Question 21

A. The definitive investigation in bladder cancer. Biopsy will allow for staging assessment and ultimately choice of treatment.

Question 22

A. This is a T2 tumour, best treated with radical cystectomy.

Question 23

A. Individuals with mild symptoms are best managed by watchful waiting as the risks of treatment usually outweigh the benefits.

Question 24

C. This patient has developed post-TURP syndrome. This is caused by systemic absorption of the irrigation fluids used during TURP and these lead to dilution of the plasma, hyponatraemia and hypothermia. Hyponatraemia can lead to seizures.

Question 25

A. A classic description of a hydrocele.

Question 26

B. Epididymo-orchitis is commonly seen in young males and is particularly tender in nature.

Question 27

B. Ciprofloxacin. This patient has prostatitis. This presents with a fever, back pain, urinary symptoms (dysuria, frequency and haematuria), haematospermia and a swollen prostate. Ciprofloxacin is a quinolone antibiotic and used because it is able to penetrate the prostate well. Doxazosin is an α-blocker, which can be used to treat BPH. Finasteride is a 5α-reductase inhibitor also used in BPH.

Question 28

E. Painless haematuria is a buzzword to associate with bladder cancer (of which TCC is the most common).

Question 29

C. A common presentation of an epididymal cyst.

Question 30

E. Acute urinary retention requires immediate urinary catheterization as complications include renal failure and hydronephrosis. Suprapubic aspiration only if symptomatic, and if urinary catheterization has failed. In the longer term, treatment depends on the underlying cause.

Question 31

E. Additional features would include swelling of the testicle. This is unlike epididymitis, where elevation may help improve the pain.

EMQ ANSWERS

Scrotal swellings
1. C   Hydrocele. A rapid onset, tense lump which is not particularly tender but is transilluminable suggests a hydrocele.
2. I   Testicular tumour. The lump arises from the testis itself and the young man has been losing weight; this is cancer until proved otherwise. The other testis must be palpated, the groin checked for lymphadenopathy (although the first point of lymph drainage for the testis is the paraaortic nodes) and tumour markers should be sent (β-HCG and alpha-fetoprotein).
3. E   Indirect inguinal hernia. Direct hernias very rarely enter the scrotum.
4. J   Varicocele. The classic statement is that when standing it feels like 'a bag of worms', and it disappears when lying down as blood is redistributed. Remember 95% are left-sided due to venous drainage into the left renal vein (where there is turbulent blood flow) as opposed to directly into the inferior vena cava on the right side (where flow is less resistant).

Lower urinary tract symptoms
1. B   BPH. This patient has a chronic history of symptoms suggestive of outflow obstruction. The tests of flow rate confirm this picture.
2. I   Stress incontinence. This woman has typical symptoms of stress incontinence (i.e., on coughing and sneezing). The risk factors for its development are three vaginal deliveries with a prolonged first labour.
3. J   Urethral stricture. This young man has symptoms of obstruction. There is a past history of a fall astride a bar as a child, which may have led to a urethral injury that was initially undetected. This has healed to form a urethral stricture.
4. E   Multiple sclerosis. This patient has symptoms of bladder instability, but the associated past medical history is that of unilateral transient blindness, which implies the possible diagnosis of multiple sclerosis.
5. F   Prolapsed intervertebral disc. This patient has a history of low back pain, which suggests the possibility of prolapsed intervertebral disc. He suddenly develops acute onset of difficulty in passing urine, which is due to a central disc prolapse compressing the spinal cord and the sacral nerve roots. This fits with an area of saddle anaesthesia and decreased anal sphincter tone.

Urological investigations
1. A   The diagnosis is a urinary tract infection most appropriately confirmed by a urine dipstick or urine microscopy and culture.
2. H   The diagnosis is renal colic. The clue is with regards to his long distance running and hence tendency to become severely dehydrated. An abdominal KUB is the most appropriate diagnostic tool.
3. D   The diagnosis is urinary tract obstruction, specifically at the bladder. An ultrasound scan will help to detect evidence of obstruction and likely hydronephrosis.
4. C   The diagnosis is most probably prostatic carcinoma. Serum PSA is likely to be notably elevated.
5. G   The diagnosis is stress incontinence most appropriately diagnosed by urodynamic studies.

Urgent urological referrals
1. I   Teratoma of testis. A painless swelling of testis is likely to be a tumour and, in a 19-year-old, the most likely diagnosis is a teratoma. Seminomas and lymphomas occur in older men.
2. K   Ureteric colic. The history is of severe, colicky loin to groin pain. Although there is some dysuria and frequency, there is no fever to suggest a urinary tract infection or pyelonephritis. The dipstick shows blood only and no evidence of infection.
3. A   BPH. This patient has acute-on-chronic urinary outflow obstruction. He has some symptoms suggestive of a urinary infection, but these are also symptoms of obstruction. As he has a long history of nocturia and poor stream and his PSA is normal, it is more likely to be BPH than cancer.
4. C   Epididymitis. This is not a simple urinary tract infection as he has testicular pain and swelling as well.

SBA ANSWERS

Question 1

A. This patient has developed Paget disease of the breast, which is caused by an underlying ductal carcinoma in-situ. It presents with a unilateral erythematous rash around the nipple, which does not respond to normal eczema treatment (such as emollients). There may also be nipple retraction and inversion, and straw-coloured discharge. Lobular carcinoma in-situ does not present with a rash around the nipple. The main differences are that it tends to be multifocal and there is no microcalcification seen on the mammogram.

Question 2

A. A classic description of localised fibroadenosis. Triple assessment would be required to establish the diagnosis.

Question 3

D. This lady has a fibroadenoma, commonly nick-named 'breast mice' due to their mobility within the breast tissue. Fibroadenomas of the breast are benign tumours characterized by an admixture of stromal and epithelial tissue.

Question 4

C. Fat necrosis is where trauma has led to fibrosis and calcification of the breast tissue. It can occur following surgery. It may be difficult to differentiate clinically from breast cancer. This is the most likely diagnosis in this patient as she has just recently had breast surgery. Recurrence of breast cancer is unlikely to occur that quickly after surgery.

Question 5

E. Breast cysts are discrete mobile lumps which produce a straw-coloured fluid on aspiration. Breast cysts can be painful and may be worrisome but are generally benign. They are most common in pre-menopausal women in their 30s or 40s. They usually disappear after menopause, but may persist or reappear when using hormone therapy.

Question 6

A. Mammary duct ectasia presents with nipple retraction as a result of fibrosis and a milky or dirty green discharge. However, formal triple assessment must be undertaken to exclude malignancy.

Question 7

B. A description of a duct papilloma. The discharge may be serous or blood stained. Intraductal papillomas of the breast are benign lesions with an incidence of approximately 2%–3% in humans. Two types of intraductal papillomas are generally distinguished. The central type develops near the nipple. They are usually solitary and often arise in the period nearing menopause. On the other hand, the peripheral type are often multiple papillomas arising at the peripheral breasts, and are usually found in younger women. The peripheral type is associated with a higher risk of malignancy.

Question 8

D. BRCA1 on chromosome 17Q and BRCA2 on chromosome 13Q are associated with breast cancer.

Question 9

A. In the UK, women between the ages of 50 and 70 are called every 3 years for screening. However, the NHS is in the process of extending the programme as a trial, offering screening to some women aged between 47 and 73

Question 10

C. Stage 3 comprises of any sized tumour, involvement of fixed ipsilateral axillary nodes or ipsilateral supraclavicular or infraclavicular nodes and no evidence of distant metastasis. It may also comprise of any sized tumour, no palpable or palpable lymph nodes and no evidence of distant metastasis.

Question 11

B. This is a stage 2 cancer with a 5-year survival rate of 71%.

Question 12

A. Ductal cancers are the most common breast cancers, with a frequency of 80%.

Question 13

D. Ultrasound helps to distinguish a solid mass from a cystic mass and is preferable to mammography in women under the age of 35 years in whom the breast tissue is very dense.

Question 14

A. This is a locally advanced breast cancer (stage 3) and is best treated with neoadjuvant chemotherapy, followed, if possible, by breast conserving surgery and axillary clearance. As it is oestrogen-receptor-negative, tamoxifen would be of no use. Herceptin would only be utilised if the cancer were HER2-positive.

Question 15

E. Paget disease of the breast is a type of cancer that outwardly may have the appearance of eczema, with skin changes involving the nipple of the breast. The condition is an uncommon disease, accounting for 1% to 4.3% of all breast cancers

Question 16

C. A classic description of a Phyllodes tumour. Histologically, the tumour would have a characteristic leaf like appearance. This is predominantly a tumour of adult women, with very few examples reported in adolescents. Patients typically present with a firm, palpable mass. These tumours are very fast-growing, and can increase in size in just a few weeks. Occurrence is most common between the ages of 40 and 50, prior to menopause.

EMQ ANSWERS

Management of breast cancer

1. B Also known as herceptin, this drug interferes with the attachment of human epidermal growth factor to HER2 and thus prevents the division and growth of breast cancer cells.
2. C Additional side effects include flushes, hot sweats and irregular periods.
3. D Such drugs prevent the conversion of androgens into oestrogen, which is needed for the growth of breast cancer.
4. B Other common side effects include diarrhoea, tumour pain and headaches.
5. A This agent is also commonly associated with tumours of the kidney.

Breast lumps

1. E Fibroadenoma. Fibroadenoma or 'breast mouse' is common in young women as a discreet highly mobile mass.
2. I Mastitis. This may precede breast abscess and is not uncommon in breastfeeding mothers.
3. D Fat necrosis. This is common after trauma, especially in the breasts. This may be seen after road traffic accidents as the seat-belt passes over the breast.
4. C Duct ectasia. This is common around the time of the menopause, and is due to a dilated, fluid-filled milk duct or ducts. These can become infected.
5. B Cyst. This is unlikely to be serious but should be aspirated if it becomes symptomatic or there are worrying features on ultrasound.

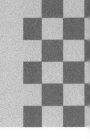

Index